Reliability Engineering Technology of Digital Diagnosis and Treatment Equipment

Xiuqing Li · Jun Gao · Wen Li

Reliability Engineering Technology of Digital Diagnosis and Treatment Equipment

中国工信出版集团
電子工業出版社
PUBLISHING HOUSE OF ELECTRONICS INDUSTRY
http://www.phei.com.cn
Springer

Xiuqing Li
Department of Engineering Physics
Tsinghua University
Beijing, China

Jun Gao
Scientific Verification and Testing
Engineering Technology Co., Ltd.
Guangzhou, Guangdong, China

Wen Li
Beijing Medical Device Inspection Institute
Beijing, China

ISBN 978-981-99-5521-3 ISBN 978-981-99-5522-0 (eBook)
https://doi.org/10.1007/978-981-99-5522-0

Jointly published with Publishing House of Electronics Industry
The print edition is not for sale in China (Mainland). Customers from China (Mainland) please order the print book from: Publishing House of Electronics Industry.
ISBN of the Co-Publisher's edition: 978-712-14-1875-4

This Springer imprint is published by the registered company Springer Nature Singapore Pte Ltd.
The registered company address is: 152 Beach Road, #21-01/04 Gateway East, Singapore 189721, Singapore

Contents

Chapter 1
Digital Diagnosis and Treatment Equipment and Its Research and Development Reliability Requirements

1.1 Overview of the Digital Medical Treatment

Digital diagnosis and treatment equipment has developed rapidly along with the comprehensive promotion and application of digital medical treatment. What exactly is digital medical treatment, and what role does it play in national health and security? Digital medical treatment is a new modern way of medical treatment by applying modern computer technology and information technology to the whole medical process, which is the development direction and management goal of public health care. The emergence of digital diagnosis and treatment equipment has greatly enriched the connotation and capacity of medical information. From the visualization of 1D information, such as Electrocardiograph (ECG) and Electroencephalogram (EEG) and other important electrophysiological information; to the visualization of 2D information, such as Computed Tomography (CT), Magnetic Resonance Imaging (MRI), Color Doppler Ultrasound, Digital X-Ray machine (DR), and other medical image information; and then the visualization of 3D information, even 4D information can also be obtained, such as: real-time dynamic display of 3D heart. The information greatly enriches doctor's diagnostic technology, promoting medical science into a brand-new visualized information age.

Digital medical is not only a simple collection of digital medical equipment, but also a new modern medical method that applies contemporary computer technology and information technology to the whole medical process. In digital medical treatment, patients can complete the treatment with the minimal process, and the accuracy of doctor's diagnosis is greatly improved. The patient medical record information file records all the current and historical health information of patients. This facilitates doctors' diagnosis and patients' self-examination to a great extent, truly realize the comprehensive data call of patients needed by remote clinic, and realize fast and effective service. Another advantage of digital medical lies in its resources sharing between medical equipment and medical experts. For medical institutions,

X. Li et al., *Reliability Engineering Technology of Digital Diagnosis and Treatment Equipment*, https://doi.org/10.1007/978-981-99-5522-0_1

the database with complete health information is more authoritative, and the establishment of health information system can greatly improve the competitiveness of them.

1.1.1 Current Situation of Digital Medical Treatment in China

The construction of digital medical treatment in China is just in its infancy. As for the hospital information system that has been built, most of them are similar to the management information system in the general sense of enterprises and institutions, and the biggest feature of digital medical treatment is to informationize clinical data, which accounts for 80% of the total information of hospital business, and support it with the core technology of medical Picture Archiving and Communication System (PACS), so as to make digital medical treatment have greater medical value. However, for a long time, people's awareness of digital medical treatment is not enough, and the technical limitations in the real-time process hinder its implementation in China. By the end of 2018, there were about 997,000 medical and health institutions in China, including 32,000 hospitals. In all these hospitals, less than 1/3 of them whose digital system has begun to take shape, and even fewer medical institutions have truly realized digitalization.

The lack of unified standardization implementation is an important factor affecting the development of digital medical treatment in China at present. According to the investigation, The problem of non-standardized communication interface is serious in the currently running Hospital Information System (HIS) products, Developers and hospitals did not refer to the corresponding international standard Health Level Seven (HL7) when building HIS, and only paid attention to the success of PACS and HIS in a single mode, but did not leave an open interface for the later PACS and HIS, which made it difficult for the current system to connect with the later systems, and it was difficult for these systems to interconnect themselves. The lack of standards in hospital business processes and confusion in sharing data standards lead to a large number of low-level repeated development of HIS, which is difficult to transplant and popularize, and difficult to share data. These problems have potential harm to the further development of digital medical treatment.

Besides Internet and database system, digital diagnosis and treatment equipment is also significant in the field of digital medical treatment. The current situation of China's digital diagnosis and treatment equipment industry is that almost all large-scale high-end equipment depend on imports. Although domestic R & D institutions aim at similar products of international advanced enterprises from time to time, High-end digital diagnosis and treatment equipment with advanced functions and performance has been developed. However, due to bottlenecks in engineering, applicability and reliability, hospitals, doctors, patients and their families can hardly trust these products. Because of the lack of evidence and conviction, it is difficult for these institutions to develop a market. The research and development of digital diagnosis and treatment equipment should not only solve the problems of existence, advanced function and performance, but also solve the problems of engineering and reliability, so that the developed products have the characteristics of safety, advanced, applicability and reliability.

Since entering the "Twelfth Five-Year Plan", the country has vigorously advocated the development of digital medical treatment, and thus China's digital medical treatment has seen a dramatic development. In November 2011, the Ministry of Science and Technology published the Twelfth Five-Year Plan for Medical Device Technology Industry (2011–2015). The plan states: "In terms of product objectives, it is necessary to create 50–80 new prevention, diagnosis, treatment, rehabilitation and emergency medical equipment products that are urgently needed clinically, focusing on the development of basic equipment and medical materials that are in large demand, widely used and mainly rely on imports, and actively develop new medical equipment products such as chronic disease screening, minimally invasive diagnosis and treatment, regenerative repair, digital medical care and rehabilitation nursing." This plays a positive role in promoting the development of medical device industry.

In 2012, the key medical device project was launched. During the 12th Five-Year Plan period, 47 projects were deployed, with an investment of 4.464 billion yuan in research and development, focusing on the development of major strategic products such as digital X-ray machines, color Doppler ultrasound, MRI and PET-CT. In 2013, the National Development and Reform Commission, the Ministry of Industry and Information Technology and relevant departments jointly organized and implemented the "Special Project for High Performance Medical Diagnosis and Treatment Equipment", focusing on supporting the upstream and downstream collaborative development of 15 types of product industry chains in the fields of imaging, advanced treatment and in vitro diagnostic equipment, and arranging 556 million yuan of central financial funds. At present, a number of major products such as 64-slice CT, 1.5 T MRI, PET-CT and implantable rechargeable bilateral brain pacemaker have successfully broken the foreign monopoly. Leading breakthroughs have been made in a number of cutting-edge technologies, such as localization and digitalization of Positron Emission Tomography (PET). On the whole, medical imaging and other industrial fields have shown a development trend of accelerating the evolution to the high end of the value chain, and the competitiveness of science and technology and industry in the field of medical devices in China has been significantly improved. The Ministry of Science and Technology, together with the Health Planning Commission and relevant local governments, jointly organized and implemented the "Demonstration Project of Innovative Medical Device Products Application". More than 10,000 sets of innovative medical devices worth nearly 500 million yuan have been demonstrated and applied in nearly 1,000 primary medical institutions in 7 provinces and cities across the country, which has played an active role in promoting the popularization of domestic medical devices and promoting the development of innovative enterprises.

Since entering the "13th Five-Year Plan", the country has deployed a pilot project of "Digital Diagnosis and Treatment Equipment Research and Development", focusing on the development trend of "digitalization, networking, and intelligence" in the new round of scientific and technological revolution in the health field and industrial revolution, and focusing on early diagnosis, precise diagnosis, minimally invasive medicine and precise treatment, with multi-modal molecular imaging, new magnetic resonance imaging system, new X-ray computed tomography, new generation of ultrasound imaging, low-dose X-ray imaging, compound endoscope Focusing on 10 major strategic products such as imaging, new microscopic imaging, large-scale radiotherapy equipment, surgical robots, and medical active implantable devices, carry out research and development of 10 types of major equipment, realize the localization of core components, and solve the constraints on industrialization to reduce the cost of equipment manufacturing; carry out cutting-edge and common technology research to lay the foundation for the development of next-generation medical devices and provide support for the overall development of the industry; carry out integrated research on several new diagnosis and treatment technologies and new service models to promote domestic medical treatment The integrated application of medical devices and the development of new medical service models; carry out application demonstration and evaluation research, improve the recognition of domestic medical devices, and promote the large-scale application of domestic innovative products. The implementation of this pilot project will build digital diagnosis and treatment equipment testing, evaluation platform and system to improve the technical standard system, develop a large number of core components and major strategic products, create dozens of industry, academia, research and innovation team and form hundreds of core patents, form clinical application solutions, evaluation and demonstration applications within the country, accelerate the integration of China's medical device field innovation chain and industry chain, significantly enhance the international competitiveness of domestic digital diagnosis and treatment equipment, and promote China's digital diagnosis and treatment equipment into the international advanced ranks as a whole.

1.1.2 Advantages of Digital Medical Treatment

The implementation of digital medical treatment can not only improve the quality of diagnosis and treatment and service efficiency of hospitals, but also have a great impact on improving the competitiveness of hospitals in the future. At the same time, the transparency of hospital management is enhanced, the trust of patients is won, and the good social image of the hospital is maintained. Its advantages are as follows:

1. **Access to Public Health Care Can Be Improved**

People can save the time of queuing for registration, pricing, inspection and taking medicine in hospitals; You can choose an expert you trust to diagnose and treat yourself; You can consult your doctor at home; You can get a doctor's health reminder at any time; More advanced equipment can be obtained for examination and diagnosis, and patients will truly become the center of hospital services in the process of examination and treatment.

2. **The Operation Mode of Hospitals Can Be Reformed**

After the implementation of digital medical treatment, the hospital will no longer be just a place to see a doctor, but will develop into a service-oriented institution integrating medical treatment, health care and health consultation. It will fundamentally change the hospital's business model, which has also led to the transformation of the hospital's business philosophy, making the hospital shift from focusing only on equipment and medical level to focusing also on the hospital's modern management level and Service Level.

3. **The Management Mode of Hospitals Can Be Changed**

After the realization of digital medical treatment, hospital administrators can free themselves from the heavy writing work, and can obtain all aspects of information from the whole hospital in real time and accurately, so as to adjust the management of the hospital to the best running state in time. The whole hospital realizes paperless office and film-free storage, which greatly reduces the cost of the hospital and improves the working efficiency of it.

4. **The Teaching and Research Work of Hospitals Can Be Improved**

Doctors can understand the flow of patients on the day through the network, and the electronic prescription and electronic application form on the network also greatly simplify the doctor's prescribing process. The image inspection data performed by advanced digital diagnosis and treatment equipment is accurate, and can also be transmitted to the diagnosis and treatment department through the network in time. In the hands of doctors, it can not only make timely diagnosis and treatment for patients, but also is especially beneficial for patients who are reexamined. Remote consultation and remote monitoring can make doctors practice medicine without leaving home, and doctors' talents can be brought into full play. Similarly, digital medical treatment endows hospitals with new connotations and opens up new ways for daily education and scientific research.

1.2 Overview of Digital Diagnosis and Treatment Equipment

1.2.1 Development History of Digital Diagnosis and Treatment Equipment

With the development of digital medical treatment, digital diagnosis and treatment equipment is becoming more and more important. If the digital diagnosis and treatment equipment providing data sources and diagnosis and treatment is unavailable and unreliable, it is futile to do digitalization (networking, informatization and intelligence) well. Digital diagnosis and treatment equipment is the most important basic equipment in the construction of medical service system and public health system, and it is also the core engine to promote a new round of healthy economic development, which is highly strategic, driving and growing.

With the rise of digital medical treatment, a large number of related digital diagnosis and treatment equipment integrating computer information system and network technology have emerged, and the research and development of digital diagnosis and treatment equipment is also one of the key research and development plans of the national "Thirteenth Five-Year Plan". Looking back at the whole development process, it has been more than 100 years since the first digital diagnosis and treatment equipment came out, in which countless landmark inventions were born.

The first X-ray computed tomography (CT) scanner for brain diagnosis was designed by British engineer G.N. Hounsfield in 1969 and made public in 1972. This is a combination of electronic technology, computer technology and X-ray technology. Its appearance is a revolutionary progress of medical digital medical equipment since the discovery of X-ray in 1895, and lays a foundation for modern medical imaging equipment science.

CT machine has the advantages of cross-sectional tomography without overlap of front and back images, and no interference from upper and lower tissues; At the same time, due to the remarkable improvement of density resolution, the difference of X-ray attenuation coefficient of 0.1–0.5% can be distinguished, which is 10–20 times higher than that of traditional X-ray examination; Quantitative analysis can also be done in digital form (CT value). In recent 3 decades, CT equipment has been updated for four generations, whose scanning time has been shortened from 3–5 min to 1–5 s, and the spatial resolution has been improved to 0.1 mm. CT equipment and technology play an important role in medical imaging diagnosis, while the diagnosis of brain, abdominal liver, gallbladder, pancreas, retroperitoneal kidney, adrenal gland and other diseases is dominant in its practical application. Ultra-high-speed CT and spiral CT were developed successively in 1980s, which further expanded and improved their clinical application scope and diagnostic effect. The birth of CT machine marked the revolutionary progress of digital medical equipment.

Magnetic resonance imaging (MRI) equipment, which was used in clinic in the early 1980s, is a brand-new non-ionizing radiation imaging equipment. MRI equipment is superior to CT because of its high-density resolution, adjustable direction and mode of gradient magnetic field, and can directly take tomographic images of transverse, coronal, sagittal sections and oblique positions. Up to now, MRI has been widely used in various systems of human body, among which central nervous system, cardiovascular system, limb joints and pelvic cavity have the best effect; In recent years, the diagnostic effect of abdomen has approached and reached the level of CT, and the resolution of brain image has been improved thousands of times under conventional scanning time, and the resolution of microscopic imaging has reached 50–10 μ m. Now it has become the most important part of medical imaging diagnostic equipment. Biological MR spectroscopy (MRS) has the function and potential to study the metabolism of substances in the body. If the combination of MRI and MRS can be applied clinically in the future, it will lead to a new breakthrough in medical diagnostics.

Multi-technology integration is an important development trend of digital diagnosis and treatment equipment. In 1950s and 1960s, ultrasound and radionuclide equipment and technology appeared one after another, and their medical applications were often systematic at that time. With the development of X-ray CT in the early 1970s, medical imaging equipment and technology entered a new stage based on the combination of computer and tomography and image reconstruction. At the end of 1970s, ultrasonic CT, radionuclide CT, MRCT and digital X-ray imaging equipment and technology gradually emerged and were applied in clinic. Although the imaging parameters, diagnostic principles and inspection methods of these devices are different, the result is to form a certain image and diagnose according to it. On this basis, medical imaging diagnostics was formed. In 1980s, Digital Subtraction Angiography (DSA) combined with Computer X-ray photography (CR) was put into use. The former has the characteristics of less invasive, real-time imaging, high contrast resolution, safety and simplicity, thus expanding the application range of angiography; The latter has the advantages of reducing exposure and strong inclusiveness, and more importantly, it can be incorporated into the Image Archiving and Communication System (PACS) as a digital image. Radiotherapy equipment, medical robots and other treatment equipment are combined with imaging equipment, which have the function of Image-Guided Radiotherapy, IGRT) and realize adaptive treatment, and have become the mainstream configuration in the market at present.

1.2.2 Characteristics of Digital Diagnosis and Treatment Equipment

Digital diagnosis and treatment equipment has the following basic characteristics:

1. **Digitalization of Diagnosis and Treatment Equipment**

The digitalization of medical treatment, first of all, is the digitalization of diagnosis and treatment equipment, which is the foundation of digital medical treatment. The so-called digital medical equipment refers to computer technology-based, signal acquisition and power input as close to the front end as possible, and process information such as control, data acquisition, processing, storage and transmission, and execution are all digitized. In addition, digital medical equipment has clearer images and more accurate quantitative measurement methods, which provides material and technical support for doctors to make more accurate diagnosis. Medical equipment working under computer software has gradually replaced conventional equipment and become the mainstream of clinical equipment.

2. **Networking of Diagnosis and Treatment Equipment**

Digital medical treatment can realize the sharing of equipment resources in hospitals, realize the transmission of images and documents, shorten the time of patient registration, payment, medicine taking and medical treatment, and reduce the probability of errors in electronic billing and electronic prescription. In telemedicine, digital medical treatment can realize distance teaching, video conference, teleconsultation, telesurgery, online inquiry and help-seeking, and online booking and registration, so as to realize the sharing of global resources.

3. **Informatization of Hospital Management**

Managers are able to know the operation of the hospital and the work of various departments at any time through the network, so that the hospital is always in the best running state. Moreover, hospitals can provide patients with all kinds of diagnosis and treatment information at any time.

4. **Personalization of Medical Service**

People can make an appointment to register through the Internet at home; People no longer need to wait for the examination results in the examination room, and various diagnosis and treatment images and data can be directly transmitted to the attending doctor through the network, so that doctors can make timely and accurate diagnosis and treatment of patients. Based on the Internet, cable television and other private health care services and public medical consultation services, the public will be reminded to carry out physical examination at any time, predict the occurrence and development of a certain disease, and recommend new treatment methods to patients, so that patients can enjoy personal doctors' medical care services without leaving home.

5. **Application and Integration of Advanced Technology**

Digital diagnosis and treatment equipment, especially major equipment, has more advanced technologies. By adopting a large number of advanced technologies in various disciplines, and even adopting multi-technology integration and integration, the detection and diagnosis ability of digital diagnosis and treatment equipment has been greatly improved, even exceeding the ability of traditional and single technology beyond imagination. Such in-depth, high-definition imaging and its image processing technology make the confirmation time of diseases, lesions and even pathology significantly earlier, and the results are more accurate, which can win precious time for patients and provide better diagnosis and treatment.

1.3 Reliability of Digital Diagnosis and Treatment Equipment

At present, China's medical equipment, especially high-end diagnostic imaging and large-scale treatment and other digital diagnosis and treatment equipment technology competitiveness is weak, high-end digital diagnosis and treatment equipment is mainly dependent on imports, according to relevant statistics show that in 2016, 90% of China's nuclear magnetic equipment, 80% of radiotherapy equipment, 80% of CT equipment, 80% of B ultrasound equipment, 70% of respiratory machines, 67% of anesthetics are dependent on imports. Especially since the "new crown" epidemic outbreak in 2020, China's high-end medical equipment procurement is heavily dependent on imports, to the most concerned EMCO (extracorporeal lung membrane oxygenation system) equipment, for example, there were only 400 units nationwide, the number is extremely scarce, and all of them are imported products, which involves the key materials Disposable lung membranes were only available from 3 M in the U.S., and the number of products was not enough to deal with major epidemics.

In recent years, with the acceleration of localization, the market share of domestic digital medical equipment has increased slightly, but in general, imported high-end medical equipment still occupies the main market. to completely change the situation and have the real core competitiveness and market trust, domestic equipment companies still need to make unremitting and arduous efforts.

1.4 Current Status of Medical Device Industry Reliability

1.4.1 Medical Device Reliability Dilemma

1. **Security is Regulated**

The International Organization for Standardization promulgated the *Application of Risk Management in Medical Devices* standard as early as 1998, standardizing enterprises' prevention and management of risks in the use of medical devices and providing tools for the realization of medical device safety. These standards were quickly adopted by European and American countries. And adopted by our country, most medical device manufacturers have carried out relevant risk analysis work. Before a medical device enters the market, it must pass the registration inspection and clinical verification, complete the registration application and obtain the registration certificate. Registration inspections usually carry out functional performance tests and general safety requirements tests (usually including safety and electromagnetic compatibility tests) based on related products. Registration inspections usually carry out functional performance tests and general safety requirements tests (usually including safety and electromagnetic compatibility tests) based on related products. At present, China's medical device registration inspection is mainly based on YY 0505–2005 *Medical Electrical Equipment Part 1–2: General Safety Requirements Parallel Standard: Electromagnetic Compatibility Requirements and Tests*, GB 9706.1–2020 *Medical Electrical Equipment Part 1: Basic Safety General Requirements for General Performance and Basic Performance*, GB/T 14,710–2009 *Environmental Requirements and Test Methods for Medical Electrical Appliances* and specific product specifications, mainly including performance, safety regulations, electromagnetic compatibility tests and some environmental adaptability tests.

As mentioned in the preface, one of the more prominent bottlenecks of China's medical devices, especially high-end diagnostic and treatment equipment, is the gap of reliability from international advanced products. The reason for this gap is very clear on the surface. China's medical device industry pays attention to and attaches great importance to safety, but there are few or no clear requirements for product reliability and reliability work, and few or no enterprises have carried out reliability work, which the product has not been tested and verified.

2. **The Foundation of Reliability Standards is Weak**

At present, standards such as YY/T 0195–1994 *Reliability Test Methods for Electrocardiographs* and GB/T 15,214–2008 *Requirements and Methods for Reliability Tests of Ultrasonic Diagnostic Equipment* can be found. In addition, Mindray is taking the lead in formulating *Medical Electrical Equipment Reliability Evaluation Method* National Standard. The "13th Five-Year" key research and development plan is still guiding some public service organizations to formulate relevant reliability and test evaluation standards, such as radiotherapy equipment, medical imaging equipment engineering and reliability technology research topics, each requiring the formulation of more than 6 relevant standards, Quality evaluation research topics such as MRI, CT, and endoscopy have also proposed standard assessment indicators.

3. **The Consciousness of Reliability Work is not Strong**

China's medical device research and development and production enterprises, especially digital diagnosis and treatment equipment enterprises, are still in a relatively preliminary stage of development. Usually, even for a long time, product function performance, regulatory requirements, and market sales are the top priorities, and they are all in a situation that cannot handle. It seems that There is no energy to care about the reliability of products; even if they have the energy to deal with it, because the reliability of medical devices is not required by regulations, the reliability of medical devices is different from other quality work. It takes a long time and costs a lot, and companies are often reluctant to invest. Therefore, there must be a common phenomenon that the failure rate of the equipment is relatively high and the life of the core components is relatively short when the equipment is in use. In fact, the economic cost of post-event failures is huge, and even the social impact is huge. This kind of state where you always feel that you have no energy in the early stage and do not care about product reliability is extremely bad. Compared with the initial investment cost, the cost of subsequent failure is even greater.

The reliability technology foundation of the medical device industry is weak. Due to the lag of standards and regulations, and the lack of research and investment of most enterprises, the reliability technology foundation of the entire medical device industry is weak, which is mainly manifested in the following aspects:

(1) Enterprise development strategies lack reliability elements, enterprise development generally has no reliability goals, and R & D products generally have no reliability indicators and requirements, which naturally lead to the lack of enterprise reliability system construction and low product reliability levels;
(2) Enterprises generaly lack reliability teams and professionals. If they do not establish reliability professional teams, it will inevitably lead to the situation that no one cares, no one manages and no one does reliability works, and the reliability level of products will certainly be low.
(3) The existing management and technical backbones generally do not master the professional knowledge and skills of reliability, and the reliability problems are seldom considered in design and verification, and the problems that arise are also managed and solved inadequately.
(4) Hardware equipment and software tools for reliability engineering are generally lacking. And the lack of tools in design leads to low efficiency and poor standardization; In the test, the hardware conditions are poor, and a large number of tests have been done, but the efficiency is still low, by which the in-depth problems cannot be fully exposed, and thus the quality of products can not be guaranteed.

At present, the main items of testing in the medical device industry are mainly on functional performances, safety requirement, and environmental adaptabilities to determine their compliance with the standards, which are necessary parts of the registration certificate application and the materials that must be submitted, to a certain extent. All of the tests and materials are to guarantee the function and performance, safety and environmental adaptability of marketed medical devices. In recent years, the reform of public service institutions for testing in the medical device industry has made its functional orientation increasingly more towards the direction of providing supervision services for government departments.

The medical device industry is in urgent need of socialized reliability professional service institutions to solve the problem of the lack of reliability service function and insufficient engineering capacity of the existing institutional testing institutions in the medical device industry. We provide reliability technical services for enterprises in the process of product development, guide them to put forward reasonable reliability requirements, introduce reliability design analysis, implement reliability testing on prototypes, carry out analysis and evaluation of service life, ensure that newly developed devices can eventually meet the requirements of registration inspection and technical review, improve the reliability level of new products developed and produced by domestic medical device enterprises, and enhance their competitiveness in the international market.

1.4.2 The Importance of Reliability to Digital Medical Equipment

1. **Complex, Multi-Functional, Advanced Technology Brings More Reliability Issues**

The medical device industry is a multidisciplinary, knowledge-intensive, capital-intensive and fast-developing high-tech industry. In particular, digital diagnosis and treatment equipment often adopts numerous cutting-edge and advanced technologies to realize its functions and performances. The equipment is complex in composition, large in scale, rich in functions and high in performance requirements. In addition, many new technologies, new processes and new materials are adopted. Each characteristic will bring negative impact on the reliability of the developed products. Therefore, the demand for reliability of digital medical diagnosis and treatment equipment is more urgent.

2. **Reliability Issues May Have Significant Impact and Advert Consequences**

As a product of modern science and technology, with the rapid development of medical diagnosis and treatment technology, the diagnosis and treatment equipment has been widely used in the prevention, diagnosis, treatment, health care and rehabilitation of diseases, and its dependence on it is getting higher and higher. In modern medical institutions, without well-functioning diagnosis and treatment equipment, various business work of hospital cannot be carried out as expected. The quality of diagnosis and treatment equipment is directly related to the effect of clinical diagnosis and treatment. The unsatisfactory application quality of diagnosis and treatment equipment, especially the low safety of them, will bring great harm to the health of medical staff and patients. The malfunction of diagnosis and treatment equipment will lead to misdiagnosis, missed diagnosis, ineffective or even harmful treatment, which may even endanger human life in serious cases. The reliability issues of diagnosis and treatment equipment may seriously shatter the confidence of hospitals and the doctors, patients and their families in using domestic medical equipments, may lead to the loss of quality cost, economic compensation and damage to the brand and reputation of enterprises, greatly affect the market development and investment return of domestic products, and then affect the technological innovation of enterprises and seriously hinder the industrial development.

It is estimated that there are at least 40,000 adverse events of medical equipment in China every year. In 2000, the State Council promulgated the *Supervision and Administration Regulation of Medical Diagnosis and Treatment Equipment*, in which it has clearly put forward that the safety and effectiveness of diagnosis and treatment equipments that have potential dangers implanted into human body for supporting and sustaining life must be strictly controlled; The Chap. 4, Article 32 of the "Regulation" stipulated that for medical equipment that cannot be guaranteed to be safe and effective, the drug regulatory department of the people's government at or above the provincial level shall revoke its product registration certificate.

3. **Reliability is an Important Means to Solve the Service Life and Availability of Diagnosis and Treatment Equipment**

Reliability is an important means to evaluate the service life of medical equipment How to realize the safety and effectiveness of medical equipment has been the focus of research and attention of manufacturers, users and regulatory authorities. Registration test and clinical verification ensure the safety and effectiveness of medical devices to a certain extent. On the basis of the existing registration test and clinical verification, in 2019, the State Drug Administration organized the formulation and release of the *Guiding Principles for Technical Review of Active Medical Device Service Life Registration*, which proposed the use of a series of reliability technologies to carry out service life analysis and evaluation. The product shall complete the specified functions under the specified condition and time, that is, the reliability of medical equipment is an important prerequisite and guarantee to realize the service life. This guiding principle will promote the application of reliability engineering technology in the research and development of medical devices, guide enterprises to carry out service life analysis, verification and evaluation more practically, and further ensure and improve the safety and effectiveness within the service life.

Reliability of diagnosis and treatment equipment used in hospitals is an important means to solve the usability issues. Due to the particularity of medical equipment in medical activities, it is required to be able to work reliably during the whole working process. Even if the product performance decreases with the increase of use time, it can still enable the availability of the equipment, and reduce the downtime in use, to avoid affecting the operation of the hospitals, the safety of patients and the effectiveness of treatment. In order to ensure the availability of medical diagnosis and treatment equipment during the service life, it is usually necessary to carry out a series of reliability engineering work, and implement reliability organization, supervision and control management in a planned and purposeful way. It is also necessary to apply reliability technology to the R & D and production of medical products, adopt appropriate reliability improvement technology to fully and quickly expose problems for enhancement, improve the maintainability and supportability of products, and take active after-sales supporting measures to enhance the reliability and maturity of medical devices.

4. **Reliability is an Important Factor to Enhance the Market Competitiveness of Domestic Medical Diagnosis and Treatment Equipment**

The reliability of medical diagnosis and treatment equipment has become an important factor affecting the market competitiveness of its industry. With the intensification of domestic market competition and the expectation of exporting domestic diagnosis and treatment equipment, the large gap in reliability level of domestic medical equipment often becomes the weakness. Although there have been a few similar domestic products for some high-quality, sophisticated and advanced digital diagnosis and treatment equipment such as MRI, CT, B-ultrasound, accelerator, etc., and although there have been many star enterprises in the field of medical equipment in China, the share of Chinese equipment in the international market is still small, and most of the domestic market is occupied by international enterprises. Taking China's import data in 2016 as an example: the import of MR machines cost 8.8 billion dollars; CT machines cost 7 billion dollars; B-ultrasound machines cost 6.5 billion dollars; linear accelerators cost 2 billion dollars. The import amount of the four major parts exceeded twice the output value of the top 20 domestic medical devices. In 2016, the proportion of domestic medical equipment was separately as follows: MR took only 10%, CT machines took 20%, B-ultrasound took 20%, and linear accelerator took 20%. Compared with some medical equipment in advanced countries, the gap in reliability of the products of most domestic medical equipment manufacturers is far greater than that in performance. In China, the per capita allocation of medical equipment is small, especially in large hospitals, where the expected frequency of equipment use is extremely high and the queue period for appointment examination is long. As hospital users, they attach great importance to the reliability of medical equipment. The lack of reliability of domestic diagnosis and treatment equipment often affects the trust of users in making purchase of the equipment, which is an important factor that leads many large hospitals in China to purchase and use similar equipment imported from abroad, and patients' families to rush to large hospitals with advanced equipment for examination and treatment. The progress of reliability technology of domestic diagnosis and treatment equipment enterprises will certainly drive the improvement of equipment reliability level, which will help to enhance the market competitiveness of these enterprises in the competition between domestic and international enterprises and in the international market.

Certainly, in order to participate in the competition in the international market, there are also a few enterprises in our country, which have begun to regard reliability as a core work in the R & D and production of medical devices, gradually integrate reliability into the R & D, production and use of medical devices, and have achieved certain results. However, in general, our medical equipment industry in order to keep up with the international standards and participate in the competition in the international market, only by continuously improving the reliability level of medical equipment can we obtain a firm status in the international market economy. Therefore, it is an urgent task for medical device enterprises in China to deeply study reliability and continuously improve product reliability.

1.4.3 Reliability Requirements Proposed by the Pilot Special Project of "Research and Development of Digital Medical Diagnosis and Treatment Equipment"

During the "13th Five-Year Plan" period, the reliability requirements of digital diagnosis and treatment equipment were clearly put forward in the special project of "Research and Development of Digital Medical Diagnosis and Treatment Equipment", and requirements are as follows:

(1) Common reliability technology is given attention to encourage quality control and inspection standardization technology research, systematically improve China's major digital medical equipment quality control and safety assurance capabilities; encourage reliability and engineering technology research, intends to establish reliability design analysis, test verification, management system of typical cases, and the formation of relevant standard specifications, to lay the foundation for the promotion and application of reliability technology for the entire industry.

(2) Each type of R & D equipment has reliability requirements for the core components and the whole machine—providing reliability design and failure model design documents for the core components and the whole machine and relevant third-party test reports, breaking the R & D mode of the medical device industry with the registration certificate as the main goal, focusing on the reliability work of the R & D process and the reliability level of the products.

Digital diagnosis and treatment equipment key R & D program in these requirements aimed at guiding the diagnosis and treatment equipment R & D enterprises from the design of the beginning to pay attention to reliability work, the research and development of product potential failure analysis more thoroughly, the product design more reliable, to carry out reliability testing to test the reliability level of new R & D products, so as to narrow the gap between China's diagnosis and treatment equipment and international advanced product reliability level.

Beijing Institute of Medical Device Testing, Guangdong Kejian Testing Engineering Technology Co., Ltd., and University of Electronic Science and Technology of China undertook the project of "Research on Reliability and Engineering Technology of Radiotherapy Equipment"; Shanghai Medical Device Inspection Institute and Machinery Industrial Instruments undertook the research on the reliability and engineering technology of imaging equipment. These two projects will study the reliability design and analysis methods, software tools and databases of digital medical equipment, research reliability testing and accelerated testing methods, build accelerated testing equipment and reliability testing platforms, and form reliability standards for relevant medical equipment.

In the research and development project of multi-mode guided stereotaxic and rotational intensity-modulated integrated radiation therapy system led by Shandong Xinhua Medical and jointly undertaken by the Shenzhen Advanced Institute of the Chinese Academy of Sciences, the National Institute of Metrology undertook the quality control method and standardization research of magnetic resonance imaging equipment; The China Institute for Food and Drug Control undertook the research on the quality evaluation method of active implanted artificial organs; the Third Military Medical University of the Chinese People's Liberation Army undertook the research on the conformity evaluation of the quality control bionic dynamic system and its clinical application software; Hubei Medical Device Quality Supervision and Inspection Center Undertook the research and development of in vivo ultrasonic diagnostic equipment to detect body membranes and quality and safety research; Taishan Medical College undertook the research and development of quality control body membranes in medical imaging and radiation therapy.

The typical program for the reliability of medical equipment is shown in Fig. 1.1.

1.5 Summary

At present, many countries in the world have taken measures to restrict the export or embargo of key components, spare parts and complete machine products to our country. Independent control, localization is increasingly becoming a major historical mission of China's major equipment enterprises. Improving the level of reliability of domestic medical equipment, narrowing the gap with the international advanced equipment of the same kind of key is an important way to win the domestic market and international market recognition of domestic medical equipment. It's hope that with the power of reliability engineering, promote China's diagnosis and treatment equipment industry reliability technology progress, improve the level of reliability of domestic diagnosis and treatment equipment products, improve the domestic diagnosis and treatment equipment enterprises and international advanced enterprise market competitiveness, help the domestic digital diagnosis and treatment equipment industry's healthy and rapid development.

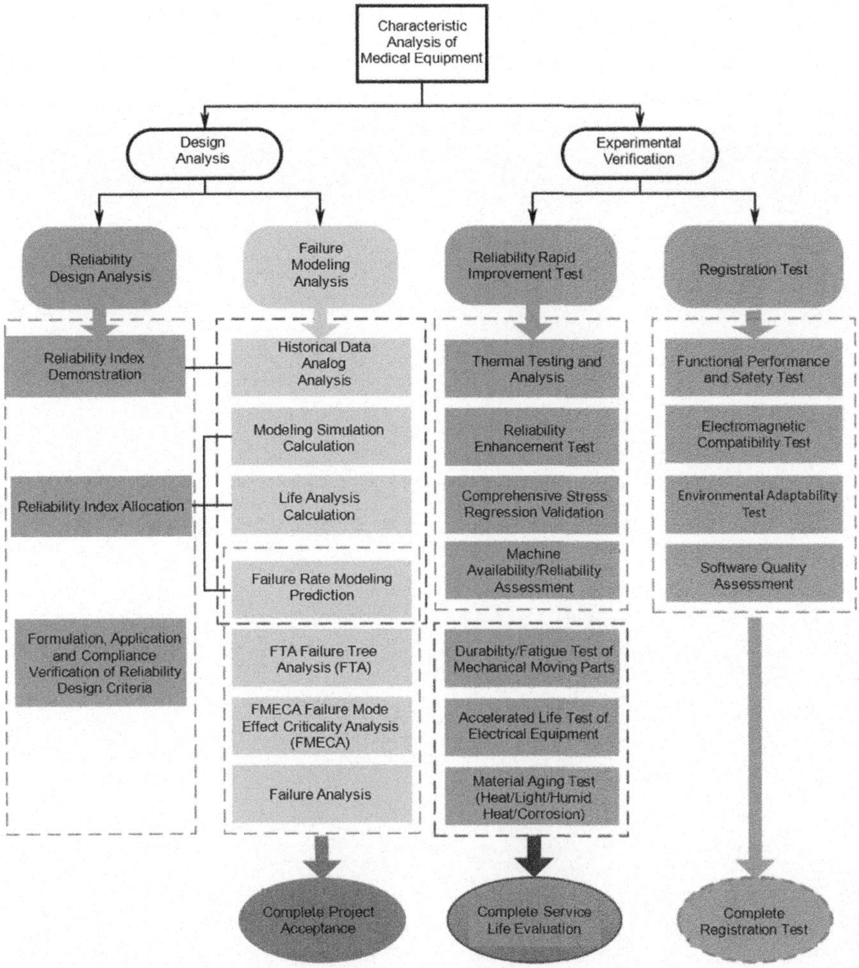

Fig. 1.1 Reliability work scheme of diagnosis and treatment equipment

Chapter 2
Overview of the Reliability Engineering of Digital Diagnosis and Treatment Equipment

In the medical device industry, the requirements for safety and effectiveness have been highly valued by most companies after years of national mandatory constraints. Medical enterprises consciously carry out relevant work to ensure that the products developed through registration inspection, clinical verification and technical review obtain the final medical device registration certificate. However, reliability is still in the initial stage of development in the medical device industry. Most R&D companies have a relatively weak foundation and are less specialized in reliability-related work. Most people only have a simple understanding of reliability—fewer failures. But they often lack professional and accurate understanding. This chapter introduces the basic concept and connotation of reliability, the relationship and difference between quality and reliability, the connotation and system of reliability engineering, and introduces the overall scheme of reliability with cases.

2.1 Basic Concept and Connotation of Reliability

2.1.1 Definition of Reliability

Reliability refers to the ability of a product to complete specified functions within a specified time and under specified conditions. The probability measure of reliability is represented by the letter (R), which is the probability that the product will complete the specified function within the specified time and under specified conditions.

When the failure obeys the exponential distribution and $\lambda(t)$ is constant, the reliability R can be calculated according to formula (2.1):

$$R(t) = \mathrm{e}^{-\lambda t} \tag{2.1}$$

The connotations of the three provisions in the reliability definition are as follows:

X. Li et al., *Reliability Engineering Technology of Digital Diagnosis and Treatment Equipment*, https://doi.org/10.1007/978-981-99-5522-0_2

(1) The specified time usually refers to the time in a broad sense, including calendar time, working hours, times of actions, mileage, etc. For medical devices, the warranty period and validity period can usually be used as the specified time;
(2) The specified conditions usually include the external environment, usage methods, maintenance conditions, etc. that the product may withstand during the entire life cycle. Harsh natural environment, bad usage methods, inappropriate maintenance, etc., may cause product failure;
(3) The specified functions usually refer to the relevant technical requirements that the product should meet, that is, the requirements for functions and performance indicators.

Reliability is often a combination of the three provisions—in the specified assessment time corresponding to the reliability index, the specified environmental stress and its comprehensive stress are repeatedly (periodically) applied to the product, so that the product simulates the actual scene and operating conditions. In principle, the functional performance of the product must be tested under different environmental conditions in each cycle, and each test must confirm whether the product is in good condition.

2.1.2 Reliability Classification

From the perspective of application, reliability can be divided into inherent reliability and service reliability. Intrinsic reliability is usually a characteristic given to a product in the process of product design and manufacturing. Inherent reliability is used to describe the level of reliability in the design and manufacture of a product. Inherent reliability only considers the failure events that the manufacturer can control in the design and production, only includes the influence of product design and manufacturing, and assumes that the use and guarantee conditions are ideal. The inherent reliability of a product cannot usually be improved without taking design and process improvement measures. Reliability in use includes the comprehensive effects of product design, installation, quality, environment, use, maintenance, etc. It can be seen that the reliability of use not only needs to consider product design and manufacturing, but also needs to consider the impact of product packaging, loading and unloading, storage, transportation, installation, use, maintenance, repair and other factors on the product. The reliability level when used in the environment is an important reflection of the true reliability level of the product.

From the perspective of design, reliability can be divided into basic reliability and task reliability. Basic reliability refers to the duration or probability of a product being free from failure under specified conditions. The basic reliability reflects the relevant requirements of the product for maintenance and guarantee, and is usually measured by the Mean Time Between Failures (MTBF). When determining the basic reliability parameters, all failure units and all failures of the product should be counted. Mission reliability refers to the ability of a product to perform specified functions in a specified mission profile. Mission reliability, which considers only the impact of failures that cause mission failure, is used to describe a product's ability to complete a mission and is usually measured by Mission Reliable (MR) and Mean Time Between Critical Failures (MTBCF).

2.1.3 Reliability Metrics

Products are generally divided into repairable products and non-repairable products. The quality problems of repairable products are usually expressed by failure. The most commonly used metric is Mean Time Between Failures (MTBF), and the metric of mission reliability is usually Mean Time Between Critical Failures (MTBCF). The quality problems of non-repairable products are usually expressed by invalidity, and the most commonly used metrics is Mean Time To Failure (MTTF).

Common reliability metrics for digital medical diagnosis and treatment equipment are as follows:

Mean Time Between Failures (MTBF)—The average working time between two adjacent failures, called Mean Time Between Failures, denoted by θ. It is a basic reliability parameter of repairable products.

Mean Time Between Critical Failures (MTBCF)—The average operating time between two consecutive failures that would result in significant loss of equipment or personnel. It is a mission reliability parameter.

Mean Time To Failure (MTTF)—The ratio of the total number of product life units to the total number of failed products under specified conditions and for a specified period of time. It is a basic reliability parameter of non-repairable products.

Failure rate (λ)—The probability of failure per unit time after which the product works up to a certain point before it fails.

Reliable (R)—A probability measure of reliability, characterized by a lifetime distribution function.

Service life—The number of life units that must be overhauled or scrapped from the beginning of use to the time when the product is unsuitable for use no matter it is technically or economically, respectively corresponding to the first refurbishment period or the total life span. The interval determines the number of overhauls.

Expected life—The period during which the intended use of the product can be maintained and the safety and effectiveness of the product can be ensured through risk management. The expiration of the validity period is the expiration of the validity period. After this time node, the safety and effectiveness of the medical device will not be guaranteed.

Availability (A)—Within a specified time interval, the ratio of the time the product is available to the specified time interval. Availability includes inherent availability, reachable availability and usage availability.

Mean Time to Repair (MTTR)—It describes the average repair time of a product from a failure state to a working state.

2.2 The Relationship Between Quality and Reliability

"Quality" refers to the degree to which a set of inherent characteristics fulfills requirements. Quality characteristics are divided into special quality characteristics and general quality characteristics. Special quality characteristics usually include product functions, performance, and technical indicators; general quality characteristics usually include product safety, reliability, maintainability, testability, and support. In the military field, general quality characteristics are usually called as the "five characteristics" of equipment (sometimes it is customary to collectively refer to it as "reliability"). In addition, it also includes product electromagnetic compatibility, environmental adaptability, software quality, etc., which are also indispensable general quality characteristics of equipment. Among them, reliability is the most common basic attribute among the general quality characteristics, and it is also the most important attribute.

It is worth mentioning that for civilian products, quality characteristics also include economy, reliability, and ease of use, and for medical equipment, there are safety and effectiveness, etc., and they have a great impact on the market. The characteristics of this aspect cannot be neglected and even must be satisfied.

2.3 Difference Between Quality and Reliability

Quality management, quality inspection, system and product quality certification are now well known to enterprises, and everyone is familiar with quality work. Almost all quality work that should be done has been done, but many enterprises cannot guarantee the reliability level of products. Everyone is very familiar with the natural enemy of reliability—failures, and they even get headaches, which become the focus of attention, because products always show unexpected failures after sale, many failures, and a high failure rate. So when it comes to reliability, everyone seems to be very familiar with and highly recognized. But when it comes to reliability technology, most people are very unfamiliar, and they don't even understand the basic concepts and methods.

The difference between reliability and quality can be expressed in one sentence—reliability is a time indicator of quality.

The quality of the development and production phase (the quality when $t < 0$) includes design quality and manufacturing quality. Manufacturing quality is reflected in strict quality management in accordance with the manufacturing and acceptance specifications confirmed during design and development or in the design and finalization stage of product development. The quality management of the product manufacturing stage is reflected in strict inspection before leaving the factory, quality inspection The results meet the requirements specified in the design, that is, qualified products. In order to improve the rate of qualified products in the product manufacturing process, the focus of quality management work should be closely around how to

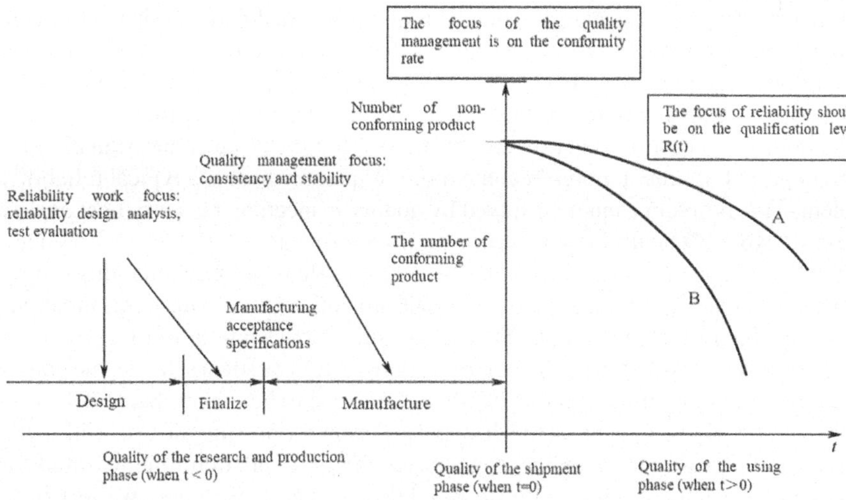

Fig. 2.1 Qualified product—time relationship diagram

maintain the consistency and stability of the production process. Technical methods include statistical process control (SPC), new and old seven quality management tools, etc.

The quality of the use stage (the quality when $t > 0$) is reflected in the ability of the product to maintain its qualified level during the user's use, which is essentially the product reliability, that is, the qualified product completes the specified quality within the specified time under the specified conditions. functional capacity. Reliability, therefore, is concerned with the ability of a product to maintain its conformance level over time. In Fig. 2.1, product A is clearly more qualified than product B, which means that product A is more reliable than product B.

The quality of the research and production stage is very important, which determines the quality of the factory time and the quality of the use stage. $t < 0$, the quality management of the manufacturing process determines the quality at $t = 0$, which can reduce the internal quality loss of the enterprise and can bring "direct" benefits to the enterprise; while the design quality of the R&D process at $t < 0$, i.e. Reliability design analysis, testing and evaluation, supervision and control directly determine the quality when $t > 0$. The ability to maintain the qualification level of qualified products, i.e. reliability, is the quality that customers are most concerned about, and is an important condition for enterprises to reduce external quality losses and improve after-sales service, and to maximize the output value of enterprises into profits, as well as an important condition for customer satisfaction.

The focus of traditional quality management is the qualified product rate at time $t = 0$. In order to improve the qualified product rate, the focus of quality management work is to ensure the consistency and stability of the manufacturing process. The focus of attention on reliability is why qualified products become "unqualified" after

$t > 0$, that is, why failures occur, and the focus of work is quality design in the research and development process. failures or defects that may occur during the use of users in the future, and preventive measures are taken during design to solve them. This is why quality management master Philip Crosby said that quality is free.

Reliability is measured and proven over time. After the product has been used for a certain period of time, failures become more frequent, which is a typical reliability problem. This problem cannot be solved by quality inspection, because most quality inspection work is usually a short-term, one-time inspection in a good environment; while reliability testing can usually help solve this problem, because reliability testing usually considers extreme and Extreme environments require long-term, hundreds of thousands of tests. For example, the average time between failures of a product is 1000 h. In order to assess this indicator, according to the statistical scheme, the cumulative operating time of the product is usually required to be higher than 1204 h and failures are not allowed (such as the decisive criterion for passing the test—allowing responsible failures If the number is increased, the accumulation time required for the test will be longer). According to reliability testing experience, we test once every 2–4 h on average. During the entire reliability testing process, the product has undergone at least 250–500 or more quality tests. Failure to pass any quality test may affect the test. Pass or not; At the same time, in the strict reliability test, the product has to withstand the extreme stress and extreme working conditions in the technical requirements for a long time, such as extreme storage and working low temperature, extreme storage and working high temperature, extreme high temperature and high humidity environment, certain temperature The rate of change, the upper and lower limits of electrical stress, the limit and various typical operating conditions, and even withstand long-term vibration and the combination of the above stresses. Therefore, in reliability testing, product problems are not only easier to expose, but also more thoroughly exposed than conventional test conditions.

It can be seen that the more in-depth difference between reliability and quality is the difference between reliability work and quality work. Reliability has its own management and technical connotations, and reliability engineering has a set of specialized management and technical methods.

2.3.1 Connotation of Reliability Engineering

Reliability engineering is a marginal discipline between management and technology, which cross-integrates many related disciplines, covers a wide range, and has a set of specialized engineering management and technical methods that are different from quality management. Reliability engineering refers to a series of work to make the product reach the reliability target. Its main work is to prevent failures, find failures in time, take effective corrective measures, try to prevent failures from recurring, and improve product reliability. Therefore, we can simply understand that reliability engineering is a discipline that fights against failures. Reliability engineering includes a series of work items including reliability engineering management, design analysis, and test verification. Each work item has its purpose, process steps, input requirements and output results. The focus of reliability engineering runs through the entire process of product development and even extends to the whole life cycle stage of a product.

Economic competition in the world today largely depends on the quality of a country's products and services. The level of quality can be said to be a comprehensive reflection of a country's economy, technology, education and management. Not only in the field of digital diagnosis and treatment equipment, but in the field of many major equipment and high-end equipment, the main gap between China and the world is more reflected in the gap in product reliability. The most direct manifestation of this gap is that many major industries do not recognize and trust domestic brands, resulting in most of the mid-to-high-end products relying on imports. This phenomenon also exists and is more serious in the field of digital medical equipment. It can be said that the brand of an enterprise is quality, and the core of quality is reliability. Under such circumstances, domestic digital medical equipment companies are required to incorporate reliability into quality objectives and business strategies, attach great importance to product reliability, and effectively narrow the gap with imported products. Only by solving this bottleneck problem and Only by proving to users in actual use can the reputation crisis of domestic products be resolved, and the brand and market share of domestic products can be improved.

The reliability work of China's military equipment, under the organization and management of the military and the requirements of laws and regulations, has been carried out relatively maturely after decades of continuous practice and is basically in line with developed countries. A number of reliability professional research institutes have been established in the field of military equipment. Institutions and enterprises having reserved a large number of reliability experts and technical backbones, the industry has formed a large number of standards, specifications, and guidance documents, and a complete reliability engineering system has been established for equipment research and development. The overall reliability level of R&D equipment has been greatly improved.

A reliability revolution broke out in many fields of China's civilian products. For example, in the early 1980s, the reliability level of China's home appliances lagged behind that of developed countries. The reliability work of the home appliance industry has been vigorously carried out, and problems have been exposed through full reliability testing, and design and process improvements have been implemented in strict accordance with reliability management requirements, and the product reliability level of the entire home appliance industry has been greatly improved. Nowadays, the home appliances we buy can be guaranteed to work without problems for 8–10 years.

Although a complete reliability engineering system has been established in the field of military industry, it has its particularity after all. For example, the customer of military industry is the army, which has characteristics of concentration, authority and initiative. The reliability of military equipment is often prioritized over cost control factors, and the promotion of reliability engineering technology is easier. Reliability work has become a mandatory work in the military field, and the implementation of reliability engineering has become a common practice in military equipment research and development.

Some industries in the field of civilian products are also similar to the military industry, especially the medical device industry. Most of the users are medical institutions such as hospitals or medical examination centers. Hospitals or physical examination centers also have the characteristics of typical large users and have the absolute right to speak. Therefore, the medical device industry has good conditions for promoting reliability engineering. Whether to implement it depends on the will of industry managers and large users, such as civil aircraft., rail transit, telecommunications, finance, environmental protection, medical equipment and other industries all have such characteristics. At present, China's civil aircraft industry attaches great importance to reliability and has basically formed a complete engineering system. Several other industries have paid attention to it but have not yet formed a reliability engineering system. Most of the other civil fields are typical market economies, customers are scattered and weak, and enterprises occupy greater dominance. Private enterprises are highly sensitive to cost. At present, most industries are still in dire straits of price competition and market share. Reliability is usually not highly valued by enterprises. Only a few enterprises with long-term development plans, especially R&D enterprises following international leading enterprises, pay attention to reliability works. Due to the characteristics of lag and difficulty in measuring reliability engineering in terms of reducing losses and bringing economic benefits, most private enterprises still lack reliability awareness and real actions. Even if there are clear reliability measures to improve product reliability, companies often have to make trade-offs from an economic point of view. Since quality problems and economic losses that may occur in the future are often not foreseeable in advance, it is usually easy to overrule during the trade-off process. A measure of reliability that incurs immediate direct costs rather than immediate direct profits.

Supported by national policies, at present, most of the powerful digital medical equipment research and development enterprises in China have participated in the pilot special project of "National Digital Medical Equipment Research and Development". The special project puts forward clear requirements for the reliability work of each project's research and development equipment, and even exploratory research and promotion of reliability engineering technology in individual important categories of equipment. Therefore, for most of our digital diagnosis and treatment equipment research and development enterprises, we can take advantage of national policies to increase efforts to establish enterprise reliability management systems and implement reliability engineering in conjunction with product development processes.

2.4 Reliability Engineering System

The specific work items of reliability engineering in the military field and the civilian field are different, but they are generally similar. In the field of military industry, the national military standard GJB 450A-2004 *General Requirements for Equipment Reliability Work* provides 32 reliability work items in 5 series. In the civilian field, reliability engineering has developed from the reliability category to the credibility category. The national standard GB/T 6992.2–1997 *Credibility Management* provides 32 reliability tasks with 6 elements. For the comparison of military standard reliability work series and the number of work items with the national standard reliability tasks and the number of work elements, please refer to Table 2.1. It is not difficult to see that whether it is a military standard or a national standard, the reliability work items They are all similar, and the purpose is to ensure that the product can meet the specified reliability index requirements and verify it.

The reliability work items stipulated in GJB 450A *General Requirements for Equipment Reliability Work* are shown in Tables 2.2 and 2.3.

It can be seen that whether according to GJB 450A—2004 or in accordance with GB 6992.2—1997, the reliability engineering system is very large. In fact, in a broad sense, reliability engineering includes the "six characteristics" of equipment (reliability, maintainability, testability, support, safety, and durability). Almost every characteristic has its own standard, and each standard contains Contains no less than 20 work items, therefore, the generalized reliability engineering work system is even larger. For the research and development of large and complex equipment, the

Table 2.1 Comparison of reliability work series/tasks stipulated by military standards/national standards

Military standard		National standard	
Serial Number—Name	Number of work items	Element Number: Name	Number of tasks
100—Reliability and Determination of Work Item Requirements	2	Element 1: Management	7
200—Reliability Management	7	Element 2: Dependability Engineering Discipline	5
300—Reliability Design and Analysis	13	Element 3: Analysis and Evaluation	9
400—Reliability Test and Evaluation	7	Element 4: Verification and Validation	3
500—Use reliability assessment and improvement	3	Element 5: Knowledge base	4
/	/	Element 6: Improvement	4
Total number of work items	32	Total number of tasks:	32

Table 2.2 Reliability work items stipulated in GJB 450A *General Requirements for Equipment Reliability Work*

Standard article number	Work item number	Work item name	Argument stage	Program stage	Engineering development and final stage	Production and use stage
5.1	101	Determine reliability requirements	√	√	x	x
5.2	102	Determining Reliability Work Item Requirements	√	√	x	x
6.1	201	Create a reliability plan	√	√	√	√
6.2	202	Create a reliability work plan	△	√	√	√
6.3	203	For research and development units, research and development units and supplier monitoring and control	△	√	√	√
6.4	204	reliability review	√	√	√	√
6.5	205	Establish failure reporting, analysis and corrective action system	x	△	√	√
6.6	206	Establish failure review organization	x	△	√	√
6.7	207	Reliability growth management	x	√	√	○
7.1	301	build a reliability model	△	√	√	○
7.2	302	Reliability assignment	△	√	√	○
7.3	303	Reliability prediction	△	√	√	○
7.4	304	Failure modes, effects and criticality analysis	△	√	√	△
7.5	305	Failure tree analysis	x	△	√	△
7.6	306	Potential pathway analysis	x	x	√	○

(continued)

Table 2.2 (continued)

Standard article number	Work item number	Work item name	Argument stage	Program stage	Engineering development and final stage	Production and use stage
7.7	307	Circuit tolerance analysis	x	x	√	○
7.8	308	Develop reliability design criteria	△	√	√	○
7.9	309	Selection and control of components, components and raw materials	x	△	√	√
7.10	310	Identify reliability critical products	x	△	√	○
7.11	311	Determine the functional testing, packaging, storage and transportation, loading and unloading, the impact of transportation and maintenance on product reliability	x	△	√	○
7.12	312	Finite element analysis	x	△	√	○
7.13	313	Durability analysis	x	△	√	○
8.1	401	Environmental stress screening	x	△	√	√
8.2	402	Reliability development test	x	△	√	○
8.3	403	Reliability growth test	x	△	√	○
8.4	404	Reliability qualification test	x	x	√	○
8.5	405	Reliability acceptance test	x	x	△	√
8.6	406	Reliability analysis and evaluation	x	x	√	√
8.7	407	Life test	x	x	√	△
9.1	501	Use reliability information collection	x	x	x	√

(continued)

Table 2.2 (continued)

Standard article number	Work item number	Work item name	Argument stage	Program stage	Engineering development and final stage	Production and use stage
9.2	502	Use reliability assessment	x	x	x	√
9.3	503	Use reliability improvements	x	x	x	√

Explanation of symbols: √ – applicable; △ —optional; ○ – applicable only when the design is changed; × —not applicable

implementation of reliability engineering will be even more complex. Usually, in the process of implementing reliability engineering, we need to grasp the key objects, select the most effective work items, and carry out them at the appropriate research and development stage. Make reliability engineering economical and efficient. The reliability work project process of each development stage is shown in Fig. 2.2.

With the gradual improvement of the reliability technology capabilities of enterprises, the scope, intensity and depth of reliability work can be continuously expanded, and the reliability engineering system in the narrow sense can be continuously expanded and improved to the reliability engineering system in the broad sense.

2.5 Reliability Engineering Master Plan Case

Combined with the development status of the domestic medical device industry, in order to better meet the development needs of the industry, the above reliability workflow can be further optimized to make it more economical, efficient and operable. Taking the 2016 national key research and development plan—digital diagnosis and treatment equipment research and development project *Volume Image Multi-mode Guided High-Intensity Accelerator Precision Radiation Therapy System* as an example, according to product development and project task requirements, *Volume Image Multi-mode Guided High-Intensity Radiation Therapy System* was formulated. The Accelerator Precision Radiation Therapy System Reliability Engineering Overall Plan guides the development unit to carry out the work of reliability engineering management, reliability design analysis and reliability test verification in the project development process, which improves the reliability, safety and usability of the product. Successfully realize product engineering and industrialization, and lay the foundation for improving market competitiveness.

Since September 2016, a domestic medical device listed company has been in the process of developing the national key research and development plan—digital diagnosis and treatment equipment research and development project "Volume

Table 2.3 Reliability work elements and tasks stipulated in GB/T 6992.2 *Credibility Management*

Credibility elements and tasks	Life cycle stage					
	C&D	D&D	MFG	INS	O&M	DIS
Element 1: Management						
Task 1: Credibility Program	xxx	xxx	xxx	xxx	xxx	xxx
Task 2: Credibility Specification		xxx	xxx	xxx		
Task 3: Process Control		xxx	xxx	xxx	xxx	
Task 4: Design Controls		xxx	xxx	xxx		
Task 5: Monitoring and Review		xxx	xxx	xxx	xxx	xxx
Task 6: Supply Chain Management			xxx	xxx	xxx	xxx
Task 7: Product Import				xxx	xxx	
Element 2: Dependability Engineering Discipline						
Task 8: Reliability Engineering	xxx	xxx	xxx			
Task 9: Maintenance Engineering	xxx	xxx	xxx			
Task 10: Maintenance Support Engineering		xxx	xxx	xxx	xxx	
Task 11: Standardization		xxx	xxx	xxx	xxx	
Task 12: Human Factors	xxx	xxx	xxx	xxx	xxx	xxx
Element 3: Analysis and Evaluation						
Task 13: Applied Environmental Analysis	xxx	xxx	xxx			
Task 14: Reliability Modeling and Simulation	xxx	xxx	xxx			
Task 15: Component Evaluation and Control		xxx	xxx			
Task 16: Design Analysis and Product Evaluation		xxx	xxx			
Task 17: Failure Cause, Effect, Effect and Risk Analysis		xxx	xxx	xxx	xxx	xxx
Task 18: Estimate	xxx	xxx	xxx			
Task 19: Trade–off Analysis	xxx	xxx	xxx			xxx
Task 20: Life Cycle Costing	xxx	xxx	xxx	xxx	xxx	xxx
Task 21: Reliability Growth				xxx	xxx	

(continued)

Table 2.3 (continued)

Credibility elements and tasks	Life cycle stage					
	C&D	D&D	MFG	INS	O&M	DIS
Element 4: Verification and Validation						
Task 22: Verify and Validate Policies		xxx	xxx	xxx		
Task 23: Credibility Verification				xxx	xxx	
Task 24: Reliability Stress Screening			xxx			
Element 5: Knowledge Base						
Task 25: Knowledge Base Creation		xxx	xxx	xxx	xxx	xxx
Task 26: Data Analysis		xxx	xxx	xxx	xxx	xxx
Task 27: Data Collection and Release		xxx	xxx	xxx	xxx	xxx
Task 28: Credibility Records		xxx	xxx	xxx	xxx	xxx
Element 6: Improvement						
Task 29: Preventive and Corrective Actions		xxx	xxx	xxx	xxx	
Mission 30: Upgrading and Retrofitting				xxx	xxx	
Task 31: Capacity Development and Enhancement	xxx	xxx	xxx	xxx	xxx	
Task 32: Management System Improvement	xxx	xxx	xxx	xxx	xxx	

Product life cycle phases: C&D—concept and definition; D&D—design and development; MFG—manufacturing; INS – installation; O&M–operation and maintenance; DIS—Disposition

Image Multi-mode Guided High-intensity Accelerator Precision Radiation Therapy System", according to the requirements of the "*Overall Plan for the Reliability Engineering of High-intensity Accelerator Precision Radiation Therapy System*", a series of reliability work including reliability design analysis and reliability test verification have been completed according to the time node: through the reliable Complete reliability design, complete reliability index demonstration and allocation, reliability prediction, failure mode, effect and criticality analysis (FMECA) and failure tree analysis (FTA), etc., form a series of guidance documents for reliability design analysis, and improve the system inherent level of reliability. Through environmental tests, safety tests, electromagnetic compatibility tests, thermal tests, reliability enhancement tests, comprehensive stress reliability tests, failure analysis, and soft system tests on the complete radiotherapy system or its core components,

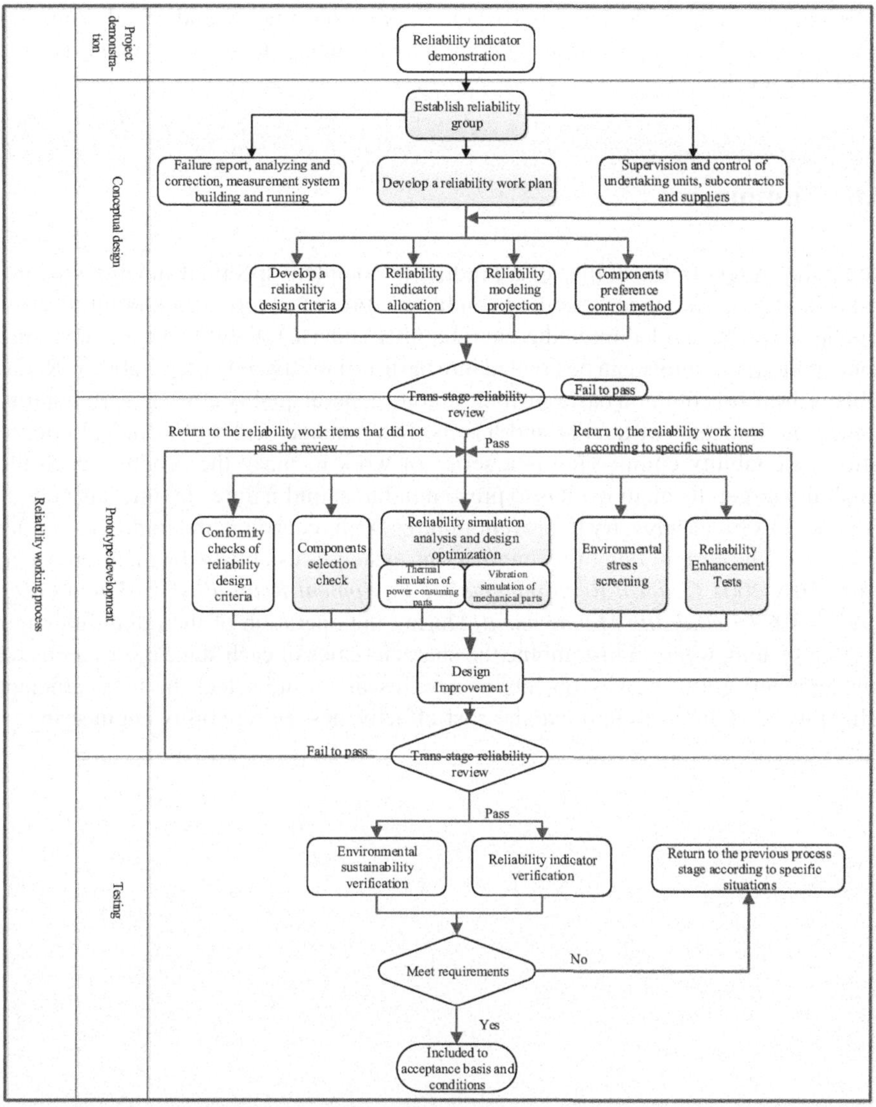

Fig. 2.2 Reliability work item flow in each development stage

radiotherapy systems have been discovered or stimulated. Various potential weak links in software and hardware, after targeted rectification of weak links, have been verified to be effective, improving product reliability, security and usability levels, and basically achieving the expected reliability goals of the project.

The implementation of reliability engineering, especially through reliability test verification, can help enterprises to quickly and fully find out the potential defects of prototypes, and implement improvements, so as to quickly and greatly improve the product's ability to withstand typical environments, technology maturity, and reliability levels.

2.6 Summary

Reliability refers to the ability of a product to complete specified functions within a specified time and under specified conditions. From the application point of view, reliability can be divided into inherent reliability and use reliability. From the design point of view, reliability can be divided into basic reliability and task reliability. Reliability is the most common basic attribute among general quality attributes. Reliability is the time indicator of quality and has its own management and technical connotations. Reliability engineering is a series of work to make the product reach the reliability target. Its main work is to prevent failures, find failures in time, take effective corrective measures, try to prevent failures from recurring, and improve product reliability. The current reliability engineering system is established with reference to GJB 450A-2004 *General Requirements for Equipment Reliability Work* and GB/T 6992.2–1997 *Reliability Management*. During the operation of the reliability engineering system, we need to combine the characteristics of each stage of research and development, grasp the key objects of new research, and select the most efficient reliability work items to improve the cost-effectiveness of reliability engineering.

Chapter 3
Reliability Design Method of Digital Diagnosis and Treatment Equipment

For digital diagnosis and treatment equipment, the reliability problem is a comprehensive system engineering problem, which is closely related to product design, manufacturing, assembly, debugging, transportation, storage, use and maintenance. Product design is only one of the links, but design is the most important link to ensure product reliability, it has laid a congenital foundation for product reliability. The reliability of digital diagnosis and treatment equipment depends on the structural form and size (type and specification) of its parts (components), selected materials and manufacturing processes, inspection standards, convenience of maintenance, and various safety protection measures, etc., and these All are determined in the design, so the design determines the reliability level of the product, that is, the inherent reliability of the product. Although the manufacture and use of digital medical equipment have an extremely important impact on its reliability, the manufacture is carried out according to the design, and the main task of manufacture and use is to ensure the realization of product reliability indicators.

Product reliability is designed, and reliability design is the most fundamental guarantee to achieve reliability. Implementing reliability design criteria in the design process of digital medical equipment is an important means to ensure product reliability. For each specific model, reliability design criteria should be formulated according to the characteristics of the model, so as to facilitate implementation. This chapter focuses on the formulation and implementation of reliability design criteria for digital medical equipment, and several commonly used reliability design methods.

X. Li et al., *Reliability Engineering Technology of Digital Diagnosis and Treatment Equipment*, https://doi.org/10.1007/978-981-99-5522-0_3

3.1 Overview of the Reliability Design

This chapter mainly starts from the reliability requirements in the national key research and development plan digital medical equipment special guidelines, focuses on the formulation and implementation of reliability design criteria and reliability design methods, and summarizes a set of reliable digital medical equipment throughout the product life cycle sexual design method.

When carrying out reliability design for digital medical equipment, the corresponding reliability design criteria should be followed. Reliability design criteria are the guidance documents for reliability design. In the design process, the necessary and appropriate methods are selected according to the actual situation and needs of the product.

Table 3.1 for the reliability design criteria of digital diagnosis and treatment equipment.

Next, through the process of formulation, implementation and application, verification and rectification of reliability design criteria for digital medical equipment, we will illustrate the criteria related to reliability design.

3.2 Development of Reliability Design Criteria

3.2.1 Purpose and Function

The purpose of formulating reliability design criteria is to guide designers in product reliability design, improve product inherent reliability, and meet reliability design requirements. Reliability design criteria have the following effects:

(1) Promote the implementation of reliability design analysis work item requirements;
(2) An important basis for continuous reliability improvement design;
(3) Ways to meet product reliability requirements;
(4) Standardize the reliability design work of designers;
(5) The benchmark for checking reliability design compliance.

3.2.2 Scope of Application

Reliability design criteria are applicable to digital medical equipment scheme design and engineering development stages, including formulation, implementation, verification and rectification of reliability design criteria.

Table 3.1 Reliability design criteria for digital medical equipment

Serial number	Design guideline name	Criterion features
1	Adopt mature technology and process	Overall control scheme of technology and process
2	Simplified design	A typical design method to achieve the purpose of improving reliability by controlling the product composition scale
3	Material selection and control	Components and raw material selection control methods
4	Derating design	A typical design method to achieve the purpose of improving reliability by reducing the working stress of components
5	Redundant design	Typical Design Approach for Improving Mission Reliability by Adding Margins
6	Fault–tolerant and error prevention design	Typical design method, by improving the diagnostic ability of hardware and software, to improve the ability of the structure to prevent errors, so as to achieve the purpose of improving reliability
7	Thermal design	A typical design method to achieve the purpose of improving reliability by eliminating or weakening the impact of internal and external thermal effects on the product
8	Environmental protection design	A typical design method to achieve the purpose of improving reliability by improving the product's internal and external resistance to environmental stress
9	EMC design	A typical design method achieves the purpose of improving reliability by improving the anti–electromagnetic interference capability of the product and reducing external electromagnetic interference
10	Circuit tolerance design	A typical design method to achieve the purpose of improving reliability by reducing the influence of component parameter drift
11	Software reliability design	Typical design methods, through software error avoidance, error detection, error correction, fault–tolerant design and other measures to achieve the purpose of improving software reliability
12	Anti–transient overstress design	Reduce safety impact through protective design
13	Human factors design	Reduce the impact of human factors on product reliability through design
14	Packaging and transportation Design	Reduce the probability of product failures during packaging, storage, loading and unloading and transportation through design
15	Reliability design of non–electronic products	Typical design approach to improve the reliability of non–electronic products

3.2.3 *Time Scheduling*

In the early stage of development, according to the reliability requirements and product characteristics stipulated in the contract, refer to relevant standards and manuals, and formulate product-specific reliability design criteria (including hardware, software and non-electronic components) on the basis of carefully summarizing engineering experience. product). In the process of product design, designers should implement the reliability design criteria, and modify and improve these design criteria during the implementation process. In order to ensure that the reliability design criteria can be effectively implemented, the research and development unit should be required to provide a compliance analysis report for the design criteria. During design review, compliance with design criteria shall be reviewed.

3.2.4 Basis for Formulation

The basis for formulating reliability design criteria is as follows:

(1) Reliability design requirements stipulated in documents such as the "Project Declaration Guide", "Project or Product Development Mission Statement" and development contracts (including work instructions) for digital medical equipment;
(2) Reliability-related design requirements proposed in relevant domestic and foreign standards, specifications and product manuals;
(3) Reliability design criteria specified in similar products;
(4) Reliability design experience and lessons accumulated by similar products and research institutes at home and abroad;
(5) Attributes of the product.

3.2.5 Dynamic Management

The development of design guidelines is a dynamic management process of continuous revision and gradual improvement. Reliability design guidelines for digital medical equipment should be developed in the program phase, and a copy of the reliability design guidelines to be used should be provided during the preliminary (initial sample) design review. As the design progresses, the guidelines are continuously improved and refined, and their contents and descriptions are finalized at the beginning of the detailed (prototype) design.

3.2.6 Documentation System

Reliability design criteria are usually design specification documents. The level of the reliability design criterion document can be divided according to the product level, that is, the leading unit should first formulate the project-oriented top-level reliability design criterion document. Supporting product development units at all levels formulate their own reliability design criterion documents according to the top-level reliability design criterion documents of the project, and all the reliability design criterion documents constitute the reliability design criterion document system, as shown in Fig. 3.1.

The reliability design rule document at the top level of the project is used to constrain the overall reliability design of the project, and the reliability design rule files of supporting products at all levels are used to constrain the reliability design of supporting products. In addition to the general terms applicable to the upper-level product reliability design criteria, the supporting product reliability design criteria should also include specific criteria closely related to product characteristics.

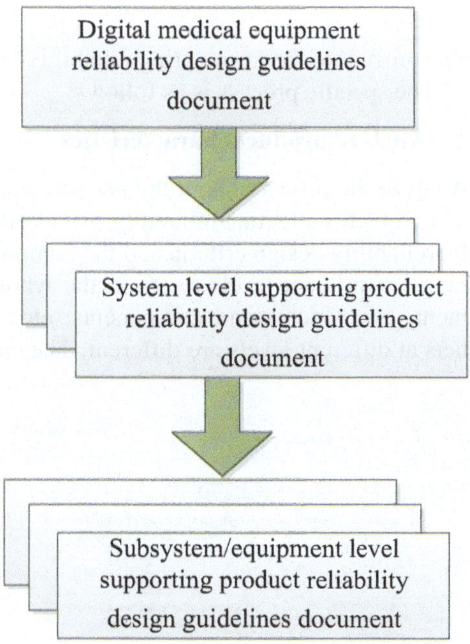

Fig. 3.1 Reliability design criteria documentation system

3.2.7 Organization and Personnel Responsibilities

The establishment of reliability design criteria should be included in the reliability management system for unified management. The research and development unit should formulate reliability design criteria based on the reliability requirements and characteristics of the product and the experience of similar products. During the product design process, designers should conscientiously implement the reliability design criteria under the leadership and supervision of the design supervisor, and modify and improve the design criteria during the implementation process. In order to ensure that the reliability design criteria can be effectively implemented, the research and development unit should provide the reliability design criteria compliance inspection report. During the review, the reliability design criteria and compliance inspection report should be taken as the content of the design review to evaluate the degree of conformity between the design and the criteria.

3.2.8 Reliability Design Criteria Formulation Procedure

The procedure for formulating reliability design criteria is shown in Fig. 3.2.

The specific process is as follows:

1. **Analyze product characteristics**

Analyze the product hierarchy and structural characteristics, as well as the factors and problems affecting reliability, and clarify the range of product hierarchy covered by reliability design criteria and the composition categories of product objects. The range of product levels refers to the whole machine, system, sub-system, equipment, components and components, etc. The reliability design criteria of products at different levels are different. The composition categories of product objects

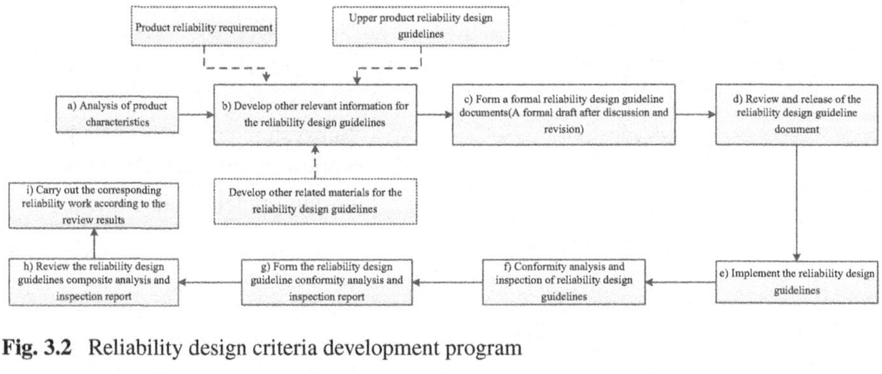

Fig. 3.2 Reliability design criteria development program

include electronic products, mechanical products, electromechanical products, software products and various combinations of these categories, etc. The reliability design criteria of different categories are different.

2. **General and specific clauses for formulating product reliability design criteria (First Draft)**

(1) Product reliability requirements are an important basis for formulating reliability design criteria. By analyzing the product reliability requirements stipulated in the development contract or mission statement, especially the reliability qualitative requirements, the scope of reliability design criteria can be clarified to avoid Omission of important reliability design terms. When formulating the reliability design criteria of supporting products, it should be extended by referring to the requirements of the "reliability design criteria of upper-level products".
(2) The terms of the general part of the reliability design criteria are generally applicable to each component unit in the product; the terms of the special part of the reliability design criteria are formulated for the specific conditions of each component unit in the product, and are only applicable to specific unit. When formulating general and specific parts of reliability design criteria, references to standards, specifications or manuals related to reliability design criteria, as well as reliability design criteria documents of related products can be collected. Among them, various reliability issues of similar products are an important means of summarizing special clauses.

3. **Form a formal reliability design criterion document (official draft revised after discussion)**

After discussions and revisions by relevant personnel (designers, craftsmen, managers, etc.), a reliability design criterion document (official draft) is formed.

4. **Evaluation and release of reliability design criteria documents**

Invite experts to review the reliability design criterion documents, and further improve the criterion documents according to their opinions. Finally, after approval by the person in charge of the project (product), release the reliability design criterion document.

5. **Implement reliability design criteria**

Product designers should carry out product reliability design according to the published reliability design criteria document.

6. **Conformity analysis and inspection of reliability design criteria**

According to the specified form, the reliability design status of the product and the reliability design criteria are compared, analyzed and checked.

7. **Formation of reliability design criteria compliance report**

Compile and complete the compliance analysis and inspection report of the reliability design criteria according to the specified format.

8. **Review reliability design criteria compliance report**

Experts are invited to review the reliability design criteria compliance analysis and inspection report.

9. **Carry out corresponding reliability design work according to the review results.**

3.3 Reliability Design Criteria

3.3.1 Adopt Mature Technology and Process

The inheritance of technologies and processes and reduce the reliability risks brought by new technologies and processes. Preference should be given to selecting design solutions (including hardware and software) and parts, components, and assemblies that have been tested, verified, and technologically mature, and fully consider the inheritance of product design.

(1) Implement standardized design and use mature standard circuits, standard modules and standard parts as much as possible.
(2) Do not adopt solutions that look advanced but immature in design.
(3) The contact design principles are as follows:

- Try to use winding, crimping, cold rolling and other processes instead of tin welding.
- Tin soldering of printed boards should adopt wave soldering process as far as possible.
- Solder joints and metallized holes on printed boards should be soldered on both sides.

(4) Reliability design of printed circuit boards, the basic principles are as follows:

- Copper-clad epoxy glass cloth laminates with stable mechanical properties and electrical properties are used as printed circuit board materials
- The wiring of the printed circuit board should adopt computer-aided design (Computer Aided Design, CAD) technology

(5) The design of printed circuit board diagrams (layout sketches, original board diagrams, machining drawings, assembly drawings, etc.) shall meet the requirements of professional standards, etc.
(6) The finalized or verified standard components, standard circuits and standard electronic function modules including microprocessors should be used.

3.3.2 *Simplifying Design*

3.3.2.1 The Purpose of Simplifying Design

Simplifying design, that is, in determining the design of the product, not one-sided pursuit of performance indicators "high and precise", in the premise of meeting the requirements of use, as far as possible to simplify the design technology, so that the product "structure" and "composition" are simplified, so as to improve the reliability of the product. "Structure simplification" means that the mechanical structure of the product should be "integrated" as far as possible, reducing the assembly level and screw connection; "Composition simplification" means reducing the number of functional units and the variety and number of components as much as possible. Since the basic reliability of a product is inversely proportional to the number of units in the product, simplifying design and reducing the size of the unit composition can improve the basic reliability of the product.

3.3.2.2 Ways of Simplifying Design

Talking about simplifying design in isolation seems too general and not practical. It is only practical to combine the simplifying design with the process of universalization, combination and serialization, which are specific applications of the principles and methods of standardization in product development activities, and is the inevitable result of standardization activities.

(1) **Universalization**

The implementation objects of generalization are usually components, components, parts, or sub-system-level products for the whole machine, which are collectively referred to as functional units. The so-called "universalization" is to directly select general-purpose units with interchangeable characteristics (both structure and function are interchangeable), and apply them to the designed products.

If there are no ready-made general-purpose units available, new general-purpose units can be purposefully and targetedly developed to meet the needs of products under development and subsequent development.

The higher the level of this kind of general-purpose unit in the whole machine product and the wider the scope of application, the more obvious the generalization effect will be.

(2) **Combination**

Combination implementation objects are generally relatively complex products, but not necessarily the final complete machine product, but can be sub-systems or equipment-level hardware products for the complete machine, or software products.

Such products usually have to complete relatively important and complex tasks. Before designing, the task must be carefully analyzed and decomposed into several relatively independent task units, and then different "general function modules" are selected to separate them. meet its mission requirements. For some special needs, there may be no ready-made general-purpose modules, so it is necessary to develop a "special-purpose module" to meet this special demand. Finally, these general and special modules are combined into an organic whole according to certain rules, then a new product is born.

(3) **Serialization**

The implementation object of serialization is usually the final product to be delivered. The "complete machine product" mentioned here can be a fairly complex large system; it can also be a small electronic component. In a word, they all have to face the market directly and are the final products that can be purchased by users.

The main parameters (structural parameters and performance parameters) of this kind of products can be divided into several grades according to the characteristics and usage requirements of the products, which are called "parameter series". Then, compile the "series type spectrum" of the product according to the parameter series. The development, production and sales of products are all carried out according to this type spectrum, which is what is commonly called "basic type serialization". The so-called "basic type" refers to the "fixed" part of the type spectrum, on which a series of new products can be derived to meet the different needs of users.

The products of each specification (grade) in the serialized products are universal within a certain range. Therefore, serialization is also generalization with an expanded scope.

3.3.2.3 Measures of Simplifying Design

Universalization is the foundation, providing standard and general-purpose functional modules for combination and serialization; combination is an application, which combines the functional modules provided by generalization into products of different levels, which can be the final product to be delivered. It can also be an intermediate product for the whole machine; serialization is the result, and various series of products are manufactured (or combined) according to the "series spectrum" of the product to meet the different needs of users. The relationship between the three can be summed up in one sentence: use common modules to combine a series of products.

When determining the product design scheme, if the "universalization, combination and serialization" principles can be seriously implemented, then the aforementioned "structural simplification" and "composition simplification" will definitely be realized. Implementing the "universalization, combination and serialization" principle can not only improve the reliability, maintainability and supportability of products, but also shorten the product development cycle and reduce the inherent cost of products.

In order to effectively implement the "universalization, combination and serialization" principle, the simplified design measures are mainly as follows:

(1) The system functions should be analyzed and weighed, the same or similar functions should be merged, and unnecessary functions should be eliminated.
(2) Under the condition of meeting the specified functional requirements, the design should be simple, and the number of product levels and component units should be reduced as much as possible.
(3) A large number of structural parts or components cannot be added for a little performance improvement. The scheme must be strictly demonstrated, and the performance index should not be too high, and reliability should be regarded as an important index;
(4) Minimize the number of parts and components that perform the same or similar functions.
(5) Parts, fasteners and connectors, pipelines, cables, etc. with a high degree of standardization should be preferred.
(6) Maximize the use of general-purpose components, parts, and components, and minimize their varieties.
(7) It is necessary to make the units with high failure rate, easy damage and criticality have good interchangeability and versatility.
(8) The finished parts of the same model produced by different factories must be able to achieve installation interchange and function interchange.
(9) To simplify the circuit design, the following principles should be followed:

- Replace medium and small-scale integrated circuits with large-scale integrated circuits as much as possible. In the design of logic circuits, in the past, the simplification work was used to reduce the number of gates or reduce the number of inputs. From the perspective of reliability, when the integration level increases, the failure rate of the device increases with the complexity of the integrated circuit. Not much. Therefore, integrated circuits with high reliability and high integration should be used as much as possible instead of silicon controlled rectifier components or small-scale integrated circuits, and the focus should be to reduce the number of devices;
- In the case of ensuring the original design function indicators, simplify the circuit design as much as possible, that is, meet the requirements of the technical indicators with the simplest circuit and the least amount of components;
- While reducing the number of components, their varieties and specifications should also be compressed to facilitate quality control, reduce the number of spare parts and facilitate maintenance;
- Software functions should be used instead of hardware functions as much as possible to simplify the circuit;
- Replace circuits composed of silicon controlled rectifier components with integrated circuits as much as possible;
- Since the failure rate of analog integrated circuits is higher than that of digital circuits, and there are problems such as characteristic drift with temperature, digital integrated circuits should be used as much as possible if digital circuits can be used instead;

- In the design, we should also pay attention to adding measures to improve circuit stability, reliability, testability and maintainability, and should not be omitted for simplification.

3.3.3 Material Selection and Control

3.3.3.1 The Purpose of Material Control

The quality and reliability of components, components, and raw materials are the basis of equipment reliability. Reasonable selection and strict control of materials is an important task to ensure equipment reliability. Through the selection and control of materials, the types of components, parts, and raw materials should be reduced as much as possible, the preferred catalog of components, parts, and raw materials should be compiled and revised, and the use of components, parts, and raw materials in the super-preferred catalog should be strictly controlled, to maintain and improve the inherent reliability of the product.

3.3.3.2 Methods of Material Selection and Control

The selection process of materials includes the selection of the performance, quality and reliability level of the selected components, and the selection of components should also meet the working environment conditions required by the equipment development contract or the development task book; understand the material production plant technology, Production line level and quality management, past use of materials, shape, structure, size and packaging of selected materials; selection, standardization, maturity and economy of materials should also be considered.

Material selection and control methods are mainly as follows:

(1) Design and selection of materials should meet the requirements of the product, pay attention to the role of lightweight materials in structural design, and pay attention to the guarantee of product reliability under various harsh environments.
(2) Material selection should not only consider the performance requirements of each part and component to meet the requirements of each sub-function of the entire product, but also consider the impact of each part and component on product performance or other components (parts) subsidiary functions.
(3) Design and material selection should follow standardization, generalization and serialization.
(4) Design and selection of materials should first select the best materials that have been included in the national standard.
(5) For the design of foreign grades of materials that may be encountered, should first be selected in the domestic grades, try to do a good job of domestic grade material substitution; for foreign grades of materials that can not be

substituted, in the design of material selection should also pay attention to the transformation of material standards.

(6) The engineering design shall conduct a comprehensive analysis of the grade, variety and specification of the material, and strive to be universal.
(7) Attention should be paid to the manufacturing and processing properties of the selected materials, including forging properties, cutting properties, heat treatment process properties, etc.
(8) Consider the maturity of material application technology.
(9) When selecting new materials, the design review should pay attention to the feasibility review of the application of new materials, and the application of important new materials must be verified.
(10) Structural materials should have high resistance to cracks during their expected structural service life, and should be resistant to brittle crack growth in the service environment.
(11) When selecting materials, the reasonable combination of material strength and plasticity should be considered; for example, if there are sharp gaps on parts bearing alternating loads, resulting in high stress concentration, it is possible that the original low-stress high-cycle fatigue of the entire structure may become localized in the gap. High-strain plastic fatigue load; the local composite strengthening method can be used to reduce or even eliminate the plastic strain at the notch and improve the local effective bearing capacity.
(12) Select mature parts and components according to the preferred list of parts and components.
(13) Necessary screening and breaking in of parts.
(14) The selected parts should meet the requirements of the use environment (anti-salt spray, anti-mold, etc.).
(15) The key components should be listed and the tolerance precision should be strictly controlled.

3.3.3.3 Selection of Components

1. **Overview**

Electronic components are the basic components of electronic and electrical systems, and are basic circuit units that can complete predetermined functions and cannot be divided. Components generally have several quality grades. At present, the quality grades of electronic components in China are divided into one, two, and three. The first category is military products, the second category is industrial products, and the third category is civilian products. Each category can be divided into several different levels. Different quality grades have different reliability levels of components; different types of components with the same quality grade have different quality requirements. Improper selection of the quality level of components will cause the system reliability level not to meet the requirements. In order to ensure system reliability, the selection of components must be controlled.

2. **Terms and Definitions**

(1) Basic failure rate of components λ_b.

The basic failure rate λ b refers to the failure rate of electronic components under the action of electrical stress and temperature stress, and is the influence factors of electronic components such as quality control level, environmental stress, application state, functional rating and type, and structure. The failure rate is only calculated under the influence of temperature and electrical stress ratio (working electrical stress/rated electrical stress).

The basic failure rate λ_b is usually expressed by the relationship model of the influence of the ratio of temperature (T) and electrical stress (S) on the failure rate of electronic components.

(2) Component failure rate λ_p

The failure rate of components refers to the failure rate of components in the application environment. Except for individual component categories, the working failure rate λ_p is related to the basic failure rate and factors such as the quality level of components other than temperature and electrical stress, environmental stress, application status, functional rating and type, structure, etc., usually $_{\text{used}}$ It is expressed by the product of the basic failure rate and the adjustment coefficient of the above-mentioned factors.

(3) Quality grade and quality factor π_Q

The quality of components directly affects its failure rate, and the degree of influence of different quality levels on the failure rate of components is expressed by the quality factor $\pi_{Q.}$ Thus, the π_Q value in the failure rate of components depends on the quality level of components. The quality level is the quality control level of components in the process of manufacturing, testing and silicon controlled rectifier before they are installed and used.

(4) General failure rate λ_G of components

The failure rate of components in a certain environmental category under the general working environment temperature and common working stress. Use this generic failure rate in component count reliability predictions.

3. **General principles for component selection**

The general principles of component selection are as follows:

(1) The technical performance, quality grade, and service conditions of components should meet the requirements of digital medical equipment.
(2) Prioritize the use of standard components that have been proven to be stable in quality, high in reliability, and promising, and prohibit the use of components that have been eliminated.

(3) The equipment design should be optimized to the greatest extent, and the types and specifications of compressed components should be reduced, and the number of manufacturers should be reduced.
(4) The use of newly developed components should be strictly controlled, and components without technical appraisal cannot be used in digital medical equipment.

Choose imported components, you should try to use components with the applicable quality and failure rate grades on the Qualified Products List (QPL) or Product Preferred List (PPL) of the producing country pieces.

4. *Questions to consider when selecting components*

When determining the type of components, it should be considered whether the components can complete the required functions in the expected working environment. When determining key components, it should be considered whether the components perform key functions and whether their failure affects safety; at the same time, consider whether the life of the components meets the life requirements of the equipment, whether they are affected by working conditions, and whether the cost is expensive. When determining the applicability of a component, it should be considered whether the component meets the relevant standards and whether it is preferred; at the same time, its delivery cycle and supply stability should be considered to confirm whether it can be purchased from multiple suppliers. When determining the applicable quality level and reliability level of components, the various stresses that components are expected to be subjected to in the circuit should be considered, and the derating factor selected for components should be specified, and the selected components should be determined through reliability prediction level of quality and reliability.

3.3.3.4 Control of Components

1. **Develop component outline**

In order to control the selection and use of standard components and non-standard components, an outline of components should be prepared. The outline should include component control items and principles, standardization of components, application guidelines for components, testing and silicon controlled rectifier of components, etc.

2. **Prepare applicable component procurement specifications**

When compiling this specification, it should be based on the following contents:

- Documents related to the selection of components in product design;
- Preferred catalog of components;
- List of qualified component production and supply units;
- Model product development and production plan;

- The requirements and documents of the superior department for the review and approval of the selected components;
- Relevant standards for procurement of components, acceptance inspection and other relevant procurement requirements.

3. **Component screening file**

Products with screening requirements for components should prepare component screening files. The content of the files includes relevant screening items and content, whether to conduct secondary screening, the arrangement and content of primary and secondary screening items, so as to control the quality and quality of selected components and reliability.

4. **Components preferences catalog**

It is very important to compile the preferences catalog of components to control the quality and reliability of the selected components. The catalog should include the following contents: component names, model specifications, main performance parameters and quantities, technical standards that components meet, quality grades, component manufacturers (preferable), comparisons between new and old and corresponding models at home and abroad, etc.

5. **Specifies the applicable derating standard**

Stipulating the applicable derating standards is convenient for designers to consider the impact of derating when selecting components, so as to make correct and reasonable choices. See Sect. 3.3.4 of this chapter for details.

6. **Application review of key components**

Critical components refer to components whose failure will seriously affect system safety, availability, mission success and difficult maintenance and high life cycle costs. The main contents of the review are: whether the selected components can meet the requirements specified in the design, whether they can meet the requirements for derating use; whether they are preferred, standard and mature components; if they are newly developed components, whether they meet the specified requirements Technical standards;

3.3.4 Derating Design

3.3.4.1 Purpose of Derating Design

Derating design refers to consciously reducing the thermal, electrical, mechanical and other stresses that components are subjected to during work in order to achieve the purpose of improving the reliability of components. Derating design is an extremely effective and simple measure to improve product reliability, so it is widely used in electronic product design.

The failure rate of electronic components is related to the environmental stress and working stress it bears. Environmental stresses include temperature, humidity, pressure, radiation, and surrounding chemicals. No matter whether the component is in working condition or not, the environmental stress it bears exists objectively. The working stress will only appear when the components are in working condition, and the working stress includes voltage, current, frequency, heat generated by the components themselves, mechanical load, etc.

3.3.4.2 Principles of Derating Design

For electronic, electrical and electromechanical components should be according to GJB/Z35-1993 *Component Derating Guidelines* for different categories of components according to different applications for derating.

The concept of derating design for mechanical and structural components is to design mechanical and structural components to withstand a load (called strength) that is greater than the load that they are subjected to in actual operation (called stress). For mechanical and structural components, stress and strength analysis should be paid attention to, and according to the specific situation, basic methods such as increasing the mean value of strength, decreasing the mean value of stress, decreasing the variance of stress and strength should be used to find out the best match of stress and strength and improve the reliability of design.

(1) Usually, components have an optimal derating range. Within this range, the reduction of the working stress of the components can significantly improve the reduction of the failure rate, and the design of the equipment is easy to realize without paying a large price in terms of the weight, volume and cost of the equipment. The derating level should be determined based on comprehensive weighing of equipment reliability requirements, design maturity, maintenance cost and difficulty, safety requirements, and constraints on equipment weight and size.
(2) Three derating levels are recommended within the best derating range:

Level I derating is the maximum derating, and it is suitable for derating design when equipment failure will endanger safety, lead to mission failure and cause serious economic loss. It is the maximum derating necessary to ensure the reliability of the equipment. If a derating larger than this is used, the reliability of the equipment will not increase much, and it is unacceptable in design. Level I derating applies to the following situations: the failure of equipment will cause casualties or serious damage to equipment and support facilities; there are high reliability requirements for equipment, and the design of new technologies and processes is adopted; due to cost and technical reasons, After the equipment fails, it is impossible or not suitable for maintenance; the system has strict restrictions on the size and weight of the equipment.

Level II derating is a moderate degree of derating, which is suitable for derating design when equipment failure will degrade work tasks and unreasonable maintenance costs will occur. This level of derating is still in the range where reducing the working stress can significantly improve the reliability of the equipment, and it is easier to achieve than the first level of derating. Level II derating applies to the following situations: equipment failure may cause damage to equipment and support equipment; high reliability requirements are required, and some special designs are used; relatively high maintenance costs are required.

Level III derating, which is the smallest level of derating, applies to situations where equipment failure will have only a minor impact on mission accomplishment and is easily repaired; this level of derating has the greatest effect on reliability growth and presents little design difficulty. Level III derating is applicable to situations where the failure of the equipment will not cause injury or damage to personnel or facilities; where the equipment is of proven standard design; where the failed equipment can be repaired quickly and economically; and where there are no major restrictions on the size and weight of the equipment.

The division of the three derating levels is shown in Table 3.2.

(3) The main derating parameters of different types of components are different:

Table 3.2 Division of the three derating levels

Derating level situation	Level I	Level II	Level III
Derating degree	Maximum	Medium	The smallest
Improved reliability	Maximum	Moderate	Smaller
Applicable situation	(1) Equipment failure leading to casualties or serious damage to equipment and support equipment; (2) High reliability requirements for equipment; (3) Adopt new technology and new process design; (4) The failed equipment cannot or should not be repaired; (5) heat dissipation difference	(1) Damage to equipment and support equipment caused by equipment failure; (2) Higher reliability requirements for equipment; (3) Some special designs are adopted; (4) The maintenance cost of the failed equipment is relatively high	(1) Equipment failure will not cause casualties and equipment damage; (2) Adopt mature standard design; (3) Failed equipment can be repaired quickly and economically
Realization of derating design	More difficult	Generally	Easy
Derating increase fee	Slightly higher	Medium	Lower

- The main derating method for resistors is to reduce the power ratio;
- The main derating method for capacitors is to reduce their operating voltage;
- The main derating method for semiconductor devices is to keep the working power consumption within the rated power consumption;
- The main derating method for digital integrated circuits is to derate through the ambient temperature and electrical load;
- Linear integrated circuits, large-scale integrated circuits and semiconductor memories also achieve derating by reducing the ambient temperature;
- For mechanical component bearings, it is based on the load ratio as the derating factor.

(4) The determination of the derating coefficient should focus on skills:

- The power derating factor of the resistor is about 0.5;
- The voltage derating factor of the capacitor is 0.4–0.5, and its failure rate is about 1/10 of the rated failure rate;
- For switches and connectors, the current derating factor should be below 0.5;
- For relays, the drop is the contact current derating;
- For digital circuits, the ratio of the actual fan-out coefficient to the rated fan-out coefficient should be less than 0.9, and the specified power supply voltage cannot be exceeded;
- The derating design cannot be used casually, and there may be dangers if the derating is insufficient or too large.

(5) The working basis of the derating value can be divided into the following three situations, which should be paid attention to in the derating design:

  - Class A: A large amount of use data has been analyzed, and a good understanding of the relationship between stress and reliability of components;
  - Class B: The available data for analysis is limited, or the structure is complex. But have a certain understanding of the stress reliability relationship of components;
  - Class C: Due to the relatively new technology or the limitation of the combination method in the equipment where the device is located, there is no derating application data for reference so far. However, engineering judgments for derating are made after studying their structure and materials.

  The basic classification of derating work is shown in Table 3.3.

(6) The basic principles of derating design can be referred to as follows:

  - Components are derated according to GJB/Z35 "Components Derating Guidelines".
  - For components in the circuit, derating must be considered, and overloading is never allowed.

Table 3.3 Derating work basis classification

Derating work basis classification	Component category
Class A	Integrated circuits, semiconductor silicon controlled rectifier devices, resistors, potentiometers, capacitors
Class B	Inductive elements, relays, switches, rotating electrical appliances, electrical connectors, cables, light bulbs, circuit breakers, fuses
Class C	Electric vacuum devices, crystals, surface acoustic wave devices, laser devices, fiber optics devices

- For components or components with high failure rate, affecting product safety, or critical or important components of reliability, derating design should be strictly carried out.
- In principle, the key parts and important parts adopt Level I derating.
- Level II derating applies to equipment designs where equipment failure would degrade the mission and incur unreasonable maintenance costs.
- Level III derating applies to equipment failures that have only a small impact on mission completion and where the equipment can be repaired economically.
- Refer to GJB/Z 35 to determine the derating parameters of related categories of components.

(7) Typical cases of transistor power derating

- The relationship between the total power dissipation allowed by the transistor and the ambient temperature (or shell temperature) can be expressed by the "power—temperature load characteristic curve".
- The ambient temperature corresponding to the maximum rated power of a low-power transistor is usually between −55 °C ~ + 25 °C. When the upper temperature limit is exceeded, the allowable total power dissipation value decreases linearly until it drops to 0. At this time, the ambient temperature (or case temperature) corresponds to the highest junction temperature of the transistor. The slope of the slope part of the curve is approximately equal to the reciprocal of the thermal resistance, which is related to the physical constants of the device.
- Figure 3.3a–c shaded parts are the allowable working areas for level I, II and III derating respectively. The derating curves are all parallel to the rating curves
- The derating of power transistors should be considered to meet the requirements of power and temperature derating guidelines at the same time, and the derating curve of the transistors is shown in Fig. 3.3d.

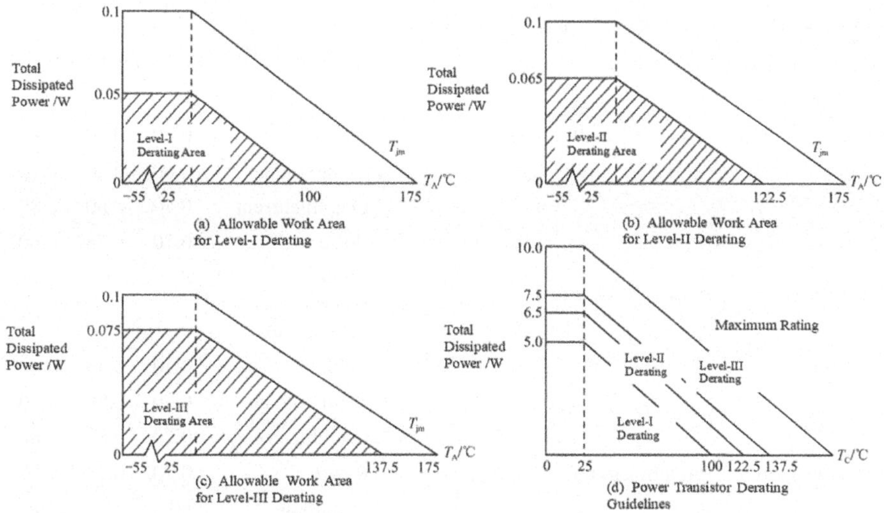

Fig. 3.3 Transistor derating curve

(8) The precautions for derating design are as follows:

- The load stress of some components cannot be derated or has a limit on the maximum derating;
- For some components, the expected derating effect cannot be obtained when the derating reaches a certain level;
- Attention should be paid to the derating of capacitors: some types of capacitors have low-level failures, that is, when the voltage across the capacitors is too low, they show open-circuit failures. That is to say, derating will not only reduce the failure rate, but will increase the failure rate.

3.3.4.3 Common Component Derating Guidelines

For the domestic components commonly used in the design of digital diagnosis and treatment equipment, they can be selected according to the derating criteria in Tables 3.4, 3.5, 3.6, 3.7, 3.8 and 3.9. For imported components, they can be selected according to the derating criteria in Tables 3.10, 3.11, 3.12, 3.13 and 3.14.

Table 3.4 Derating guidelines for integrated circuits

Type of components			Derating parameter	Derating level		
				I	II	III
Integrated circuit	Analog circuit	Amplifier	Voltage	0.70	0.80	0.80
			Input voltage	0.60	0.70	0.70
			Output current	0.70	0.80	0.80
			Power	0.70	0.75	0.80
			Maximum junction temperature (°C)	80	95	105
		Comparators	Voltage	0.70	0.80	0.80
			Input voltage	0.70	0.80	0.80
			Output current	0.70	0.80	0.80
Integrated circuit	Analog circuit	Comparators	Power	0.70	0.75	0.80
			Maximum junction temperature (°C)	80	95	105
		Voltage regulator	Voltage	0.70	0.80	0.80
			Input voltage	0.70	0.80	0.80
			Input/Output voltage difference	0.70	0.80	0.85
			Output current	0.70	0.75	0.80
			Power	0.70	0.75	0.80
			Maximum junction temperature (°C)	80	95	105
		Analog switch	Voltage	0.70	0.80	0.85
			Input voltage	0.80	0.85	0.90
			Output current	0.75	0.80	0.85
			Power	0.70	0.75	0.80
			Maximum junction temperature (°C)	80	95	105
	Digital circuit	Bipolar circuitar	Frequency	0.80	0.90	0.90
			Output current	0.80	0.90	0.90
			Maximum junction temperature (°C)	85	100	115
	MOS circuit		Voltage	0.70	0.80	0.80
			Output current	0.80	0.90	0.90
			Frequency	0.80	0.80	0.90

(continued)

Table 3.4 (continued)

Type of components		Derating parameter	Derating level		
			I	II	III
		Maximum junction temperature (°C)	85	100	115
	Hybrid integrated circuit	Thick film power density (W/cm^2)	7.5		
		Film power density (W/cm^2)	6.0		
		Maximum junction temperature (°C)	85	100	115
	Large scale integrated circuit	Maximum junction temperature (°C)	Improved heat dissipation to lower junction temperature		

Note

(1) The power supply voltage of the analog circuit should not be lower than the recommended normal working voltage after derating, and the input voltage should not exceed the power supply voltage under any circumstances. The input voltage of the voltage regulator is generally the power supply voltage;

(2) The derating of the bipolar output current will reduce the fan-out, which may lead to an increase in the number of devices used, which in turn will reduce the expected reliability of the device. This should be prevented when derating;

(3) The power supply voltage of MOS-type digital circuits should not be less than the recommended normal operating voltage after derating; the input voltage should not exceed the power supply voltage under any circumstances, only applicable to buffers and flip-flops, derating from the maximum value of IOL; working Devices in the particle radiation environment need to be further derated;

(4) Due to the characteristics of its function and structure, the internal parameters of large-scale integrated circuits usually allow a small range of variation. Therefore, its derating should focus on improving the heat dissipation method of the package to reduce the junction temperature of the device. When using large-scale integrated circuits, under the premise of ensuring the normal function of the device, its input frequency, output current and operating frequency should be reduced as much as possible

3.3.5 Redundant Design

3.3.5.1 Purpose of Redundant Design

In order to improve the reliability of a system, the system is composed with additional working units or backup units so that even if one of them fails, the whole system will still perform the required tasks. Redundant design is one of the design methods to obtain high task reliability, high safety and high survivability of the system or equipment, using multiple less reliable subsystems or equipment to form a system with high task reliability or safety.

Table 3.5 Derating guidelines for semiconductor discrete devices

Type of components		Derating parameter		Derating level		
				I	II	III
Semiconductor discrete devices	Transistor	Reverse voltage	General transistor	0.60	0.70	0.80
			Gate-source voltage of power MOSFET	0.50	0.60	0.70
		Electric current		0.60	0.70	0.80
		Power tube safe working area	Collector—emitter voltage	0.70	0.80	0.90
			Collector maximum allowable current	0.60	0.70	0.80
		Maximum junction temperature T_{jm} (°C)	200	115	140	160
			175	100	125	145
			≤150	T_{jm} − 65	T_{jm} − 40	T_{jm} − 20
	Microwave transistor	Maximum junction temperature		Same transistor		
	Diodes (except reference tubes)	Reverse voltage (not applicable to Zener tube)		0.60	0.70	0.80
		Electric current		0.50	0.65	0.80
		Power		0.50	0.65	0.80
		Maximum junction temperature Tjm (°C)	200	115	140	160
			175	100	125	145
			≤150	Tjm −60	Tjm −40	Tjm −20
	Microwave diode	Maximum junction temperature		Same diode		
	Silicon controlled rectifier	Voltage		0.60	0.70	0.80
		Electric current		0.50	0.65	0.80
		Maximum junction temperature Tjm (°C)	200	115	140	160
			175	100	125	145

(continued)

Table 3.5 (continued)

Type of components		Derating parameter		Derating level		
				I	II	III
			≤ 150	*Tjm* −60	*Tjm* −40	*Tjm* −20
	Semiconductor optoelectronic devices	Voltage		0.60	0.70	0.80
		Electric current		0.50	0.65	0.80
		Maximum junction temperature *Tjm* (°C)	200	115	140	160
			175	100	125	145
			≤150	*Tjm* −60	*Tjm* −40	*Tjm* −20

Note

(1) The worst combination of transistor DC, AC and transient voltage or current shall not be greater than the limit value after derating (including inductive load). Suitable for Gate-source voltage derating for power MOSFETs;

(2) The diode reverse voltage derating is not applicable to the Zener tube and the reference tube, and the transient peak surge voltage and transient peak surge current should also be derated according to this table. This table is not applicable to the reference tube, only For junction temperature derating;

(3) Due to the influence of distribution parameters, microwave transistors and microwave diodes cannot be considered as independent variables, but the derating of junction temperature should be carried out according to the derating criterion of junction temperature

Redundant design is one of the main ways to improve system mission reliability. Most systems can be simplified into a series system composed of several working units, and the reliability of each working unit in the series system is higher than the reliability of the system; when the actual reliability of a certain unit is lower than the reliability required by the system, if the requirements cannot be met through other methods of improving the design, only redundant design can be effective.

In the product design, mission interruption and personnel injury due to any single point of failure should be avoided. If this single point of failure mode affecting personnel or safety cannot be eliminated by design, it must be designed to be insensitive to failure (that is, robust design) Or use fault-tolerant design techniques. Redundant technology is the most commonly used fault-tolerant technology, but the redundant design must be comprehensively balanced, and the reliability obtained by redundancy should not be increased by the conversion devices, error detectors and other external devices required to form a redundant layout offset by the failure rate.

3.3.5.2 Classification of Redundant Design Methods

There are many forms of redundancy, which can be classified according to different requirements.

1. **According to redundant resources**

Table 3.6 Resistor and potentiometer derating guidelines

Type of components		Derating parameter		Derating level I	Derating level II	Derating level III
Fixed resistor	Synthetic resistor	Voltage		0.75	0.75	0.75
		Power		0.50	0.60	0.70
		Ambient temperature		Derating according to component load characteristic curve		
	Thin film resistors	Voltage		0.75	0.75	0.75
		Power		0.50	0.60	0.70
		Ambient temperature		Derating according to component load characteristic curve		
	Resistor network	Voltage		0.75	0.75	0.75
		Power		0.50	0.60	0.70
		Ambient temperature		Derating according to component load characteristic curve		
	Wire–wound resistors	Voltage		0.75	0.75	0.75
		Power	Precision	0.25	0.45	0.60
			Power type	0.50	0.60	0.70
		Ambient temperature		Derating according to component load characteristic curve		
Potentiometer	Non–wound potentiometer	Voltage		0.75	0.75	0.75
		Power	Synthesis, thin film fine-tuning	0.30	0.45	0.60
			Precision plastic type	do not use	0.50	0.50
		Ambient temperature		Derating according to component load characteristic curve		
	Wire–wound potentiometer	Voltage		0.75	0.75	0.75
		Power	Normal type	0.30	0.45	0.60
			Unsealed power type	–	–	0.70
			Fine tuning wire wound	0.30	0.45	0.50
		Ambient temperature		Derating according to load characteristic curve		

(continued)

Table 3.6 (continued)

Type of components	Derating parameter	Derating level		
		I	II	III
Thermistor	Power	0.50	0.50	0.50
	Ambient temperature (°C)	*TAM*—15	*TAM*—15	*TAM*—15

Note
(1) The maximum rated ambient temperature T_{AM} of the thermistor is determined by the detailed specifications related to the component;
(2) The failure rate of the non-wire wound potentiometer is high, and the contact resistance becomes larger. It is not used in the case of level I derating, and a fixed resistor is used instead;
(3) Non-sealed power potentiometers are not used for wire-wound potentiometers I and II derating

(1) Hardware redundancy: hardware (components, components, equipment or subsystems) is used as a resource for redundant design.
(2) Software redundancy: Usually used in computer systems, software for failure detection and diagnosis, software for redundant management and system recovery, and other key software are compiled and stored in memory.
(3) Time redundancy: Redundancy is generated by repeatedly executing a certain program or the entire program.
(4) Information redundancy: also known as functional redundancy or analytical redundancy, it uses the functional relationship between various sensor signals or various system information to generate redundant information.

2. **According to the operation mode of the redundant system**

(1) Working reserve: It means that in the redundant layout, there is no distinction between the working part and the redundant part, all of which are connected to the system and are in working state. When a working channel fails, no other devices are needed to complete the failure detection and channel Converted redundant structure.
(2) Non-working reserve: Refers to the redundancy structure in which the redundant part does not work and is in a reserve or waiting state. When the working channel fails, other devices or labor are required to complete the failure detection and channel conversion redundant structure. According to the state of the redundant part before participating in the work, it can be divided into:

- Hot reserve—the redundant part is in working state but not connected to the system, once the working channel fails, it will take over the work immediately;
- Cold reserve—the redundant part does not work at all during the reserve or waiting process, and only starts and connects to work when the working channel fails;

Table 3.7 Guidelines for capacitor derating

Type of components		Derating parameter	Derating level		
			I	II	III
Fixed glaze type		DC working voltage	0.50	0.60	0.70
		Ambient temperature (°C)	*T*AM—10	*T*AM—10	*T*AM—10
Fixed mica type		DC working voltage	0.50	0.60	0.70
		Ambient temperature (°C)	*T*AM—10	*T*AM—10	*T*AM—10
Type of components		Derating parameter	Derating level		
			I	II	III
Fixed ceramic type		DC working voltage	0.50	0.60	0.70
		Ambient temperature (°C)	*T* AM—10	*T* AM − 10	*T* AM—10
Fixing paper/Plastic film		DC working voltage	0.50	0.60	0.70
		Ambient temperature (°C)	*T* AM—10	*T* AM − 10	*T* AM—10
Electrolytic capacitor	Aluminum electrolysis	DC working voltage	–	–	0.75
		Ambient temperature (°C)	–	–	*T* AM—20
	Tantalum Electrolysis	DC working voltage	0.50	0.60	0.70
		Ambient temperature (°C)	*T* AM—20	*T* AM—20	*T* AM—20

(continued)

Table 3.7 (continued)

Type of components	Derating parameter	Derating level		
		I	II	III
Trimmer capacitor	DC working voltage	0.3 ~ 0.40	0.50	0.50
	Ambient temperature *T* AM (°C)	*T* AM—10	*T* AM—10	*T* AM—10

Note

(1) The maximum rated ambient temperature T_{AM} of fixed paper/plastic film capacitors, fixed glass glaze capacitors, fixed mica capacitors, fixed ceramic capacitors, and point solution capacitors is determined by the relevant detailed specifications of the components;

(2) The value of the piston type variable capacitor in the fine-tuning capacitor is 0.40, and the maximum rated ambient temperature T_{AM} is determined by the relevant detailed specifications of the components

Table 3.8 Derating guidelines for inductance components

Type of components	Derating parameter	Derating level		
		I	II	III
Inductive element	Hot spot temperature *T* HS (°C)	*T* HS—(40 ~ 25)	*T* HS—(25 to 10)	*T* HS —(15 to 0)
Inductive element	Working current	0.6 ~ 0.7	0.6 ~ 0.7	0.6 ~ 0.7
Inductive element	Transient voltage/current	0.90	0.90	0.90
Inductive element	Dielectric withstand voltage	0.5 ~ 0.6	0.5 ~ 0.6	0.5 ~ 0.6
Inductive element	Choke coil working voltage	0.70	0.70	0.70

Note Inductive element T_{HS} is the rated hot spot temperature and is only applicable to choke coils

- Warm reserve—between hot reserve and cold reserve, such as electronic tubes, which are always in a heating state during the waiting process, so as to ensure that they can be connected to work immediately if the working channel fails.

3. **According to the form of redundant structure**

   1. A redundant structure with no voting and no conversion. When any component in this structure fails, no external components are required to complete the failure detection, judgment and conversion functions, such as simple parallel, hybrid parallel, double parallel systems, etc.
   2. Redundant structure with voting but no conversion. In this structure, if a channel fails, an external component is needed to detect and make a judgment

Table 3.9 Relay derating guidelines

Type of components	Derating parameter			Derating level I	II	III
Relay	Continuous contact current	Small power load (<100 mW)		No derating		
		Resistive load		0.50	0.75	0.90
		Capacitive load (maximum inrush current)		0.50	0.75	0.90
		Inductance load	Inductor rated current	0.50	0.75	0.90
			Resistor rated current	0.35	0.40	0.75
		Motor load	Motor rated current	0.50	0.75	0.90
			Resistor rated current	0.15	0.20	0.75
		Filament load	Bulb rated current	0.50	0.75	0.90
			Resistor rated current	0.07~0.08	0.10	0.30
Relay	Contact power (for reed mercury type)			0.40	0.50	0.70
	Coil pull-in voltage	Minimum holding voltage		0.90	0.90	0.90
		Minimum coil voltage		1.10	1.10	1.10
	Coil release voltage	Maximum allowable value		1.10	1.10	1.10
		Minimum allowable value		0.90	0.90	0.90
	Ambient temperature (°C)			T AM −20	T AM −20	T AM −20
	Vibration limit			0.60	0.60	0.60
	Working life (number of cycles)			0.50	–	–

(i.e., vote), but there is no need to switch channels. Such as majority voting logic system, *r* out of *n* system, etc.

3. There is a redundant structure for switching. If this structure fails, it needs to be switched to another working channel. Such a redundant structure is adopted in the non-working reserve as mentioned above.

Table 3.10 List of derating guidelines for imported components

Type of components			Derating parameter	Derating level		
				I	II	III
Integrated circuit	Analog circuit	Bipolar circuit	Voltage	0.7	0.8	0.8
			Input voltage	0.6	0.7	0.7
			Frequency	0.75	0.8	0.9
			Output current	0.7	0.75	0.8
			Fan−out	0.7	0.75	0.8
			Maximum junction temperature (°C)	85	110	125
		MOS circuit	Voltage	0.7	0.8	0.8
			Inp−+0ut voltage	\0.6	0.7	0.7
			Frequency	0.8	0.8	0.8
			Output current	0.7	0.75	0.8
			Fan−out	0.8	0.8	0.9
			Maximum junction temperature (°C)	85	110	125
	Digital circuits	Bipolar circuit	Frequency	0.8	0.9	0.9
			Output current	0.8	0.9	0.9
			Maximum junction temperature (°C)	85	100	115
		MOS circuit	Voltage	0.7	0.8	0.8
			Frequency	0.8	0.8	0.8
			Output current	0.7	0.75	0.8
			Fan−out	0.8	0.8	0.9
			Maximum junction temperature (°C)	80	110	125
	Hybrid integrated circuit		Maximum junction temperature (°C)	Below the temperature recommended for the process used		

(continued)

Table 3.10 (continued)

Type of components			Derating parameter	Derating level		
				I	II	III
	Memory	Bipolar circuit	Frequency	0.8	0.9	0.95
			Output current	0.7	0.75	0.8
			Maximum junction temperature (°C)	125	125	125
Integrated circuit	Memory	MOS circuit	Frequency	0.8	0.8	0.9
			Output current	0.7	0.75	0.8
			Maximum junction temperature (°C)	125	125	125
			Maximum write cycle (EEPROM)	13000	105000	300000

Figure 3.4 shows the classification by redundant system operation mode and redundant structure.

Table 3.15 lists the characteristics, scope of application and mathematical models of several typical redundant structures.

3.3.5.3 Redundant Design Method

1. **Overview**

In addition to selecting the redundancy type according to the product type, constraints and the purpose of redundancy, the task of redundancy design should also include determining the redundancy level, redundancy configuration and redundancy management scheme.

2. **Determining the Level of Redundancy**

Redundancy level, also known as fault tolerance criterion, refers to the ability of the system to maintain work or maintain safety even when some equipment in the redundant system is in failure. If the redundancy level is Fail—Work (FO for short), it means that the system can still perform tasks normally when the product fails, which puts higher requirements on the redundancy design; if the redundancy level is Fail—Safe (FS for short),), that is, the product fails and the system cannot continue to work normally, but safety can still be guaranteed. Fail—safety is the minimum requirement for redundant design. If the redundancy level is failure—work/failure—work (FO/

Table 3.11 List of derating guidelines for imported components (continued 1)

Type of components			Derating parameter	Derating level		
				I	II	III
Integrated circuit	Microcircuit	Bipolar circuit	Voltage	3%	5%	5%
			Frequency	0.75	0.80	0.90
			Output current	0.70	0.75	0.80
			Fan−out	0.70	0.75	0.80
			Maximum junction temperature (8BIT) (°C)	80	110	125
			Maximum junction temperature (16BIT) (°C)	70	110	125
			Maximum junction temperature (32BIT) (°C)	80	110	125
		MOS circuit	Voltage	3%	5%	5%
			Frequency	0.80	0.80	0.80
			Output current	0.70	0.75	0.80
			Fan−out	0.80	0.80	0.90
			Maximum junction temperature (8BIT) (°C)	125	125	125
			Maximum junction temperature (16BIT) (°C)	90	125	125
			Maximum junction temperature (32BIT) (°C)	60	100	125
Discrete semiconductor device	Silicon bipolar transistor		Power consumption	0.50	0.60	0.70
			Collector − emitter voltage	0.70	0.75	0.80
			Collector current	0.60	0.65	0.70
			Breakdown voltage	0.65	0.85	0.90
			Maximum junction temperature T jm (°C)	95	125	135
	GaAs MESFET		Power consumption	0.50	0.60	0.70
			Breakdown voltage	0.60	0.70	0.70
			Maximum channel temperature (°C)	85	100	125
	Silicon MOSFET		Power consumption	0.50	0.65	0.75
			Breakdown voltage	0.60	0.70	0.70

(continued)

Table 3.11 (continued)

Type of components		Derating parameter	Derating level		
			I	II	III
		Maximum junction temperature (°C)	95	120	140
	Silicon bipolar RF pulse transistor	Power consumption	0.50	0.60	0.70
		Collector – emitter voltage	0.70	0.70	0.70
		Collector current	0.60	0.60	0.60
		Breakdown voltage	0.65	0.65	0.65
		Maximum junction temperature (°C)	0.85	0.85	0.85

FO), it means that the system has the ability to work with double failures, that is, the system can still work normally even if two failures occur, and other redundancy levels can be deduced by analogy.

For a redundant system, the appropriate redundancy level must be determined as needed at the early stage of design. For example, Table 3.16 lists the general and minimum requirements for the redundancy levels of various components of a control system.

3. **Determine the redundancy configuration scheme**

The redundant configuration mainly involves the selection of the redundant number, the setting of the voting/monitoring surface and the selection of the signal transmission mode.

(1) Selection of redundant numbers

The number of redundancy should be determined after comprehensive weighing of mission reliability, safety, weight, volume, cost, and redundancy management level. At present, most of the redundancy at the sub-system level or component level of digital diagnosis and treatment equipment adopts double redundancy, triple redundancy and quadruple redundancy. It should be noted that the higher the number of redundancy is not, the higher the task reliability must be. As the number of redundancy increases, the corresponding detection, judgment isolation and conversion devices will inevitably increase, which will lead to a decrease in the reliability of system tasks. Therefore, the design should ensure that the increase in task reliability brought about by redundancy will not be offset by the increase in the failure rate of these devices required for redundant layout.

(2) Setting of voting/monitoring surface

Redundant systems are often composed of multi-level and multiple redundant components. It is more reasonable to set up the voting/monitoring surface at which level or levels. The general setting principles are:

Table 3.12 List of derating guidelines for imported components (continued 2)

Type of components			Derating parameter		Derating level		
					I	II	III
Discrete semiconductor device	GaAs type RF pulse transistor		Power consumption		0.50	0.60	0.70
			Breakdown voltage		0.50	0.60	0.70
			Maximum channel temperature (°C)		85	100	125
	Signal/Switching diodes		Reverse current		0.50	0.60	0.75
			Reverse voltage		0.70	0.70	0.70
			Maximum junction temperature (°C)		95	105	125
	Power rectifier diode		Reverse current		0.50	0.65	0.75
			Reverse voltage		0.70	0.70	0.70
			Maximum junction temperature (°C)		95	105	125
	Microwave/Schottky /PIN diode		power consumption		0.50	0.60	0.70
			reverse voltage		0.70	0.70	0.70
			Maximum junction temperature (°C)		95	105	125
	TVS diode		power consumption		0.50	0.60	0.70
			Average current		0.50	0.65	0.75
			Maximum junction temperature (°C)		95	105	125
	Zener diode		Power consumption		0.50	0.60	0.70
			Maximum junction temperature (°C)		95	105	125
	Reference diode		Maximum junction temperature (°C)		95	105	125
	Silicon controlled rectifier		Voltage		0.60	0.70	0.80
			Electric current		0.50	0.65	0.80
			Maximum junction temperature (°C)	T jm = 200	115	140	160
				T jm = 175	100	125	145
				T jm ≤ 150	T jm −65	T jm −40	T jm −20
	Optoelectronic devices	Transistor	Maximum junction temperature (°C)		95	105	125
		Avalanche diode	Maximum junction temperature (°C)		95	105	125

(continued)

Table 3.12 (continued)

Type of components			Derating parameter	Derating level		
				I	II	III
		Photodiode /PIN tube	Reverse voltage	0.7	0.7	0.7
			Maximum junction temperature (°C)	95	105	125
		Injection laser diode	Output Power	0.5	0.6	0.7
			Maximum junction temperature (°C)	95	105	110
Resistor	Synthetic resistor		Power	0.50	0.50	0.50
			Maximum temperature derating (°C)	30	30	30
	Power wire–wound resistors		Power	0.50	0.50	0.50
			Maximum temperature derating (°C)	125	125	125

(1) Meet the system reliability index requirements. Generally, the reliability of the multi-level setting of the voting/monitoring surface will be higher than that of the single-level setting. Because the redundant system is divided into several levels, it will increase the number of survival channels. However, multi-stage setups are limited by the detection rate of conversion component failures.
(2) To meet the fault-tolerance requirements of the component level (replaceable failure unit level) failure—work. Some redundant systems, especially digital systems, require components to also have double failure—work fault-tolerance and require signal selection (voting) and failure monitoring between component levels.
(3) Satisfy the consistency requirements of the signal.
(4) Meet the requirements of multi-modal control.
(5) Meet the requirements of reducing failure spread and failure transient effects.

3. **The choice of signal transmission method**

In a redundant configuration, signal transmission is carried out by information exchange and transmission between components and channels. There are several ways of signal transmission:

(1) Direct transmission: In the redundant system, each signal channel is independent of each other, and the signals are processed separately and then sent to the signal selector of each channel for voting. With this transmission method, if a working unit (such as a sensor, an electronic circuit) fails, the channel will be declared invalid, so it is unfavorable from a reliability point of view.
(2) Cross-transfer method: Fig. 3.5 shows an example of the signal cross-transfer method. Cross pass is a powerful means to improve system reliability (can be increased by 5–10 times), and can make the failure monitoring coverage rate reach 100% level.

Table 3.13 List of derating guidelines for imported components (continued 3)

Type of components			Derating parameter	Derating level		
				I	II	III
Potentiometer			Power	0.50	0.50	0.50
			Maximum temperature derating (°C)	45	35	35
Capacitor	Film, porcelain, mica, glass glaze		DC working voltage	0.50	0.60	0.60
			Maximum rated ambient temperature (°C)	$T_{AM}-10$	$T_{AM}-10$	$T_{AM}-10$
	Electrolysis container	Non−solid tantalum	DC working voltage	0.50	0.60	0.60
			Maximum rated ambient temperature (°C)	$T_{AM}-20$	$T_{AM}-20$	$T_{AM}-20$
		Solid tantalum	DC working voltage	0.50	0.60	0.60
			Maximum working temperature (°C)	85	85	85
		Aluminum electrolysis	DC working voltage	–	–	0.80
			Maximum working temperature (°C)	–	–	$T_{AM}-20$
	Porcelain variable		DC working voltage	0.30	0.50	0.50
			Maximum rated ambient temperature (°C)	$T_{AM}-10$	$T_{AM}-10$	$T_{AM}-10$
	Piston variable		DC working voltage	0.40	0.50	0.50
			Maximum rated ambient temperature (°C)	$T_{AM}-10$	$T_{AM}-10$	$T_{AM}-10$
Inductive element			Hot Spot Temperature (T_{HS})	$T_{HS}-40$	$T_{HS}-25$	$T_{HS}-15$
			Working current	0.60	0.60	0.60
			Dielectric withstand voltage	0.50	0.50	0.50
Relay			Contact current – Resistive load	0.50	0.75	0.75
			Contact current – Capacitive load	0.50	0.75	0.75
			Contact current – Inductive load	0.35	0.40	0.40
			Contact power	0.40	0.50	0.50
			Ambient temperature (°C)	$T_{AM}-20$	$T_{AM}-20$	$T_{AM}-20$

(continued)

Table 3.13 (continued)

Type of components	Derating parameter		Derating level		
			I	II	III
Switch	Contact current	Resistive load	0.50	0.75	0.75
		Capacitive load	0.50	0.75	0.75
		Inductive load	0.35	0.40	0.40
	Contact power		0.40	0.50	0.50
Electrical connector	Operating voltage		0.50	0.70	0.70
	Working current		0.50	0.70	0.70
	Temperature (°C)		$T_{AM} - 50$	$T_{AM} - 25$	$T_{AM} - 25$

3. Input/output interface transmission type: This method is suitable for computer systems. When a central processing unit fails, the relevant information will not be lost, and the heavy redundant management tasks can be assigned to the input/output interface. (I/O) processing machine to complete, thus greatly reducing the computing burden on the central processing unit.

4. **Determine how to manage redundancy**

The redundant management method is the core of the redundant design, and the advantages and disadvantages of the redundant management method play a decisive role in the reliability, weight, volume and cost of the redundant system. The same number of redundancy, but with different redundancy management, can get very different reliability.

The redundant management method needs to study the work coordination between multiple channels, failure detection and isolation, etc., mainly involving two issues of signal selection (voting) and monitoring technology:

(1) Signal selection is done by the voting machine according to the prescribed voting form, which is usually done with software in digital systems. Signal selection improves the consistency of signals across channels and is used in conjunction with crossover transmission to improve system reliability. Most voting machines can only be used for digital circuits; analog circuits mostly use average or median selectors.
(2) Monitoring technology Any multi-redundancy solution needs to take certain failure monitoring measures to detect and isolate failures. There are two main types of monitoring: comparative monitoring and self-monitoring. Due to the relatively intuitive and simple monitoring and high coverage, both analog and digital systems are used more. Self-monitoring does not need to use external similar data as a benchmark, and fully relies on its own means to monitor its

Table 3.14 List of derating guidelines for imported components (continued 4)

Type of components		Derating parameter		Derating level		
				I	II	III
Rotating electrical machine		Working temperature (°C)		$TM-40$	$TM-25$	$TM-15$
		Bearing load		0.75	0.90	0.90
Light bulb	Incandescent lamp	Operating voltage		0.94	0.94	0.94
	Neon/Argon	Working current		0.94	0.94	0.94
Circuit breaker		Electric current		0.75	0.80	0.80
Fuse		Electric current		0.50	0.50	0.50
The crystal		range of working temperature		Less than the range specified in the technical conditions		
		Driving power		no derating		
Electric vacuum device		Output Power		0.80	0.80	0.80
		Reflected power		0.50	0.50	0.50
		Duty cycle		0.75	0.75	0.75
Surface acoustic wave devices		Input power	Input power greater than 500 MHz	Reduce +13dBm		
			Input power is less than 500 MHz	Reduce +18dBm		
		Working temperature (°C)		125		
Fiber and cable		Tension	Specified value of optical fiber tensile test	20%		
			Optical cable tensile strength rating of	50%		
		Bending radius		200%		

own failures, which is its advantage. However, the self-monitoring technology is more complicated and the coverage rate is lower.

In the design of redundancy management, the following principles should also be followed:

(1) Some redundant management systems are directly responsible for the key functions of ensuring system safety. Therefore, the hardware and software of the redundant management system must be fully analyzed, tested and confirmed.
(2) Redundancy management should be carried out automatically, without the need for the user to reset or restart.
(3) The number of monitors should be at least, and they should be installed only when FMECA or FMET shows that it is necessary.

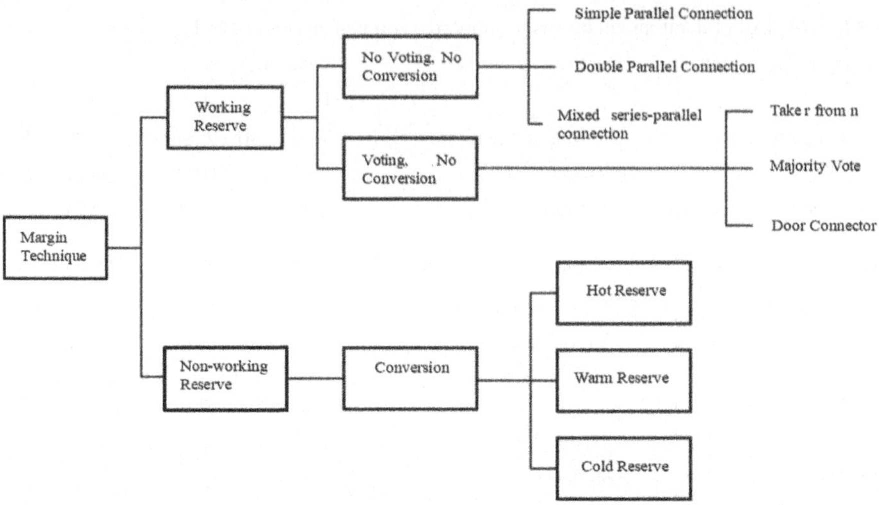

Fig. 3.4 Classification by redundant system operation mode and redundant structure

(4) It should have a low false alarm rate.

3.3.5.4 Redundancy Design Principles

1. Redundancy design requires the use of multiple sets of subsystems, equipment or components. Therefore, it pays a price in terms of weight, volume, maintenance complexity, cost, etc., and inevitably reduces the basic reliability of the system. Only when it is confirmed that the use of better components and derating design methods cannot meet the system task reliability and safety requirements, or when the cost of improving components is higher than the cost of using redundant technology for the system or equipment, the redundant design is adopted.
2. The effect of redundant systems on improving mission reliability or safety is not directly proportional to the number of redundancy. For a simple parallel redundant system, as the number of redundancy increases, the speed of improvement of mission reliability or safety will be slower and slower. The reliability of a single unit (no redundancy) and a simple parallel redundant system with $n = 2$ *to 5 at different times* (t/T_{BF}) is shown in Fig. 3.6. Figure 3.7 shows the relationship between the multiplier of system *TBF improvement and the number of redundancy*. In the figure, TBF is set as the unit value when $n = 1$. When the number of units connected in parallel in the system is *n*, the improvement factor of *TBF is* M_n, and the relative increment is ΔM_n.
3. A system can be divided into different levels such as sub-systems, equipment, components, modules, circuits and components, and which level to adopt redundancy design depends on the actual situation. Generally speaking, it is better to use redundancy in low-level parts. But the lower the level, the more complex the

Table 3.15 Characteristics, scope of application and mathematical models of several typical redundancy structures

Redundant structure	Model picture	Characteristics	Application scope	Mathematical model assumption	Mathematical model	Note
Simple parallel collection	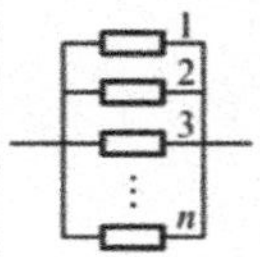	Simple, much improved reliability but difficult to prevent fault propagation	For electrical and non-electrical products, available for analog and digital circuits	Exponential distribution	$R_s(t) = 1 - (1 - e{-}^{\lambda t})^n$ $(T_{BF}) = \int_0^{\infty} R_s(t)\mathrm{d}t = \frac{1}{\lambda} + \frac{1}{2\lambda} + \cdots + \frac{1}{n\lambda}$ ..	n, number of units. λ, failure rate. Rs(t), system reliability (TBF)a, mean time between failures of the system
Series-parallel connection	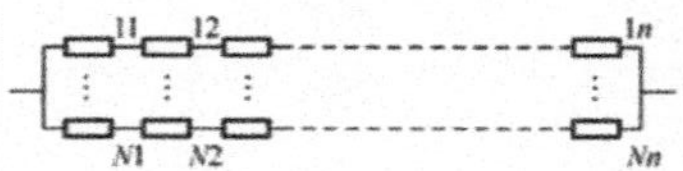	Significantly improved reliability in a short mission time	Mainly used at the component level where short-circuit fault mode protection is required	/	$R_{sp}(t) = 1 - \left[1 - R^n(t)\right]^N$	n series and N parallels. R(t), unit reliability
Parallel-series connection	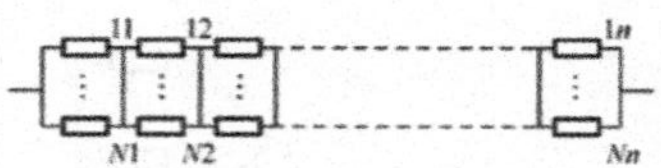	Significantly improved reliability in a short mission time	Mainly used at the component level where open-circuit fault mode protection is required	/	$R_{ps}(t) = 1 - \left[1 - R^N(t)\right]^n$	n series and N parallels. R(t), unit reliability

(continued)

Table 3.15 (continued)

Redundant structure	Model picture	Characteristics	Application scope	Mathematical model assumption	Mathematical model	Note
Take r from n (*r/n*)	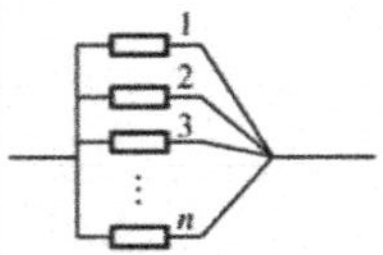	Formal output results fault <r	For continuous or intermittent work	Exponential distribution	$(T_{BF})_{\alpha} = \frac{1}{n\lambda} + \frac{1}{(n-1)\lambda} + \ldots + \frac{1}{r\lambda}$	r, the minimum number of units necessary to make the system work properly. n, the number of unit
Majority vote	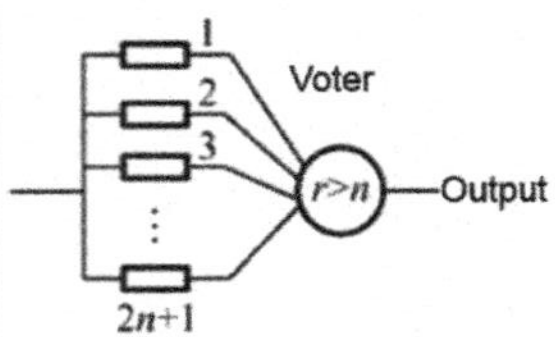	Improved short-term mission reliability, with output only when the number of failed units is less than the number of active units	Generally used in conjunction with logic circuits for continuous or intermittent operation, such as data acquisition systems	2n+1 units n=2,1...... r>n voting machine reliability is 1	$R(t) = \sum_{i=0}^{n} C_{2n+1^{i}}^{e-\lambda t(2n+1-i)(1-e-\lambda t)i}$	r, the minimum number of units necessary to make the system work properly. λ, failure rate. 2n+1, number of units

(continued)

Table 3.15 (continued)

Redundant structure	Model picture	Characteristics	Application scope	Mathematical model assumption	Mathematical model	Note
Tri-mode Redundant Voting System (T_{MR})	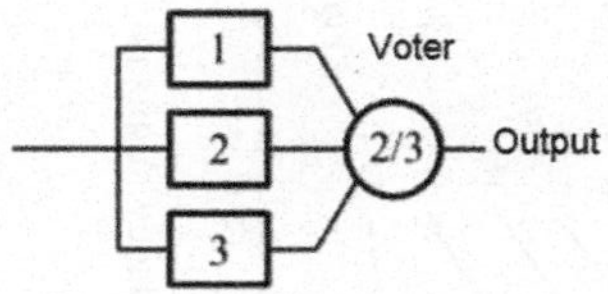	Reliability increased a lot when λt is relatively small, take 2 out of 3	Achieve single-failure-working redundancy levels	Exponential Distribution	$R_{TMR} = e^{-2\lambda t}(3 - 2e^{-\lambda t})$	λ, failure rate. RTMR, system reliability
Non-working Reserve System (Bypass System)	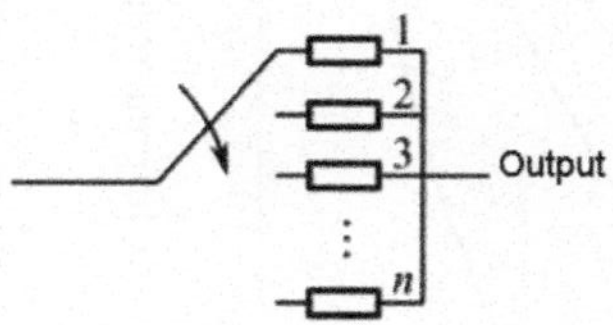	Failure monitoring and switching devices are key and effective for intermittent failure modes	Control systems that do not require a high degree of continuity of operating conditions and have only a single output	Exponential distribution, the same unit composition monitoring switching device reliability is 1	$R_s(t) = e^{-\lambda t}\left[1 + \lambda t + \frac{(\lambda t)^2}{2!} + \cdots + \frac{(\lambda t)^{N-1}}{(n-1)!}\right]$ $(T_{\text{BF}})_\alpha = \frac{n}{\lambda}$	λ, failure rate. n, number of identical units Rs(t), system reliability

Table 3.16 General requirements and minimum requirements for redundancy levels of various components of a certain control system

Part name	Part type	General requirements	Minimum requirements
The key components	Electrical and electronic components	Failure—work/ failure—work	Failure - Work/Failure – Safe
	Hydromechanical components	Failure—Work/ Failure—Safe	Failure—Safe
	Mechanical components	According to damage tolerance requirements	According to damage tolerance requirements
Non-critical components	Electrical and Electronic Components	Failure—Safe	—

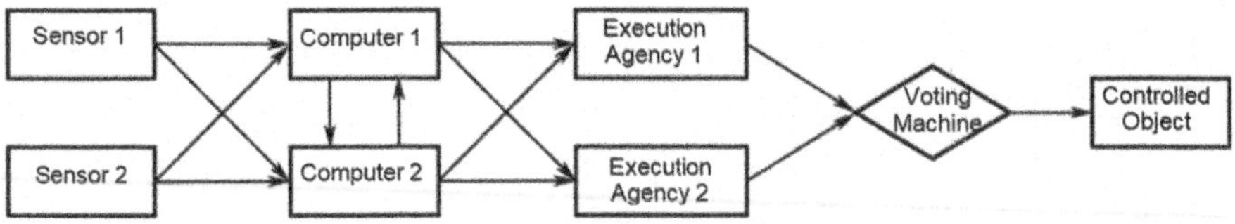

Fig. 3.5 Example of signal cross transmission mode

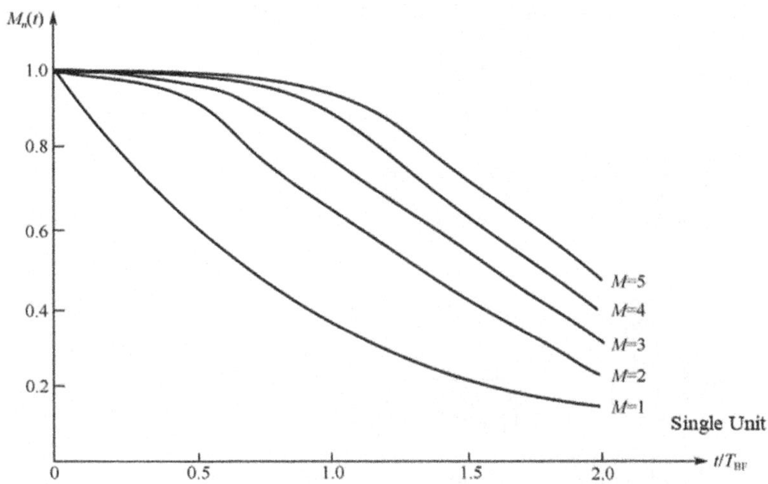

Fig. 3.6 Reliability of simple parallel systems with different redundancy numbers

implementation of fault tolerance, so it should be considered comprehensively. Figure 3.8 has two redundant configurations each consisting of 2 n units. The first type is connected in series first and then connected in parallel, which is a

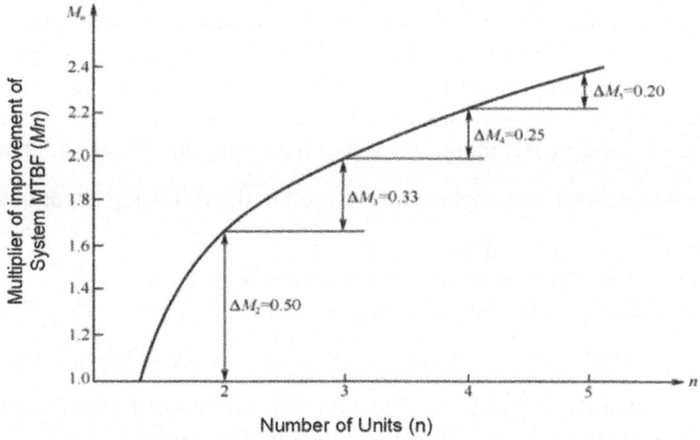

Fig. 3.7 The relationship between redundant number and MTBF increase multiple

subsystem-level redundant system; the second type is connected in parallel first and then connected in series, which is a redundant system at the unit level.

The reliability of subsystem-level redundant system is

$$R_{SS} = R_0^n(2 - R_0^n) \tag{3.1}$$

The reliability of the unit-level redundant system is

$$R_{SU} = R_0^n(2 - R_0)^n \tag{3.2}$$

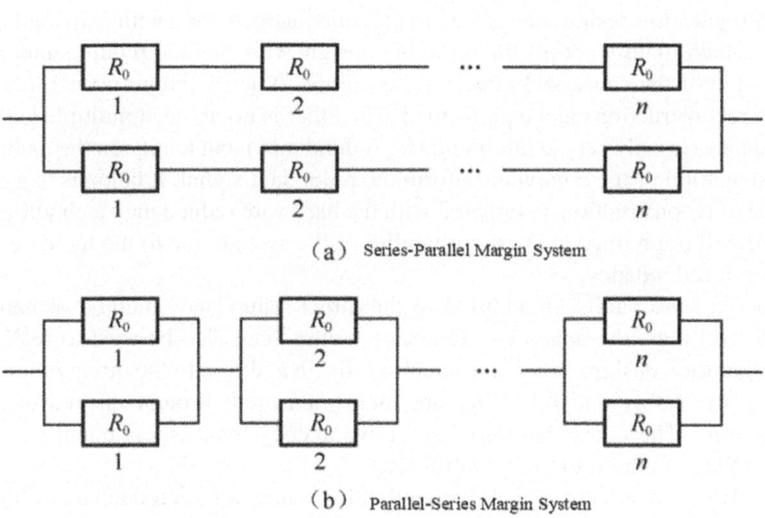

Fig. 3.8 The impact of different redundancy configurations on reliability

Obviously, the reliability of the unit-level redundant system is higher than that of the subsystem-level redundancy. But what kind of redundant configuration to use also depends on its failure distribution. If the unit short-circuit rate is high, it is more favorable to use the subsystem-level redundant system; on the contrary, if the open-circuit rate is high, it is more appropriate to use the unit-level redundant system.

(4) The working reserve model cannot be used in the following situations:

- Insufficient power supply;
- Unit heating has a great impact on system work;
- A failed unit cannot be effectively isolated.

(5) The non-working reserve model cannot be used in the following situations:

- The reliability of the failure detection and conversion device is not high, that is, its unreliability exceeds 50% of the unreliability of the unit;
- Work requires legacy systems, such as computer systems.

(6) If the failed redundant unit can be repaired in time when it is not working, and can be reused as the redundant unit of the system after repair, the number of redundant units will be greatly reduced. In the case of certain redundant units, will greatly improve the mission reliability and safety of the system.

3.3.5.5 Development Direction of Redundancy Design

Redundancy technology is currently developing in the direction of system reconfiguration, analytical redundancy and non-similar redundancy. The so-called "reconstruction" is a redundant management measure adopted to transfer the system to a new working structure when the redundant system fails. There are two main methods of reconfiguration design: one is the direct redundancy method with hardware redundancy, which mainly adopts the re-layout design. This method requires more prior knowledge of the cause and effect of the failure. When a failure occurs, real-time system reconstruction can be performed. The other is not to need multiple hardware redundancy (or only set the minimum two redundancy), but to rely on the mathematical calculation of the computer to form the redundant signal. It belongs to a design method of reconstruction. Compared with the hardware redundancy technology, this method will not reduce the basic reliability of the system due to the increase of the number of redundancy.

When a sensor fails, in addition to the direct redundancy method of hardware repeated settings, the analytic redundancy method can also be used to realize the reconfiguration design. When the actuator fails, in addition to the direct redundancy method, the safety and reliability are mainly ensured through the redistribution of functions. The redistribution of executive agency functions is mainly achieved through the reconfiguration of control laws.

In addition, in order to achieve high reliability, a non-similar redundant technology in which a redundant system is composed of completely different hardware and software is currently being vigorously developed.

3.3.6 *Fault-Tolerant and Error Prevention Design*

3.3.6.1 The Purpose of Fault-Tolerant and Error Prevention Design

Fault-tolerant technology refers to the system's tolerance to failures, that is, when one or more key parts of the system in working state fail or make errors, it can automatically detect and diagnose, and take corresponding measures to ensure that the system maintains its specified functions. It is a technology that keeps its functionality within acceptable limits. fault-tolerant technology is essential for the design of high-reliability systems, and is currently being developed rapidly.

Taking error prevention design measures for product interfaces and operating positions can reduce the possibility of errors in human–computer interaction operations.

3.3.6.2 Fault-Tolerant Design Method

The contents of the fault-tolerant technology are shown in Fig. 3.9. It mainly consists of the following two parts:

(1) System failure detection and diagnosis: the purpose is to automatically discover system failures, and determine the location, type, and consequences of the failure. At the same time, failures are automatically isolated, namely:

- failure detection: Once a failure occurs in some key parts of the system, it should be detected automatically and timely, and an alarm signal will be given;
- Failure diagnosis: find the source of the failure based on the detected system failure information, determine the type of failure and the magnitude of the consequences of the failure, and perform failure isolation.

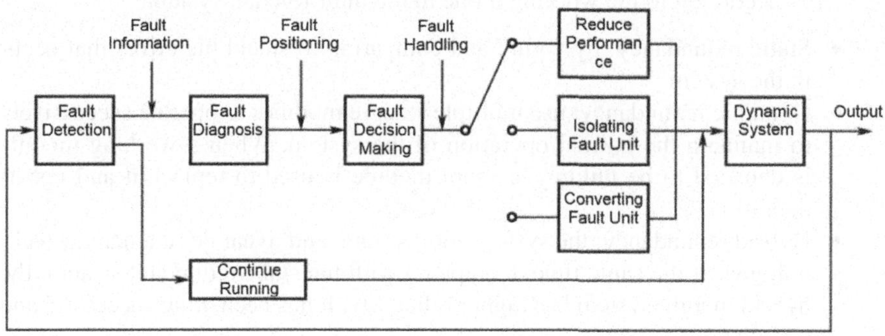

Fig. 3.9 Contents of fault tolerance technology

For the fault detection and diagnosis of digital systems, the excitation check method or the parity check method is often used for self-checking, and the comparison method is also commonly used, that is, using redundant hardware, redundant information, redundant time and redundant software to conduct comparisons or votes to detect and diagnose system failures.

There are many failure detection and diagnosis methods for dynamic systems, among which the voting method is the most widely used because of its advantages of simplicity, high detection accuracy, easy real-time control and is suitable for nonlinear systems and parameter uncertainty systems. The so-called "voting method" is to use hardware redundancy and analysis redundancy to vote to detect and diagnose failures.

(2) System fault decision-making: it is to adopt a corresponding fault-tolerant processing plan and put it into practice according to the location, type and magnitude of the failure consequences. For example: take measures to reduce system performance in the presence of failures to ensure that system reliability is within the allowable range; or isolate failure units and reorganize the system structure so that it can complete system functions; or use redundant resources Replace the failure unit so that the system continues to work normally.

The implementation of fault-tolerant technology mainly has the following methods:

(1) Fault-tolerance of information: it is to detect or correct errors in the operation or transmission of information, and to achieve the purpose of fault tolerance by adding a part of information.
(2) Fault-tolerance of time: that is, the high reliability of the computer system is exchanged for the sacrifice of time. There are two specific ways: one is to increase the reliability of the system by reducing the speed of the machine to a limited extent; the other is to eliminate the impact of transient errors by repeatedly executing instructions or programs.
(3) Fault-tolerance of hardware or fault-tolerance of structure: it is the most commonly used redundancy technology, and it can be divided into the following types according to the working mode in the fault-tolerant system:

- Static redundancy: by voting and comparing to shield the errors that occur in the system.
- Dynamic redundancy: use multiple reserve modules to operate successively to maintain the normal operation of the system. When a working module is detected to be failurey, a spare module is used to replace it and restart operation.
- Hybrid redundancy: the system adopts static and dynamic redundancy technologies at the same time. Compared with the static redundant system, the hybrid margin system has higher reliability. It has been quite successful and widely used.

(4) Fault-tolerance of software: that is, to improve the reliability of software by adding programs.

3.3.6.3 Error Prevention Design Method

The error prevention design method is mainly as follows:

(1) Active function protection: early warning function is designed to provide timely and accurate early warning before errors occur, so as to avoid, transfer or reduce the risks caused by errors.
(2) Sound and light alarm: the sound and light alarm function is designed. When an error occurs in the man–machine interface or the internal interface of the product, the device will send out a sound and light alarm to remind the operator.
(3) Error prevention of interface: the man–machine interface, various interfaces inside the product, and the operation of the product should be as simple as possible to reduce the possibility of human error.
(4) Error prevention of color: For different interfaces, connectors with different appearance and colors are used, and the color of the connectors matches the interface to reduce the probability of errors.
(5) Warning signs: to paste obvious warning signs on the interfaces that are prone to errors.
(6) Error prevention of operation: preventive measures should be taken for operations that are prone to human errors. For parts, groups, and components that are similar in shape but different in function, they should be structurally designed so that they cannot be installed with each other, such as electrical connections with the same dimensions. Devices should be equipped with anti-mis-insertion positioning pins, including measures such as setting different color dot marks; for devices that may cause operational errors, there should be marks for the operation sequence number and direction.
(7) Error prevention identification: under the conditions of product use, storage and transportation, any error prevention identification marks must be clear, accurate, and durable, and the size and position of the identification marks must be appropriate so that operators and maintenance personnel can easily identify them.

3.3.7 Thermal Design

3.3.7.1 Purpose of Thermal Design

Heat is an important environmental factor that affects the reliability and life of electrical and electronic equipment. Every 10 °C increase in temperature reduces the life span by half, which is an image to describe the relationship between heat and life span. Unreasonable thermal design can lead to reduced accuracy of instruments and equipment; can lead to non-electronic products moving part of the jam, resulting in serious accidents; may lead to electronic equipment dead, increased failure rate, shortened life; local overheating may damage the device itself or even affect the normal work of the surrounding devices with relatively low heat resistance or overheating stress. Typical component failure rate curve with temperature change is shown in Fig. 3.10.

The main purpose of thermal design is to reduce the working temperature of the product through reasonable heat dissipation design, avoid failure caused by high temperature, and improve the reliability of the product.

The goals of thermal design include:

(1) Reducing the heat generated inside the device (line) should be an indicator of circuit design;
(2) Reducing thermal resistance is one of the purposes of electronic equipment structural design;
(3) Reduce the overall temperature and local hot spot temperature;
(4) To ensure stable electrical performance, the thermal design prevents components from working under high temperature conditions, so as to avoid parameter drift and maintain stable electrical performance;
(5) Improve the reliability of electronic equipment;
(6) Extend the service life.

The thermal design should first determine the design target according to the allowable heat generation requirements of the product and the environmental conditions of the product. The thermal design target is generally the allowable maximum temperature of the internal components of the product, which can be obtained by using the method of reliability prediction according to the reliability requirements of the equipment and the failure rate assigned to the components. Determine the thermal design scheme based on thermal design objectives, product structure, volume, weight and other requirements and thermal design engineering experience.

The main contents of a complete electronic equipment-level thermal design plan include: selection and design of cooling methods, installation and layout of components, design of circuit board heat dissipation structure, and chassis heat dissipation structure design. The thermal design solutions at the component level and circuit board level can be tailored as needed. For example, the component level mainly

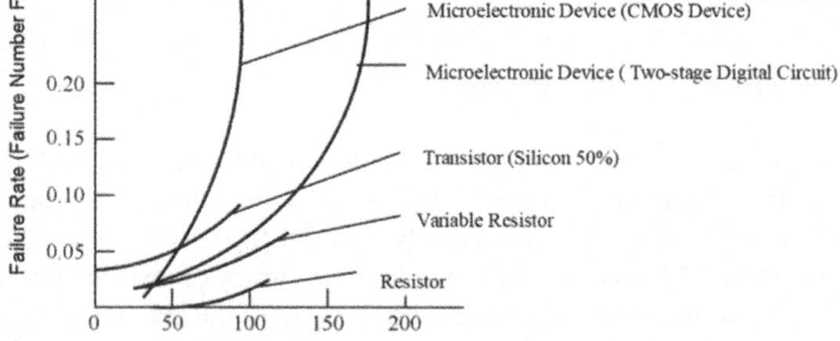

Fig. 3.10 Typical component failure rate—temperature change curve

considers the thermal installation of components, the design of high-power devices plus radiators, etc., and the circuit board level mainly considers the installation and layout of components on the circuit board, and the heat dissipation structure design of the circuit board. After the thermal design scheme is determined, the thermal design of the product starts according to the scheme.

Thermal analysis is performed after thermal design. In order to prevent the designed product performance and reliability from being destroyed by inappropriate thermal characteristics, thermal analysis must be performed on thermally sensitive products. Perform analysis to verify that no components are exposed to temperatures beyond those determined by the line stress analysis and worst case analysis. Based on the thermal analysis results, it is judged whether the thermal design objectives and related reliability requirements are met.

If the thermal analysis meets the requirements, the principle prototype is manufactured, and then the thermal test is carried out on the principle prototype, and whether the thermal design meets the requirements is judged according to the thermal test results.

If the thermal test meets the requirements, the thermal design method, thermal analysis and thermal test results will be sorted out to form a thermal design report for the product. If it is found that the results of thermal analysis and thermal testing do not meet the thermal design requirements, a trade-off analysis is performed to improve the design.

The general procedures for thermal design, thermal analysis, thermal testing, and thermal improvement are shown in Fig. 3.11.

3.3.7.2 Basic Requirements for Thermal Design

The basic requirements for thermal design are as follows:

1. **Thermal design should meet the requirements of product reliability**

   High temperature will have a serious impact on most components, which will lead to the failure of components, and then cause the failure of the entire product. Therefore, when conducting thermal design, the maximum allowable operating temperature (including after derating) should be initially determined for key and high-power components, and determine the failure rate of components according to the working temperature, and then calculate the reliability of the product. If the product reliability meets the requirements, this temperature is the maximum allowable working temperature of the components. In the thermal design, the operating temperature of the components is controlled below this value.
2. **The thermal design should meet the thermal environment requirements of the product's intended operation**

   Thermal environments in which electronic products are expected to operate include:

   - Limits for ambient temperature and pressure (or altitude);
   - Rate of change of ambient temperature and pressure (or altitude);

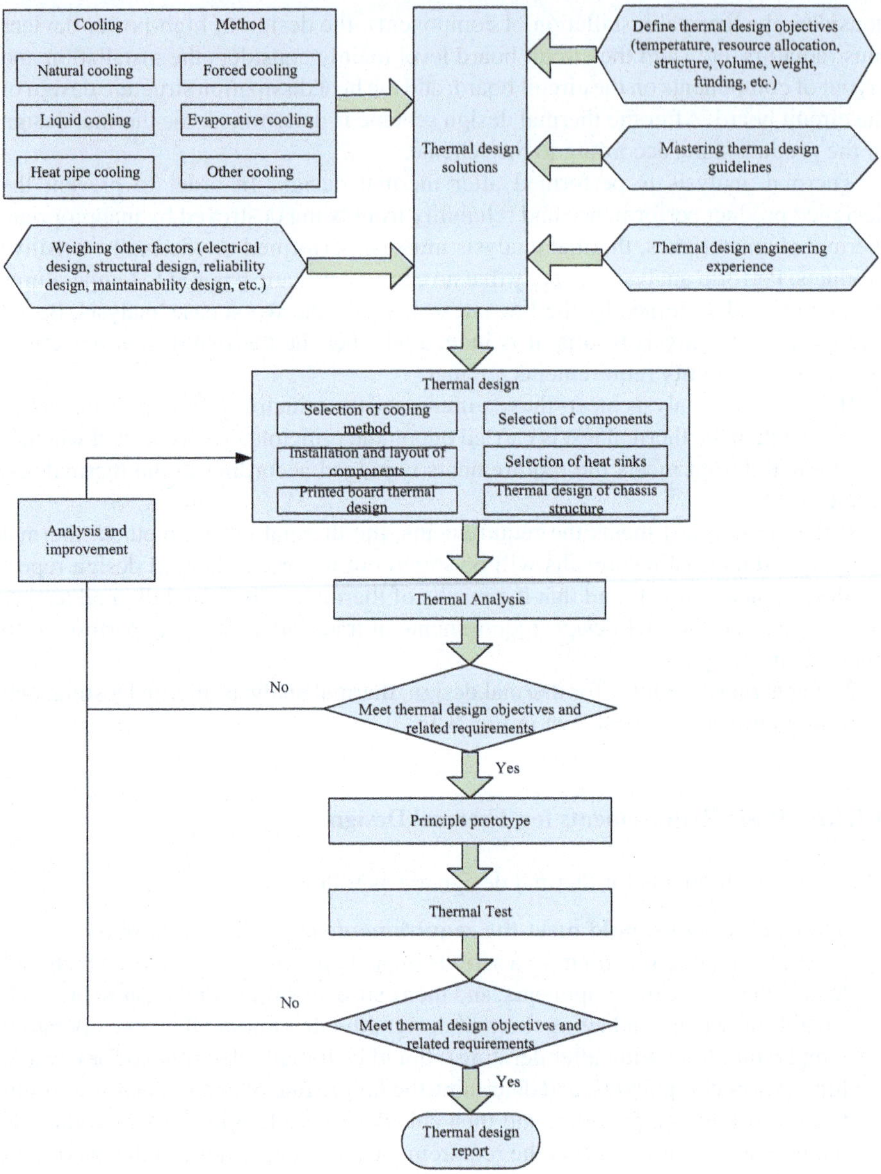

Fig. 3.11 General procedures for thermal design, thermal analysis, thermal testing, and thermal improvement

- Radiative heat loads from the sun or other surrounding objects;
- Available heat sinks;
- The coolant temperature, pressure and allowable pressure drop used.

3. **The thermal design should meet the constraints imposed on the cooling system**

   - Restrictions on the power source used by the cooling system (AC or DC and strategy);
   - Vibration and noise restrictions on forced cooling equipment;
   - Limitations on the air outlet temperature of forced air cooling equipment;
   - Structural restrictions on the cooling system (including installation conditions, sealing, volume and weight, etc.).

4. **Thermal design should be done simultaneously with other designs (electrical design, structural design, reliability design, etc.)**
   When conflicts arise, a trade-off analysis should be carried out and a compromise should be resolved. However, the electrical performance must not be compromised, and the reliability requirements must be met to minimize the life cycle cost of the equipment.
5. **Thermal design should be combined with maintainability design**

   - During equipment maintenance or testing, there should be good cooling measures;
   - When performing maintenance on the cooling system, it should have good safety and accessibility;
   - The installation position of air or other coolant filters should be set in a place that is convenient for maintenance and replacement;
   - Fresh water for ships—air heat exchangers must be easy to disassemble and clean;
   - The pipeline connection of the liquid cooling system shall adopt a quick automatic sealing joint device to prevent the coolant from overflowing.

6. **Choice of cooling method**
   The simplest and most effective cooling method should be selected according to factors such as heating power, ambient temperature, allowable working temperature, reliability requirements, volume, weight, economy and safety.
7. **The thermal design should meet the requirements for the specified conditions**

Such as requirements for the power supply used (AC, DC power capacity), requirements for vibration and noise, requirements for coolant inlet and outlet temperature, and requirements for structure (installation conditions, sealing, volume and corrosion of coolant, etc.).

(1) Larger errors are allowed in thermal design, but sufficient design margin should be guaranteed.
(2) Thermal design should ensure that electronic products should have auxiliary cooling measures in case of emergency, so that key components or equipment

have the ability to continue to work when some components of the cooling system are damaged or fail to work.
(3) The thermal design scheme should be formulated according to the specific conditions (equipment level, circuit board level, component level), and implemented according to the thermal design scheme.

3.3.7.3 Thermal Design Method

The heat dissipation design method can refer to GJB/Z 27-1992, mainly as follows:

(1) The main methods of heat dissipation design include: conduction heat dissipation design, convection heat dissipation design, radiation heat dissipation design and heat resistance design to improve the heat conduction system.
(2) Conduction and heat dissipation design: if materials with high thermal conductivity are selected, the contact area with heat-conducting parts is increased, and the heat conduction path is shortened as much as possible. There should be no heat insulation or heat insulation parts in the heat conduction path;
(3) Convective heat dissipation design: If the temperature difference is increased, the temperature of the surrounding convective medium is reduced, and the contact area between the fluid and the solid is increased; the flow velocity of the surrounding medium is increased to make it take away more heat, etc.
(4) Radiation heat dissipation design: such as covering the heat dissipation coating on the surface of the heating element to increase the blackness coefficient; increasing the surface area of the radiator, etc.

Commonly used cooling methods include natural cooling, forced air cooling, liquid cooling, evaporative cooling, etc. The design requirements of common cooling methods are shown in Table 3.17.

The selection of the cooling method should be carried out simultaneously with the simulation test research of the electronic circuit to ensure that the electronic product can not only meet the electrical performance requirements, but also meet the reliability thermal design indicators. When choosing a cooling method, the following factors should be considered: heat flux density, volume power density, total power consumption, surface area, volume, working environment conditions and other special conditions of the product. The procedure for cooling method selection is shown in Fig. 3.12.

The heat flux density and volume power density of commonly used cooling method are shown in Figs. 3.13 and 3.14 respectively.

3.3.7.4 Natural Cooling Heat Dissipation Design

Commonly used natural cooling methods for electronic components are shown in Table 3.18.

Table 3.17 Design requirements for common cooling methods

Cooling method	Design requirements
Natural cooling	Maximize the use of heat conduction, natural convection and radiation cooling; Shorten the heat transfer path and increase the heat transfer or heat conduction area; Reduce the contact thermal resistance during installation, and the arrangement of components is conducive to the convection heat transfer of fluid; Adopt heat−dissipating printed circuit board, edge rail with small thermal resistance; The distance between printed circuit board assemblies is controlled at 19–21 mm; Increase the surface blackness of the chassis and enhance radiation heat transfer
Forced air cooling	The air used to cool the internal components of the equipment must be filtered; The direction of forced air flow should be consistent with the direction of natural convection air flow; The difference between the inlet air temperature and the outlet air temperature generally does not exceed 14 °C; Cooling air inlet and outlet locations should be far away; Try not to open the ventilation holes on the top of the chassis; For air−cooled electronic equipment working in hot and humid environments, direct contact between humid air and components should be avoided, and air−core printed circuit boards or chassis cooled by air−cooled cold plates can be used; Minimize airflow and fan noise; When large cabinets are forced to cool by air, try to avoid air leakage from the gaps in the cabinets
Liquid cooling	The coolant is preferably distilled water, and deionized water should be used for special requirements; Ensure that the coolant does not boil at the highest operating temperature and does not freeze at the lowest operating temperature; The thermal expansion of the coolant should be considered, and the chassis should be able to withstand a certain pressure; The coolant for direct liquid cooling should be compatible with electronic components; It should be equipped with temperature, pressure (or flow) control and protection devices, and equipped with coolant filtering devices; In order to improve the degree of convective heat transfer, a turbulence device can be installed in the appropriate position of the equipment
Evaporative cooling	The boiling point temperature of the coolant is lower than the minimum allowable operating temperature of the heating components in the equipment; When direct evaporative cooling, the installation of electronic components should ensure that there is enough space to facilitate the formation and movement of air bubbles; The coolant should have low viscosity, high density, large volume expansion coefficient, good thermal conductivity, and sufficient insulation performance; The closed evaporative cooling system has a condenser, and its secondary cooling can be air−cooled or liquid−cooled; The cooling system should be easily maintained

Table 3.18 Common natural cooling methods for electronic components

Serial number	Type	Components	Rule requirements
1	Semiconductor device		The area of semiconductor devices is small, natural convection and its own radiation heat transfer do not play a major role, and heat conduction is the most effective heat transfer method for such devices
1.1		Power Transistor	Power transistors are characterized by generally large and flat mounting surfaces. In order to reduce the interface thermal resistance between the shell and the radiator, insulating gaskets with good thermal conductivity (such as thermally conductive silicone rubber sheets, polytetrafluoroethylene, beryllium oxide ceramic sheets, mica sheets, etc.) and thermally conductive insulating glue should be selected. And the contact pressure should be increased
1.2		Semiconductor integrated circuit	The characteristic of semiconductor integrated circuits is that there are many leads, and the surface area available for natural convection heat transfer is relatively large. With an appropriate radiator for integrated circuits, a better cooling effect can be obtained
1.3		Rectifier and semiconductor diode	The thermal design of rectifiers and diodes is similar to that of transistors. The diode can be directly installed on the heat sink with electrical insulation to reduce the interface thermal resistance. When the heat sink is at the same potential as the diode, the maintenance personnel must be protected from electric shock criticalitys
1.4		Semiconductor microwave device	Semiconductor devices such as microwave diodes and varactor diodes are generally packaged in a cavity or housing with low internal thermal resistance. The operational reliability of these devices depends on the control of their thermal resistance. And they are sensitive to temperature, appropriate heat conduction measures should be taken to reduce the surface temperature of the shell

(continued)

Table 3.18 (continued)

Serial number	Type	Components	Rule requirements
1.5		Plastic packaged semiconductor device	Due to the low thermal conductivity of potting and packaging materials, plastic packaged devices mainly rely on the heat conduction of plastics and connecting wires to dissipate heat. Sometimes a metal heat conductor is also added to this kind of component. At this time, the heat dissipation is mainly carried out by metal heat conduction, so the thermal design is based on metal heat conduction. In addition, some electronic components or components that need to withstand strong vibration and impact, which are potted with synthetic resin, can add aluminum particles to the resin to form good thermal conductivity
2	Resistor		The natural cooling method of the resistor is to rely on the natural convection of the resistor and the metal heat conduction between the resistor itself and the circuit board or heat sink. Metal thermal clips are used on resistors with higher power, but tight contact should be ensured
3	Transformer		The key issue in the design of transformer natural cooling is how to reduce the thermal resistance of the heat transfer path. Thick wires should be used and have good thermal contact with the mounting components. The installation surface should be flat and smooth. Metal foil can be added at the contact interface to reduce the interface thermal resistance. If the transformer has a shield, try to make the shield and the base have good heat conduction. Install copper tape between the shell or core and the frame to help enhance thermal conductivity
4	Passive component		Passive components include capacitors, switches, connectors, fuses, and structural elements. They do not generate heat themselves, but will deteriorate and fail due to high temperature. They can receive heat from nearby active devices by three modes of heat transfer (conduction, convection, and radiation). Measures of thermal shielding and thermal isolation should be adopted in the design to avoid the thermal impact of high-power active devices as much as possible, and ensure that their failure rate is lower than the value required by reliability design

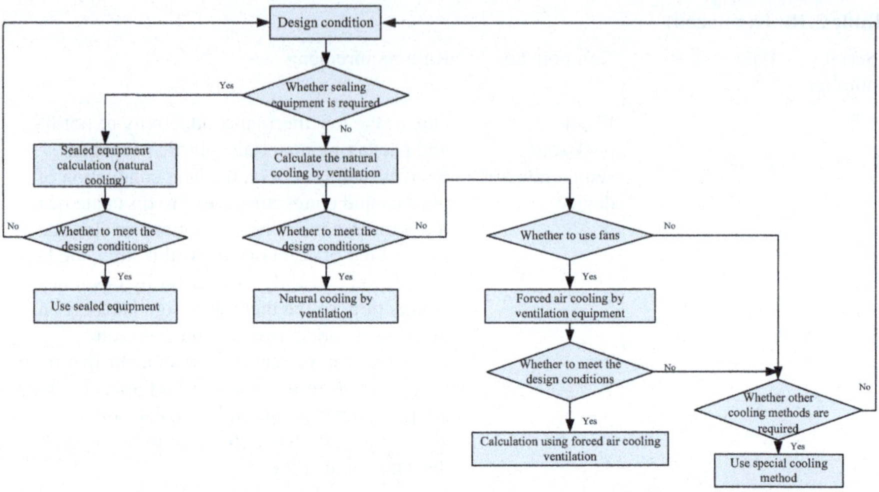

Fig. 3.12 Program for cooling method selection

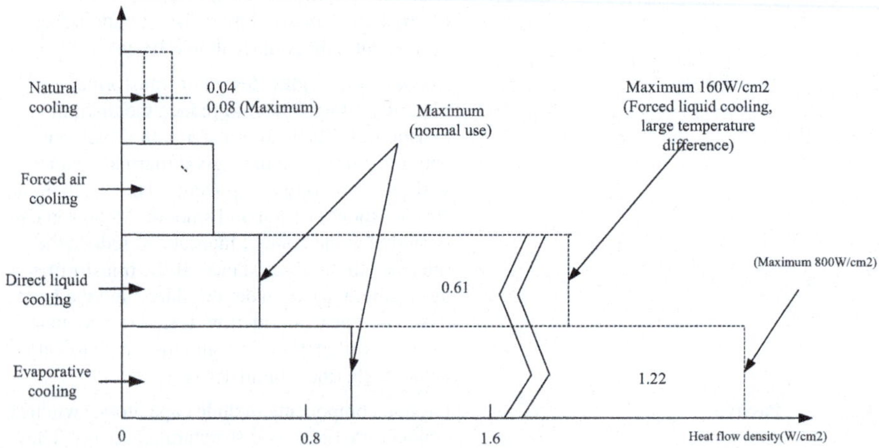

Fig. 3.13 Heat flux density of commonly used cooling methods (temperature rise is 40 °C)

Methods of installing natural cooling and heat dissipation of commonly used electronic components is illustrated in Table 3.19

Table 3.20 for the natural cooling and heat dissipation design methods of circuit boards and mechanical structures.

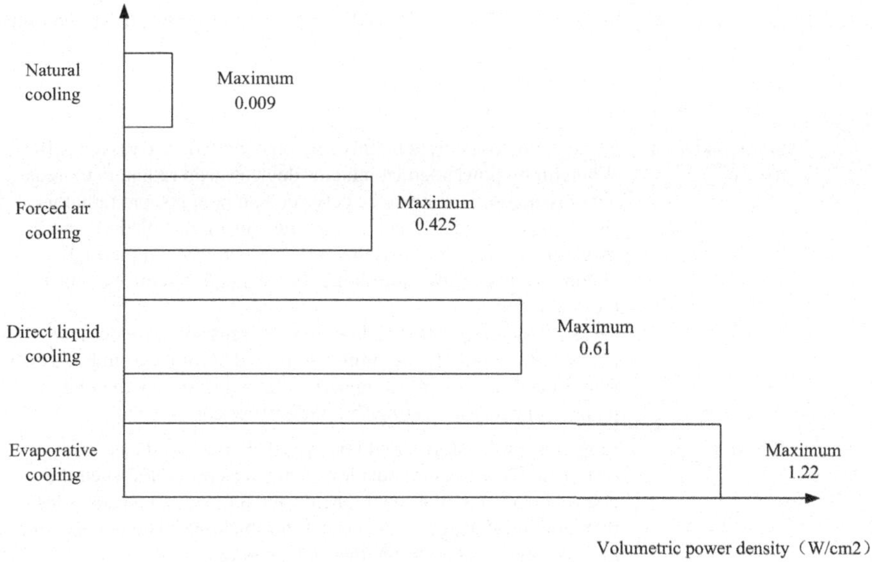

Fig. 3.14 Volume power density of commonly used cooling methods (temperature rise 40 °C)

3.3.7.5 Thermal Installation Technology

Where an electronic device is placed in an operating environment has a large impact on how it transfers heat. Electronic equipment with good thermal design performance, if the thermal installation is improper or the installation environment does not meet the technical conditions, it will cause the equipment to overheat and affect its thermal reliability. The installation of electronic components inside the equipment should meet the thermal installation requirements of low thermal resistance to ensure its good heat transfer performance and reliability.

The thermal environment specified in the technical conditions refers to the thermal environment existing around the equipment. The thermal design should ensure that the equipment can work normally in this link.

1. **Thermal installation technology of electronic equipment**
   (1) The equipment with natural cooling on the outer surface of the equipment is generally designed to be placed on the table or on a stand alone. When this type of equipment is installed in the same cabinet as other equipment, the natural convection cooling path for the equipment will change. The air temperature in the cabinet increases, creating additional thermal resistance and overheating the equipment. In this case, auxiliary cooling should be provided.
   (2) Small equipment using forced air cooling, when they are placed side by side or stacked, will cause the hot air discharged from one equipment to enter the cold air inlet of the other equipment, and after circulation, the temperature

Table 3.19 Methods of installing natural cooling and heat dissipation of commonly used electronic components

Serial number	Type	Rule requirements
1	Semiconductor device	Semiconductor devices mainly rely on conduction to dissipate heat; When high–power semiconductor devices need radiators to assist heat dissipation, the distance between components and radiators should be reduced as much as possible during installation, and insulating liners with good thermal conductivity and thermally conductive insulating glue should be installed to reduce contact thermal resistance; The installation position of low–power transistors, diodes and integrated circuits should minimize heat absorption from large heat sources and heat–generating parts of metal heat–conducting paths, and heat–insulating shielding plates can be used
2	Resistor	Large power resistors should be installed on a metal base and installed in a horizontal position as much as possible; when the distance between other components and the power resistor is less than 50 mm, it is necessary to heat the shielding plate between the high power resistor and the thermal element; Do not install power resistors directly on terminals or circuit boards without a heat sink; The length of the resistor lead wire should be shorter so that the contact with the circuit board can play a role in heat dissipation. And preferably slightly bent to allow thermal expansion and contraction; When resistors are installed in rows or rows, consider the limitation of ventilation and the influence of mutual heat dissipation, and combine them appropriately
3	Transformer and inductor	It should be mounted in a location that minimizes thermal interaction with other components, preferably in a separate corner of the enclosure or in a separate enclosure
4	Passive element	Try to install in the lowest temperature area; When it must be installed in the active area, heat shielding and heat isolation measures should be taken

of the air will rise greatly Exceeds the expected ambient temperature. At the same time, when the equipment is installed, its air inlet and air outlet should not be blocked. The direction of the exhaust port should not affect the operation of personnel.

(3) When multiple devices are installed in the same space and consume heat, the space will be overheated.

(4) The equipment shall not be installed in an environment exceeding the specified humidity, or make the equipment work under conditions lower than the air dew point.

5. The equipment shall not be installed to work under harsher conditions than the expected thermal environment. For example, the device should not be

Table 3.20 Natural cooling heat dissipation design methods for circuit boards and mechanical structures

Serial number	Type	Method	Rule requirements
1	Circuit board	Structural design	(1) Lay metal strips on the ordinary circuit board to form a heat−conducting strip circuit board (see Fig. 1 below); (2) Lay metal plates on ordinary circuit boards to form heat−conducting plate circuit boards (see Fig. 2 below); (3) A metal sandwich heat−dissipating circuit board with a heat−conducting metal core sandwiched between ordinary circuit boards (see Fig. 3 below) 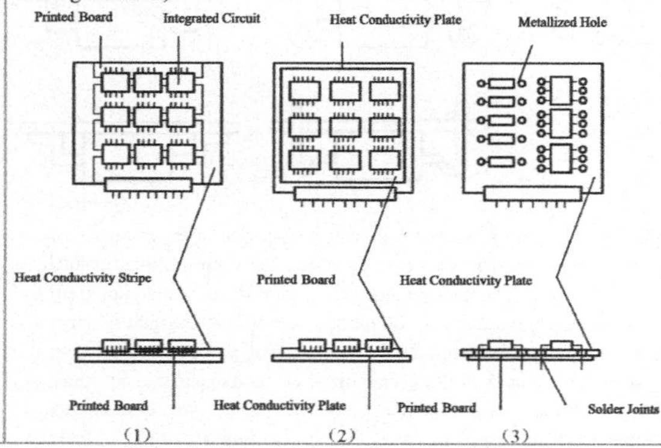

(continued)

Table 3.20 (continued)

Serial number	Type	Method	Rule requirements
1.1		Balance temperature	(1) To reduce the thermal resistance from the component housing to the circuit board, the components can be directly glued to the circuit board or thermal strip (or board) with thermally conductive insulating glue. If no bonding is used, the gap between the components and the circuit board or the thermal strip (or board) should be minimized; (2) When installing high–power components, if you want to use insulating sheets, you should use insulating sheets with sufficient compression resistance, high dielectric strength and thermal conductivity, such as thermally conductive silicone rubber sheets. In order to reduce the thermal resistance of the interface, a thin layer of thermal paste should also be applied to the interface; (3) Electronic components on the same circuit board should be arranged according to their calorific value and heat resistance. Electronic components with poor heat resistance should be placed at the most upstream (at the entrance) of the cooling airflow, and electronic components with good heat resistance Components are placed in the most downstream (exit); (4) In the case of mixed installation of large–scale and small–scale integrated circuits, the large–scale integrated circuits should be placed upstream of the cooling airflow as much as possible, and the small–scale integrated circuits should be placed downstream, so that the temperature rise of the circuit board components tends to be uniform; (5) Since the thermal expansion coefficients of components and circuit boards are inconsistent, some structural measures to eliminate thermal stress should be taken under temperature cycle and high temperature conditions. Cylindrical components such as axial leads (such as resistors and diodes) should provide a minimum strain of 2.6 mm during lap welding and socket welding, as shown in the figure (a) below; components with higher mounting density, Since the components are closely arranged and the surrounding space is small, a ring structure is allowed, as shown in the figure (b) below; large rectangular components (such as transformers, choke coils, etc.), usually have thicker leads, and should have larger strain, as shown in the figure (c) below 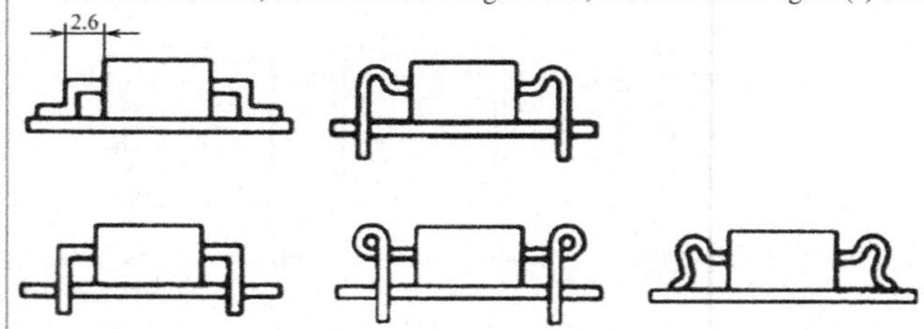 (a) (b) (c)

(continued)

Table 3.20 (continued)

Serial number	Type	Method	Rule requirements
	Edge–rail thermal design		(1) Improve the surface roughness and flatness of the contact surface between the guide rail and the chassis. The higher the precision, the smaller the thermal resistance of the guide rail. However, the higher the precision, the higher the processing cost will increase accordingly. Usually, the surface roughness only needs to reach 3.2 μm.; (2) The material of the guide rail is made of soft, high thermal conductivity metal such as phosphor bronze, beryllium bronze, red copper or aluminum alloy, which can be closely attached to the mating material under a certain pressure to obtain a small thermal resistance.; (3) Use wedge–shaped guide rails. The structure of commonly used edge guide rails is shown in the figure below; among them, the thermal resistance of G –type, B –type and U –type guide rails is relatively large, and the thermal resistance will change greatly with the change of altitude; the wedge–type guide rail not only has a thermal resistance value Small, and the thermal resistance value is almost unchanged with the change of altitude, and it also has good anti–vibration and shock resistance, especially suitable for harsh environments 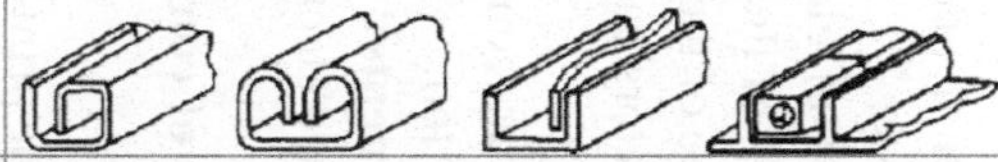
	Chassis		(1) The chassis (chassis) has a good thermal connection with the base and bracket. Most of the thermal resistance in the thermal path exists at the junction interface. All metal–to–metal contact surfaces must be clean, smooth, and the contact area should be as large as possible with high contact pressure; (2) The inner and outer surfaces of the case (casing) are painted, and ventilation holes are opened on the top, bottom or both sides of the case near the heating element. The temperature change of the device; (3) The size of the casing opening should be compatible with the flow rate of the cooling air in and out, and the pressure drop should be smaller than the buoyancy pressure of the hot air (4) The arrangement principle of the ventilation holes should make the air inlet and outlet holes as far away as possible. The air inlet holes should be opened at the lower end of the side of the chassis close to the bottom plate, and the air outlet holes should be opened at the upper end of the side of the chassis close to the top plate. The shape and size of the ventilation hole can be determined according to the application site, electromagnetic compatibility and reliability requirements of the equipment

installed in a poorly ventilated room, on the chimney side of a ship or next to a steam pipe, or next to an engine or other heat source.

2. **Principles of thermal installation of electronic components**
   (1) Heat-sensitive components should be placed in the cold area (such as the bottom) of the equipment, and should not be placed directly on the heating components.
   (2) The arrangement of components should be classified according to their allowable temperature, and the components with higher allowable temperature should be placed above the components with lower allowable temperature.
   (3) Components with high heat generation should be installed as close as possible to the surface with the lowest temperature (such as the inner surface of the metal shell, metal base and metal bracket, etc.), and there should be good contact heat conduction with the surface.
   (4) The thermal resistance of the installation interface and heat transfer path should be reduced as much as possible.
   (5) Electronic components with leads should make use of the heat conduction of the leads as much as possible. Thermal stress should be prevented during thermal installation, and structural measures should be taken to eliminate thermal stress.
   (6) The orientation of the installation of electronic components should conform to the flow characteristics of the airflow and the principle of improving the degree of turbulence of the airflow. In order to improve the heat dissipation effect, turbulators can be installed at appropriate positions.
   (7) The mounting plate of electronic components should be placed vertically to facilitate heat dissipation.
3. **Installation of common electronic components**
   The installation methods of commonly used electronic components are shown in Table 3.21.
4. **Requirements for installation and layout of components on printed circuit boards**

The cooling of the components installed on the printed circuit board mainly relies on heat conduction to provide a low thermal resistance path from the components to the printed circuit board and the side wall of the chassis. The installation precautions are as follows:

(1) In order to reduce the thermal resistance from the component shell to the printed circuit board, the components can be directly bonded to the printed circuit board or the thermal strip (board) with thermally conductive insulating glue. If it is not used for bonding, it should be minimized The gap between components and printed circuit boards or thermal strips (plates);
(2) When installing high-power components, if you want to use insulating sheets, you should use insulating sheets with sufficient compression resistance, high

Table 3.21 Installation methods of common electronic components

Type of components	Installation methods
Resistor	High−power resistors generate a lot of heat. Not only should attention be paid to their own cooling, but also consideration should be given to reducing heat radiation to nearby components. Resistors with a length of more than 100 mm should be installed horizontally, if the distance between the components and the power resistor is less than 50 mm, the shielding plate needs to be heated between the high−power resistor and the heat−sensitive components
Semiconductor device	The installation position of low−power transistors, diodes and integrated circuits should minimize heat absorption from large heat sources and heat−generating parts of metal heat−conducting paths, and heat−insulating shielding plates can be used. For components with power equal to or greater than 1W and with extended convection surface heat sinks, the mounting method and orientation with the best natural convection cooling effect shall be adopted
Transformer inductor	The power transformer is an important heat source. When the temperature of the core device is relatively high, special attention should be paid to its thermal installation. The installation position should minimize the interaction with other components. It is best to install it in the shell a separate corner of the or mounted in a separate housing
Conduction cooling components	It is best to install the components on separate heat−conducting components. If they are installed on a common heat−dissipating metal conductor, there may be obvious thermal interaction
Non−heating components	Placed in the lowest temperature area, usually near the part with the lowest thermal resistance between the heat sink
Temperature sensitive components	Thermal shielding and thermal isolation measures are adopted between the heating components, specifically: (1) Connect the thermal path directly to the heat sink as much as possible; (2) Heating the shielding plate to form a hot zone and a cold zone

dielectric strength and thermal conductivity, such as thermally conductive silicone rubber sheets. In order to reduce the thermal resistance of the interface, a thin layer of thermal paste should also be applied to the interface;

(3) Components on the same printed circuit board should be arranged according to their calorific value and heat resistance. Components with poor heat resistance are placed at the most upstream (at the entrance) of the cooling airflow. Good components are placed in the most downstream (exit);

(4) In the case of mixed installation of large-scale and small-scale integrated circuits, the large-scale integrated circuits should be placed upstream of the cooling airflow as much as possible, and the small-scale integrated circuits should be placed downstream of the cooling airflow, so that the printed circuit board The temperature tends to be uniform;

(5) Due to the wide working range of electronic equipment, the thermal expansion coefficients of component leads and printed circuit boards are inconsistent.

Under the conditions of temperature cycle changes and high temperatures, some structural measures to reduce thermal strain should be taken.

3.3.7.6 Thermal Design of the Chassis

The task of chassis thermal design is to use various necessary heat dissipation methods to dissipate the heat generated by the product to the maximum extent under the premise of ensuring that the product withstands various external environments and mechanical stresses, so as to meet the temperature requirements specified by the electronic components in the product.. Commonly used enclosures mainly include sealed enclosures, ventilated enclosures, and forced air-cooled enclosures. The forced air-cooled enclosures can be further divided into two types: forced ventilation inside the enclosure and cold plate type forced air cooling. See Table 3.22 for the characteristics of the sealed chassis, ventilated chassis, and forced air-cooled chassis.

Precautions for thermal design are:

(1) The system thermal design of electronic equipment should be carried out simultaneously with the circuit and structural design;
(2) When designing the circuit, the heat generated by the circuit should be minimized;
(3) Reduce the number of heating elements;
(4) Select components and raw materials with good heat resistance and thermal stability;
(5) Adopt the derating design method, etc.;
(6) The cooling method should be reasonably selected during structural design;
(7) Optimal design of heat transfer channels;
(8) Minimize thermal resistance and friction heating components.

Remedies for thermal design are:

(1) Enhance the heat dissipation capacity, replace with the same type of radiator with stronger heat dissipation capacity, and use a heat dissipation method with stronger heat dissipation capacity;
(2) Change the internal layout, disperse multiple hotspots, adjust the location of devices that are not resistant to hotspots, and adjust the location of devices with high hotspots;
(3) Change the structural size and material, change the chassis or local structure, size, material and flow channel layout, so that the heat can be dissipated more easily and the heat can be dissipated faster;
(4) Replacement of more heat-resistant devices, for devices whose temperature is too high or the temperature is too high after being affected by heat, replace with more heat-resistant or higher-quality devices;
(5) Take derating measures, and for devices with excessive heat generation, reduce the heat generation through derating design.

Table 3.22 Features of sealed chassis, ventilated chassis, and forced air cooling chassis

Chassis type	The main methods of heat dissipation	Main design elements	Features	Scope of application
Sealed chassis	Heat dissipation from the chassis surface and heat conduction to the chassis	The surface area of the chassis and the installation of the chassis, etc., are generally considered to design heat sinks on the outside of the chassis to increase the effective heat dissipation area of the chassis	Poor heat dissipation	Applied to electronic products with low system power consumption and low heat dissipation requirements
Ventilated chassis	Chassis surface cooling and natural ventilation cooling	Chassis surface area equal to vent area	Relatively good heat dissipation	The power consumption of the system is small, and the heat dissipation through the ventilation holes can meet the temperature requirements
Forced ventilation inside the box	Chassis Surface Cooling and Forced Air Cooling	Select suitable fans and set up reasonable air ducts, including ventilation paths, distribution and control of airflow, influence of air exit/ entrance obstacles, distance between fans and vents, ventilation inlet and outlet design, use of air filters, etc	Good cooling performance	It has a strong heat dissipation capability and is suitable for systems with large power consumption. There are strict requirements on the temperature, humidity and quality of cooling air
Cold plate forced air cooling chassis	Chassis surface cooling, cold plate cooling and forced air cooling	Aluminum plate is generally used for the cover plate, bottom plate and partition material of multi−layer cold plate. The thickness of the cover plate and bottom plate is generally 3~6 mm, the thickness of the partition is 0.4~2 mm, and the shape of the ribs, rib spacing, rib height and rib thickness are selected according to the working environment conditions of the cold plate	Good heat dissipation performance, able to reduce various pollution, compact structure	High heat transfer efficiency, no pollution, simple structure, widely used in thermal design of electronic products, especially electronic products whose volume and weight are strictly limited

3.3.8 Environmental Protection Design

3.3.8.1 The Purpose of Environmental Protection Design

The failure of the product is often related to the environment in which it is located. When the product works in harsh environments such as shock, vibration, humidity, high and low temperature, salt spray, mold, nuclear radiation, etc., some of the units cannot withstand the impact of this environmental stress and cause failures. Therefore, it is necessary to adopt an environmental protection design to improve its reliability. In environmental protection design, in addition to considering the protection of the external environment, we should also pay close attention to the internal environment generated by the product itself. In addition, since various environmental factors are likely to act on the product at the same time, various environmental factors will also affect each other and further deteriorate the environment. Therefore, the principle of comprehensive management should be adopted for environmental protection to grasp the main contradiction. Firstly, start with the environmental factors that have the greatest impact on product reliability, and take corresponding protective measures; at the same time, various protective design measures must be comprehensively weighed before making a decision. For example, in order to prevent vibration and moisture, silicone rubber is poured into the equipment, but it will make it difficult to dissipate heat inside the equipment, resulting in deterioration of the temperature environment. Therefore, silicone rubber can be used only when the temperature resistance of the product allows it.

3.3.8.2 Classification of Environmental Protection Design Methods

The correct environmental protection design includes: temperature protection design; moisture-proof, salt spray and mildew-proof "three-proof" design; shock and vibration protection design, wind and sand protection, pollution prevention, electromagnetic interference protection, static protection, etc. In addition, special attention should be paid to the design of comprehensive environmental protection. For example, the use of an overall sealed structure can not only play the role of "three defenses", but also protect the electromagnetic environment.

For the main environmental factors that may be encountered by digital diagnosis and treatment equipment, their impacts and typical failure modes, they are shown in Table 3.23.

3.3.8.3 Environmental Protection Design Method

1. **Temperature Protection Design**

Temperature is the direct medium for the chemical and physical effects of substances, because most of the chemical and physical properties of materials change with

Table 3.23 Environmental factors and their effects and typical failure modes

Protection item	Main impact	Typical failure mode	Protective measures
High temperature	Thermal expansion forms internal stress; thermal aging and softening affect material properties; viscosity changes affect lubrication performance; temperature changes cause performance changes of components, etc	Structural damage, increased mechanical stress; reduced strength, increased wear, reduced lubrication function; deterioration of mechanical and electrical properties	Carry out thermal design, rationally select materials and lubricants, and adopt heat dissipation or cooling devices
Low temperature	Different shrinkage; lubricant solidification, water vapor condensation, freezing; hydraulic system leakage and solidification; embrittlement, property deterioration	Structural damage; lubricating function reduction; function reduction, performance deterioration; material and component characteristics deterioration	Carefully select materials and leave gaps; reasonably select lubricants; use low-temperature sealing materials, etc.; remove moisture and provide water outlet holes
Humidity	Moisture will deteriorate the performance of components, chemical reaction and corrosion will reduce the strength, circuit short circuit, rust, etc	Reduced electrical and mechanical strength, structural damage, affected function, changes in electrical conductivity	Improve protective coating, drying device, sealing, etc., and choose moisture-resistant materials
Shock, vibration, noise	Mechanical stress and fatigue damage the structure of the parts, cause resonance, damage the seal, and cause the product to work abnormally	The strength is reduced, the function is affected, the structure and components are loose and damaged	Eliminate or reduce shock source, vibration source and sound source, shock vibration isolation, vibration damping buffer design
Static electricity	Casualties, etc	Flammable items burning	Grounding, preventing charge accumulation, high voltage isolation
High pressure	Structural rupture; seal failure; function affected	Container explodes; causes leak; does not function properly	Overvoltage protection; structural strength design
Low pressure	Expansion, air leakage; unstable chemical properties; reduced dielectric strength of air	Reduced mechanical strength; changes in electrical properties; insulation breakdown	Structural sealing, anti-leakage, electrical equipment arc suppression measures to prevent breakdown

(continued)

Table 3.23 (continued)

Protection item	Main impact	Typical failure mode	Protective measures
Electric (lightning) strike	Magnetic induction, electrostatic induction, causing fire, explosion, casualties, etc	Damage to lines and equipment, burns to the human body, ignition of flammable items	System/equipment grounding wire, shell grounding, preventing charge accumulation, high voltage isolation
Explode	Potential source of accident; cause structural damage; incapacity	Structural damage; fire, casualties	Flammable and explosive substances, and safety design is carried out
Mold	Deteriorates materials and reduces performance; changes electrical insulation properties	Functional affected; Electrical performance degraded	Choose materials that do not grow mold; avoid high temperature and humid conditions; use antifungal agents to treat
Salt spray	Constitutes chemical reaction conditions, causing metal galvanic corrosion, mechanical strength reduction, flux corrosion, circuit corrosion, etc.	Increased wearout, loss of strength, change in performance, affected function, material deterioration	Reduce galvanic corrosion, surface treatment or coating barrier layer, avoid moisture accumulation, etc.

temperature; the chemical reactions of substances are obviously affected by the temperature of the reacting substances. Higher temperatures tend to increase the failure rate of products, while lower temperatures can lead to new failure modes. Sudden changes in temperature often increase mechanical stress, thereby reducing strength and sealing failure. Therefore, temperature protection should be divided into high temperature protection and low temperature protection, and the influence of temperature shock should also be considered.

The best way to design for high temperature protection is to use good thermal analysis, thermal design. This has been introduced in Sect. 3.3.7 and will not be repeated.

Low temperature protection methods are shown in Table 3.24.

The impact of temperature shock is mainly due to thermal expansion and contraction, which leads to problems in the fit and sealing of parts, and sometimes excessive internal stress leads to structural damage. The main method of temperature shock protection is to take temperature insulation measures, carefully select the material of the product, and leave appropriate gaps between moving parts.

The temperature protection design measures mainly include the following:

(1) Improve efficiency and reduce power consumption of heating devices, such as selecting low-power integrated circuits and devices with low saturation voltage drop.

Table 3.24 Low temperature protection methods

Influence	Protective measures
Different shrinkage	(1) Carefully select materials; (2) Provide proper clearance between movable parts; (3) The control cable adopts spring tensioner and deep pulley; (4) The shell is made of heavy heat dissipation material
Lubricated and solidified	(1) Choose an appropriate lubricant; (2) Use silicon grease compound; (3) Eliminate the use of liquid lubricants as much as possible
Hydraulic system leaks	Use low temperature sealing and packaging materials such as silicone rubber
Freezing of the hydraulic system	Use suitable cryogenic hydraulic fluids
Damage caused by condensation of moisture and freezing	Exclude moisture by: providing outlet holes, adequate water drainage, elimination of moisture pockets, proper heating, sealing, drying air
Reduced material properties and reduced component reliability	Carefully select materials and components to provide satisfactory low temperature properties

(2) The high-power tube used in the power supply should be installed separately, and the mechanical cooperation with the cooling plate should be closely matched. The components with high heat generation are not allowed to be densely installed, and their layout, arrangement, and installation should be conducive to heat dissipation.
(3) Make full use of the metal chassis for heat dissipation.
(4) Cooling measures such as forced air cooling, liquid cooling and heat pipe cooling shall be adopted for components and assemblies with large heat generation.
(5) For products exposed to direct sunlight, a sunshade should be added.
(6) Pay attention to the installation position and blowing direction of the heater in the shelter or compartment to avoid overheating and damage to the walls and floors.
(7) Avoid using liquid lubricants as much as possible.
(8) Anti-fog measures should be taken for optical equipment working in a low temperature environment.
(9) Vehicles, power supply equipment, etc. must have low-temperature start-up measures, and use antifreeze and suitable low-temperature hydraulic oil.

2. **Moisture-proof design**

Moisture is often a solvating agent for various impurities that can cause various chemical damages to products. Especially when choosing an inappropriate combination of two materials, moisture often accelerates the electrochemical corrosion, degrades the performance of the material, and promotes the growth of mold.

The moisture- proof design measures mainly include the following:

(1) Use waterproof and anti-corrosion materials;
(2) Provide drainage dredging system or dehumidification device to remove moisture accumulation;
(3) Adopt a drying device to absorb moisture;
(4) Apply a protective coating to prevent corrosion;
(5) Hydrophobic treatment to reduce the water absorption of the product or change its hydrophilic property;
(6) The equipment and components are sealed, and put in a desiccant to keep the internal air dry;
(7) Impregnation, filling certain insulating materials with high-strength and good insulating properties, such as gaps, small holes, capillaries, etc. in various coils;
(8) Pouring and potting, heat and melt with epoxy resin, wax, silicone rubber, etc., inject into the component itself or the space between the component and the shell, and the pores of the lead hole, and solidify and seal itself after cooling.

On the other hand, designers must take into account that various adverse effects may be caused due to the adoption of the above protective measures. For example: seals, protective coatings, etc. may seal moisture inside the product, or cause condensation to make the effects of moisture more serious.

3. **Anti-salt spray design**

Salt spray is a good conductor, which will reduce the insulation resistance, accelerate the galvanic corrosion of metals, and cause electrolytic corrosion of metals.

The anti-salt spray design measures mainly include the following:

(1) Selection of anti-salt spray materials;
(2) Use non-metallic protective sleeve;
(3) Provide drainage dredging system or dehumidification device to eliminate moisture accumulation;
(4) Adopt a drying device to absorb moisture;
(5) Set a barrier layer such as paint between the metal surface and the liquid surface to eliminate the conductive channel formed by two different metals passing through the liquid;
(6) Plating a metal layer that can reduce the potential difference on corrosion-prone metals and hard-to-corrosion metals or areas;
(7) Eliminate electrical contact and insulate different metals. For example, steel is made of French blue, and aluminum is anodized to form an oxide film on the metal surface to prevent metal corrosion;
(8) Seal with an alkali-resistant organic insulator;
(9) Use tin or iron-plated components, avoid magnesium.

4. **Anti-humidity, anti-salt spray and anti-mold design**

The anti-mold design measures mainly include the following:

(1) Choose materials that do not grow mold. Such as wool, cotton, feathers, leather, etc. can provide nourishment for mold. Some synthetic materials are originally resistant to mold, but are also susceptible to mold erosion due to the application of plasticizers or hardeners;
(2) Treat parts or equipment with antifungal agents;
(3) The equipment and components are sealed, and put in a desiccant to keep the internal air dry;
(4) Treat parts or equipment with antifungal agents;
(5) Before sealing, the material is irradiated with ultraviolet rays of sufficient intensity to prevent and inhibit mold.

5. **Shock and vibration resistant design**

Excessive vibration and shock will degrade product performance, work unstable, and even cause mechanical damage and structural damage (such as fracture, deformation, wear, open welding, etc.), so corresponding vibration and shock control must be taken during product design measure. The following protective design methods are generally adopted in engineering:

(1) Source elimination design. That is to take measures to reduce the vibration (shock) intensity of the vibration source (shock source) itself. For example, the vibration of the rocket engine is a main source of vibration. The engine designer first devotes himself to eliminating unstable combustion through research, design and testing, and secondly changes the arrangement and flow of nozzles at the head of the thrust chamber to reduce the source of vibration. Reduce the level of engine vibration.
(2) Vibration isolation design. Vibration isolation design is the most widely used in vibration control. The specific method is to add a flexible link (commonly known as a vibration isolator) between the vibration source and the object to be isolated, so as to reduce the impact of the vibration source on the vibration isolation object. Vibration isolation design can be divided into two categories: one is to reduce the transmission of force excitation, often called the first type of vibration isolation (referred to as force isolation), and the other is to reduce the transmission of motion excitation, often called the second type Vibration isolation (abbreviated as spacer).

Table 3.25 lists the commonly used types of vibration isolators and vibration isolation materials, some of which are also used in vibration damping design and buffer design.

3. Vibration reduction design. The so-called vibration reduction is to use various forms of damping to convert part of the vibration energy of the vibrating body into heat energy and dissipate it quickly, so as to achieve the purpose of reducing the vibration value. In engineering, vibration isolation design and vibration reduction design are often integrated and used at the same time, so as to obtain the best effect. The types, damping principles and damping characteristics of commonly used shock absorbers are shown in Table 3.26.

Table 3.25 Commonly used vibration isolators and types of vibration isolation materials

Type	Characteristic	Application	Precautions
Rubber vibration isolator	High bearing capacity, high stiffness, damping coefficient of 0.15 ~ 0.3, creep effect, can be made into various forms, and stiffness in three directions can be freely selected	When the load is large, it is made into a pressure-bearing type, and when the load is small, it is made into a shear-bearing type. Used in conjunction with metal springs, it has a better effect of isolating high frequencies, and is often used for active vibration isolation	The pressure−bearing vibration isolator should ensure that the rubber expands freely to the surroundings, and the relative deformation should be controlled at 10–20%
Metal spring	High bearing capacity, large deformation, small stiffness, damping coefficient of 0.01, lower lateral stiffness than vertical stiffness, easy to shake	It is used for the second type of vibration isolation and the first type of vibration isolation for equipment with large excitation force. Because it is easy to shake, it is not suitable for vibration isolation of precision equipment	When greater damping is required, dampers can be added or combined with materials with greater damping (such as rubber)
G type vibration isolator	It is a finalized product of the shear-type rubber vibration isolator, and its lateral stiffness is larger than the vertical stiffness	Used for vibration isolation of resistance equipment and constant temperature equipment of precision instruments and meters, precision machine tools	Select the model of the vibration isolator according to the size of the static load, and then check whether it meets the vibration isolation requirements, avoid eccentric force during installation, and control the ambient temperature at—5 ~ 50 °C
Air spring	The stiffness is determined by the internal energy of the compressed air, and the damping coefficient is 0.15 ~ 0.5	Class II vibration isolation for precision instruments and equipment with special requirements	The air pressure is required to be stable, so a constant pressure air source is required
Cork	Light weight, certain elasticity, damping coefficient 0.08 ~ 0.12, creep effect	Used as the first type of vibration isolator or combined with rubber metal spring as auxiliary vibration isolator	The stress is controlled at about 1 kg/cm^2, to prevent the cork from expanding freely around, the cork should be coated with paint to prevent it from absorbing water and oil

(continued)

Table 3.25 (continued)

Type	Characteristic	Application	Precautions
Foam rubber	Small stiffness and high elasticity, the damping coefficient is 0.1 to 0.15, the bearing capacity is small, the performance is unstable and easy to change	Used for very small instruments and meters as the second type of vibration isolation	The allowable stress is very low, and the relative deformation should be controlled within the range of 20% ~ 35%. It is strictly forbidden to expose to the sun and rain, and prevent contact with acid, alkali, oil
Foam plastic	Low bearing capacity, low stiffness, unstable performance, easy aging	Used for very small instruments and meters as the second type of vibration isolation	The use stress of foam plastics should be controlled at about 0.2 kg/cm^2
Felt	Large damping, easy to harden and lose elasticity under repeated dry and wet action	for shock isolation	In application, generally take its thickness as 0.65 ~ 7.6 cm
Other material	Sawdust, glass fiber, yellow sand and other irregular vibration isolation materials	For shock isolation and vibration isolation between floors and equipment	These vibration isolation materials should be placed in suitable containers
Wire rope isolator	Has good elasticity and damping, high load-bearing capacity	Widely used for vibration isolation of various equipment, it is a relatively new type of vibration isolator in the world at present, and there are small batches of products in China	/

4. Vibration-absorbing design. That is, the vibration energy of the vibration-absorbing object is transferred to the auxiliary mass by using the additional auxiliary mass spring system, so as to achieve the purpose of reducing the vibration value of the vibration-absorbing object. The auxiliary mass spring system is called a dynamic shock absorber, and appropriate damping is usually added in the application, and its specific structure needs to be determined according to the actual situation.
5. Buffer design. Its purpose is to make the shock first pass through the buffer and then act on the product, so that the response value of the product to the shock (such as transmission force, acceleration, relative displacement, etc.) drops below the allowable value. It can be seen that the core problem is the design of the buffer. Because vibration and shock often exist at the same time, the design calculation

Table 3.26 Types, damping principles and damping characteristics of commonly used shock absorbers

Type	Principle of vibration reduction	Damping characteristics
Solid friction damper	Use the friction generated between the moving part and the damping part and between the damping part and the fixed part to consume vibration energy	Frictional damping
Liquid damping shock absorber	Using the viscosity of the fluid to apply damping to the vibrating body	Viscous damping
Electromagnetic damping shock absorber	Use the damping formed by the interaction between the eddy current generated when the metal moving part vibrates in the magnetic field and the magnetic field to reduce vibration	Electromagnetic damping
Shock absorber	When incomplete elastic bodies collide with each other, their vibration energy will be lost	Shock damping

of the buffer is often used as a supplement to the design of the vibration isolator, so that the hardware has both functions of vibration isolation and buffering.

6. Rigid anti-vibration design. Products with good rigidity and anti-vibration design still have good anti-vibration performance even if they are rigidly fixed on the bracket without vibration isolation device or vibration damping device. Rigid anti-vibration design principles are:

   - Find out the dynamic environment of each part of the product, and install the equipment that is sensitive to vibration and impact as much as possible in the part with the least stress in the dynamic environment;
   - Improve the installation rigidity of silicon controlled rectifier electrical components, shorten the length of leads as much as possible, avoid cantilever installation, pay attention to veneer welding, and seal them on the mounting board with epoxy or polyurethane glue;
   - Integrated circuit components must be installed on the surface to reduce the installation height of integrated circuits;
   - The equipment frame, printed board, plug, etc. are installed firmly to prevent the fasteners from loosening;
   - Try to reduce the vibration response on the printed board. In addition to using constrained damping processing technology, the vibration response of the printed board can also be improved by changing the size of the printed board, the installation form, and the arrangement of components on the printed board.

3.3.9 *Electromagnetic Compatibility Design*

3.3.9.1 The Purpose of Electromagnetic Compatibility Design

Electromagnetic compatibility refers to the coexistence state in which systems, subsystems, and equipment can coordinate and complete their respective functions in a common electromagnetic environment. Electricity and magnetism are interrelated, and every electronic device inevitably has electromagnetic compatibility problems. Therefore, in order to make electronic devices operate reliably, electromagnetic compatibility technology must be studied. Through the electromagnetic compatibility design, the anti-electromagnetic interference ability of the product can be improved, the external electromagnetic interference can be reduced, and the product failure caused by the interference can be avoided, thereby improving the reliability of the product.

In order to achieve electromagnetic compatibility, the following five issues must be studied in depth:

(1) Research on electromagnetic disturbance sources. Including the frequency domain and time domain characteristics of electromagnetic disturbance sources, the mechanism of generation and the research of suppression measures.
(2) Research on the propagation characteristics of electromagnetic disturbance. That is to study how electromagnetic disturbance is transmitted from disturbance source to sensitive equipment, including the research on conduction disturbance and radiation disturbance.
(3) Research on the anti-interference ability of sensitive equipment. This anti-interference ability is often characterized by electromagnetic susceptibility or immunity. The smaller the electromagnetic susceptibility level, the lower the immunity and the worse the anti-interference ability.
(4) Research on measuring equipment, measuring methods and data processing methods. Due to the complexity of electromagnetic disturbances, there are many requirements for measurement and evaluation. For example, the receiver must have multiple detection methods, multiple measurement bandwidths, large overload coefficients, and strict intermediate frequency filtering characteristics. It also requires the propagation characteristics and theory of the measurement site. The values match up very well. How to evaluate the measurement results is also a key issue, which requires the application of mathematical tools such as probability theory and mathematical statistics.
(5) Research on electromagnetic compatibility within and between systems. Research in this area requires extensive theoretical knowledge and rich practical experience.

3.3.9.2 Classification of Electromagnetic Compatibility Design Methods

Electromagnetic compatibility design can be mainly divided into two types: suppression design for conducted interference and suppression design for radiated interference. Among them, conducted interference refers to the electromagnetic disturbance transmitted along the conductor, and radiated interference refers to the electromagnetic disturbance radiated by devices, components, connecting lines, cables or antennas, and equipment or systems.

The basic idea of suppressing conducted interference is "draining" (bypass). The interference noise is introduced into the ground wire, where it is converted into heat energy and dissipated; it is not allowed to enter the input terminal of the amplifier, and form interference after being amplified.

The basic idea of suppressing radiation interference is "isolation". Measures such as space isolation, time isolation or frequency isolation are used to isolate the source of radiation interference from the interference sensor.

3.3.9.3 EMC Design Measures

Electromagnetic compatibility design generally needs to be designed from the aspects of suppressing interference sources and cutting off interference propagation channels. The main design measures are as follows:

(1) In the design of electrical and electronic equipment and systems, the system electromagnetic compatibility design requirements should be met.
(2) The signal and the power circuit should avoid sharing the ground wire, and the signal should be effectively shielded to avoid the influence of electromagnetic interference, or reduce its influence to an acceptable level.
(3) For high voltage and strong radiation parts, there should be obvious signs or instructions, and effective protection or shielding measures should be taken.
(4) It is forbidden to connect the ends of the power line and signal line to the adjacent jacks of the connector.
(5) The input/output of the circuit cannot be adjacent.
(6) Carry out electromagnetic compatibility design according to relevant requirements to ensure that the product is compatible with the external environment and the internal circuits of the product are compatible at all levels.
(7) All grounding leads should be as short, thick and straight as possible, and directly grounded, and non-conductive substances are not allowed between their contact surfaces; the grounding of small signal circuits should be separated from other groundings; large transient currents may occur The circuit should have a separate grounding system.
(8) Good conductors (steel, aluminum) should be used as shielding materials for high frequency electric fields, and magnetically permeable materials (electrical pure iron, high magnetic rate alloys) should be used as shielding materials for low frequency magnetic fields.

(9) Multi-layer shielding is adopted to improve the shielding effect and expand the frequency range of shielding.
(10) After giving priority to taking good grounding and shielding measures, filter technology is only used when necessary.
(11) The filter should be able to withstand the specified input current and peak voltage fluctuations to ensure its reliable operation; when selecting filter components, their impedance network must match the signal parameters of the input filter; the filter should try to Close to the filtered line, connect with short wire or shielded wire.
(12) The printed circuit board should take decoupling measures to suppress external conduction interference.
(13) The electrical lap should meet the relevant requirements, and the metal surfaces that need to be lapped must be in close contact; it is best to use the same material, otherwise, in order to ensure compatibility of different materials and prevent lap corrosion, insert gaskets or The protective layer.
(14) Electric connector leakage and high-frequency leakage should be prevented.
(15) When necessary, measures such as adjusting component layout, wiring arrangement, and circuit layout can be adopted to meet electromagnetic compatibility requirements.
(16) The grounding design should pay attention to the design points of protective grounding design, working grounding design and shielded cable grounding design.
(17) Shielding design should pay attention to the key points of electric field shielding design, magnetic field shielding design, electromagnetic field shielding design, and shielding case design.
(18) Filter design should pay attention to power filter design, line noise filter design composed of ferrite magnetic ring, and isolation transformer design points.
(19) The interference suppression of signal lines should pay attention to the design points of interference suppression of analog signal lines and digital signal lines.

3.3.10 Circuit Tolerance Design

3.3.10.1 Purpose of Circuit Tolerance Design

In actual work, sometimes this situation is encountered. During the long-term operation of the product, its characteristic parameters will drift. When the parameter drift exceeds the allowable range, the specified function cannot be completed. The failure at this time is called drift failure.

In order to prevent drift failure and keep the product in a normal state throughout its life and under specified environmental conditions, in addition to selecting components with better quality, tolerance design should also be carried out in circuit design. From the design point of view, measures to adapt to parameter drift are taken to allow the parameters of the components used to change within a certain range, while still ensuring that the performance indicators meet the specified requirements. Tolerance analysis technology is a method to predict the stability of circuit parameters. By analyzing the parameter deviation of circuit components, the influence of circuit performance tolerance is analyzed within the specified range of use conditions.

3.3.10.2 Classification of Circuit Tolerance Design Methods

The tolerance analysis of electronic products can be carried out directly, or the mathematical model of the product can be established first, and then the theoretical calculation and analysis can be carried out. The tolerance analysis methods include worst case test method, worst case analysis method, Monte Carlo method, The adjoint network method and the step-moment method, except the worst-case test method, are all theoretical calculation and analysis methods. The various analysis methods are briefly described below.

1. **Worst case test**

Make the circuit under the conditions of the upper and lower limits of main factors such as atmospheric pressure, power supply voltage, grid frequency, component parameters, signal source amplitude and frequency, etc., and test the actual parameter deviation of circuit performance through experiments. This method does not need to establish a mathematical model of the circuit, but it must be tested on an actual circuit, and the results of the test are used as test data. Generally, this analysis method is used when the reliability of the circuit is high and the cost is not strictly limited.

2. **Worst case analysis**

According to the circuit mathematical model established, it is a non-probability statistical method to analyze the deviation of circuit performance parameters under the worst combination of circuit component parameters. It designs circuits according to the possible limit values of component performance parameters. If the parameters obtained in the worst case fall within the allowable range, it means that the designed circuit can be guaranteed to have sufficient tolerance and drift reliability.

Due to the difference in specific algorithms, the worst case analysis method is divided into linear expansion method and direct substitution method. The linear expansion method is suitable for circuits with low analysis precision requirements, and the direct substitution method is suitable for circuits with high analysis precision requirements. Generally speaking, the worst-case analysis method is simple and intuitive, and it is a very conservative and foolproof design method, so it is often used in some important circuit or component designs. The disadvantage is that it will greatly increase the requirements for components, thereby increasing costs.

3. **Monte Carlo method**

Monte Carlo method is a computer simulation method. Its theoretical basis is the law of large numbers in probability theory. The procedure for simulating with the Monte Carlo method is: first, according to the distribution of each component, a number is randomly selected to form a random array; then it is substituted into the characteristic equation to calculate the characteristic value; Whether it falls within the given value range. If so, record as success; otherwise, fail. Then extract and calculate, generally more than hundreds of times, and finally count the probability of success. If the probability of success exceeds the required value, it means that the component is selected properly; otherwise, re-select the component and calculate again until the requirement is met.

The Monte Carlo method is applied to very complex circuits. If the distribution of components conforming to the measured data of the components can be given, and the required characteristic values can be accurately defined, even if the form is very complicated, it is not difficult to use the Monte Carlo method for calculation, and this method can finally give the characteristic value distribution, which cannot be achieved by other methods.

4. **Accompanying network method**

The adjoint network method is a method for circuit tolerance analysis by calculating the branch voltage and current of the original circuit network and its accompanying network to obtain the sensitivity and deviation of the circuit output response to the branch components. This method needs to establish the current and voltage equations of the branch circuit and the impedance matrix and admittance matrix of the accompanying network to form a mathematical model of the circuit. The parameter value of each component of the circuit is the deviation of the rated value, and the analysis result obtained by solving the equation is the deviation of the circuit output parameter. The adjoint network method is only suitable for linear and time-constant circuits, and can analyze more complex circuits of this type, but the calculation is complicated, and computer-aided analysis can be used.

5. **Step-moment method**

The step-moment method is a probability statistics method to analyze the deviation of circuit performance parameters according to the mean value and variance of the parameter values of circuit components. According to the mean value and variance of the circuit components, the method calculates the mean value and variance of the circuit performance parameters, and analyzes the probability of the allowable deviation of the circuit performance parameters. This method needs to establish a mathematical model between the parameters of the circuit components and the output parameters of the circuit, and deduce the relationship between the mean value of the parameters of the circuit components and the mean value of the circuit output parameters according to the mathematical model, as well as the parameter variance of the circuit components and the circuit The relationship between the variances of the output parameters is computed accordingly. The order-moment method is suitable for linear circuits or nonlinear circuits, but it requires the random drift of the parameters of the circuit components within a small range around the nominal value, and it is assumed that the circuit performance parameters are approximately normal distribution, so it is subject to certain restrictions in use. limit.

The scope of application of the above tolerance analysis methods is different, among which the worst case test method is applicable to all circuits, the worst case analysis method and Monte Carlo method are applicable to all analog circuits, and the adjoint network method and order moment method are applicable in linear analog circuits. Due to the high cost and complicated implementation of the worst-case test method, this method is generally not used unless there are special requirements. Therefore, the worst-case analysis method and the Monte Carlo method are first selected when performing tolerance analysis. At present, there are specialized tool software to support the worst-case analysis method and Monte Carlo method.

3.3.10.3 Circuit Tolerance Design Measures

For circuit tolerance design, please refer to GJB/Z 89—1997 "Guidelines for Circuit Tolerance Analysis". Tolerance analysis and tolerance design should be carried out for key circuits according to needs. The main design measures are as follows:

(1) The object of circuit tolerance analysis should select circuits that seriously affect safety, circuits that complete tasks, expensive circuits, circuits that are difficult to purchase and manufacture, and circuits that require special protection.
(2) When designing the circuit, there must be a certain power margin, usually 20–30% of the margin, and 50–100% of the margin can be used in important places, and places with higher stability and reliability are required. The amount should be larger.
(3) Temperature compensation should be performed on components whose parameters change with temperature to keep the circuit stable.
(4) Correctly select components with stable electrical parameters to avoid drifting failures in the circuit.
(5) The requirements for critical values of input and output signals should be relaxed reasonably.
(6) Redundant contacts should be added to the contacts of connectors, switches, and relays to work in parallel.
(7) The reserve design should adopt functional redundancy as much as possible, and the failure of redundant components will not affect its main function.
(8) When information transmission is not allowed to be interrupted, work reserves should be adopted.
(9) Use feedback technology to compensate (or suppress) the impact of parameter changes to ensure stable circuit performance.
(10) The components of the redundant system and the main system cannot pass through the same connector.

3.3.11 Software Reliability Design

3.3.11.1 Purpose of Software Reliability Design

Failure of the software in use will lead to the failure of the mission, and even lead to catastrophic consequences. Therefore, possible failures should be analyzed during the software design process, and necessary measures should be taken to avoid introducing defects that cause failures into the software, so as to provide a basis for formulating failure correction measures and provide reference for avoiding similar problems. These works will greatly improve the reliability of the software in use and reduce various losses caused by software failure.

Software reliability design is an important design characteristic of software. Only when reliability characteristics are designed into software, can software have the required reliability level. To ensure the reliability of software, we must first ensure that all work is carried out in strict accordance with software engineering specifications during the software development process. In addition, we should also ensure that software development realizes " industrialization".

3.3.11.2 Classification of Software Reliability Design Methods

There are four main types of software reliability design:

(1) Software error avoidance design. Software error-avoidance design is a design method to make software products avoid errors or make fewer errors during the design process. The design principle of error avoidance design is to control and reduce the complexity of the program.

(2) Software error checking design. Software error detection design refers to a design method in which some special functions are given to the program in the design, so that the program can automatically find errors during operation. Error detection design can be divided into passive error detection and active error detection in two ways.

(3) Software error correction design. Software error correction design refers to a design method that empowers the program to self-correct errors and reduce the degree of error damage in the design. The premise of correcting errors is that the cause and location of software errors have been accurately found out (failure detection and failure location are collectively called failure diagnosis), and the program has the ability to modify and eliminate erroneous statements. At this stage, it is limited to reducing the harmful effects caused by software errors, or limiting the harmful effects to a smaller range. failure isolation techniques are often used.

(4) Software fault-tolerant design. Software fault-tolerant design refers to a design method in which a program is endowed with a special function in the design, so that the system still has the ability to operate normally even if the program

has been triggered by an error. fault-tolerant design can be divided into time-tolerance, structure-tolerance, and information-tolerance.

3.3.11.3 Software Reliability Design Measures

1. **Software error avoidance design**

Software error avoidance design embodies the idea of prevention first, and is the primary method of software reliability design. The design of software error avoidance should start from multiple places such as development methods and tools, and error avoidance should be carried out at all stages of the product. In-depth study of user needs, early intervention, selection of good development methods, such as structured methods, object-oriented methods, component-based development methods, rapid prototyping methods, etc., to carry out software error-avoiding design to avoid requirements errors.

The design criteria for software error avoidance design are mainly as follows:

(1) Modularization and module independence. Modularization is based on the fact that it is easier to solve a complex problem after it is divided into several manageable small problems. The independent procedures of modules can be measured by two qualitative criteria, namely cohesion and coupling. Coupling measures how tightly different modules depend on each other, and cohesion measures how closely each element in a module is combined with each other.
(2) Abstraction and progressive refinement. Abstraction is to extract the essential characteristics of things without considering their details for the time being. Every step of the software engineering process is a refinement of the abstraction level of the software solution.
(3) Information concealment. The principle of information hiding points out that modules should be designed and determined in such a way that the information contained in a module cannot be accessed by modules that do not need the information, that is, "only need to know". If the vast majority of data and procedures are hidden from other parts of the software, errors introduced inadvertently during modification are less likely to propagate to other parts of the software.
(4) Information localization. Localization refers to physically placing closely related software elements close to each other.
(5) Carefully use structures and techniques that are prone to introducing defects.

2. **Software error checking design**

Software error detection design can be divided into passive error detection and active error detection in two ways. Among them, passive error detection refers to setting detection points in several parts of the program and waiting for the appearance of error symptoms; active error detection refers to actively checking the status of the program.

(1) Passive error detection

Passive error detection should follow the two detection principles of mutual suspicion and immediate detection. When designing any unit or module, it is assumed that there are errors in other units or modules. When error symptoms appear, they should be detected as soon as possible to limit the damage of the error and reduce the difficulty of troubleshooting. Passive error detection also has some negative effects. For example, the set "acceptance criterion" cannot completely match the expected correct result, resulting in misjudgment or missed judgment.

The implementation methods of passive error detection are mainly as follows:

1. Watchdog timer. Transitioning the system to a defined safe state when a potentially unsafe system state occurs or is possible to transition to such a state.
2. Cycle waiting times control.
3. Design for processing with hardware, such as power failure, electromagnetic interference, system instability, interface failure, interference signal, and wrong operation.
4. Check the data against known data limits.
5. Test according to the constant relationship between variables.
6. Check the validity of all multivalued data.
7. Conduct consistency check on redundant input data.

(2) Active error detection

Active error detection is mainly realized through software BIT. Through the software BIT, the code in the ROM is checked, the RAM is checked to ensure the correct operation code, the correctness of the memory is checked to ensure the correct operation, and the key and important functions and logic functions are typically compared. According to statistics, the combination of software BIT and hardware watchdog timer can generally detect 98% of failures. Proactive error detection can be scheduled as a periodic task, or it can be performed as a low-priority task.

3. **Software error correction dsign**

Software error correction design usually adopts failure isolation technology. The principle of least authority is the main idea to realize failure isolation. In order to limit the spread of failures, strict definitions and restrictions are required on processes and data. For example, the failure isolation methods for the operating system mainly include:

(1) Do not allow one user's application to reference or modify other user's applications or data;
(2) An application is absolutely not allowed to reference or modify the code of the operating system or the data inside the operating system;
(3) Protect the application program and its data so that it will not be accidentally changed due to the error of the operating system;
(4) The application program must not terminate the system work, nor induce the operating system to change other application programs or data.

4. **Software fault-tolerant design**

Software fault-tolerant design is divided into three methods: time fault tolerance, structural fault tolerance, and information fault tolerance. The design methods are mainly as follows:

(1) Time tolerance. Time fault tolerance refers to a means of obtaining high reliability of the software system at the cost of sacrificing time. It includes two commonly used and effective methods: repeated execution of instructions and repeated execution of programs. In the case of unsuccessful reexamination, the usual processing method is to issue an interrupt, transfer to the error handling program, or recalculate the program, or reassemble the system, or give up the program processing.
(2) Structural fault tolerance. The basic idea of structural fault tolerance comes from redundancy technology in hardware reliability, including static redundancy and dynamic redundancy. Mutual shielding of failures between redundant versions cannot be completely relied on back-to-back programming (random differences), and different programming (forced differences) should be implemented consciously, including different personnel independent of each other, different algorithms, different programming languages, different Compilers, different design tools and methods, etc.
(3) Information fault tolerance. Information error tolerance includes error detection and error correction. Generally, parity codes can be used for non-critical information. A certain distance should be kept between key and important information and other information, and system failure will not be caused by one or two errors. If there is an error in safety–critical information, it should be able to be detected and returned to a specified state (eg safe state).

3.3.12 Anti-transient Overstress Design

Anti-transient overstress design is also an important method to ensure the stability and reliability of the circuit. Attention must be paid to the corresponding protection design, for example: add a capacitor between the protected wire and the ground wire that absorbs high frequency; use diode or Zener tube protection to prevent the voltage from exceeding the rated value (clamp value); use series resistance To limit the current value, etc.

The design of anti-transient overstress mainly needs to consider the following aspects:

(1) Select components with overload capacity that meets the requirements.
(2) Take transient suppression measures for known transient sources in the line. For example, the inductive load back EMF can be suppressed by a series network of resistors and diodes connected in parallel with the inductive load.

(3) For silicon controlled rectifier components that may be subject to strong transient overload, protective measures for transient overload should be taken for themselves.
(4) Minimize the static charge generated by friction as much as possible.
(5) Electronic components should strictly implement the requirements of GJB/Z105-98 "Electrostatic Discharge Control Manual for Electronic Products" on the classification indicators of electrostatic discharge sensitive components, components and equipment. Printed Circuit Board (PCB) It is necessary to do a good job in the electromagnetic compatibility design of the anti-static electromagnetic field effect.

3.3.13 Design Related to Human Factors

In addition to the failure of the equipment itself, human error actions can also cause system failure. Human factor design is the application of ergonomics and reliability design to reduce equipment or system failures caused by human factors. The skills of the personnel who use, operate and maintain the product should generally be designed with the average level in mind, and their physical strength should be considered with the level that more than 95% of the personnel can achieve.

Design related to human factors mainly needs to consider the following aspects:

(1) The working space should conform to the size of the human body and the type of work.
(2) Body posture, physical strength and movement should be suitable for operation to improve sustainable working ability.
(3) Operation and maintenance personnel should not be required to do things that his coordinating function does not allow.
(4) Natural or artificial lighting required for the completion of operations, controls, training and maintenance shall be provided.
(5) Human health should be fully considered in terms of environment, safety and technical documents, emphasizing people-oriented comprehensive design ideas.
(6) The selection, shape and arrangement of control and adjustment components shall be suitable for the relevant body parts and their movements, and the requirements for sensitivity, accuracy, speed and force shall be considered, and the design details shall be suitable for human operation reliability.
(7) The size of the console, the color of the indicator light, the size of the handle and various operating forces should be designed according to the best state of the person.
(8) The working environment of the product should be designed according to the physiological characteristics of human sensory organs, executive organs and nervous system, and the external factors that are prone to work fatigue should be reduced as much as possible, so that operators can use and read in the most comfortable state. and respond.

3.3.14 Packaging and Transportation Design

The purpose of packaging and transportation design is to put forward reliability design constraint requirements for packaging, storage, loading and unloading and transportation methods by considering possible failures in the process of product packaging, storage, loading and unloading and transportation.

1. **Packaging design**

    (1) The packaging of the product should be coordinated with the intended transportation and storage methods of the product.
    (2) The packaging of the product should be easy to unpack, clean and reseal.
    (3) The packaging of the product should be convenient for loading, unloading, storage, transportation and management, and under normal loading, unloading, storage and transportation conditions, it is guaranteed that from the date of delivery to the scheduled storage and transportation period, the product will not be damaged due to poor packaging. Corrosion, mildew, failure (failure), damage and loss.

2. **Transportation design**

    (1) In the case of ensuring the task requirements, the transportation mode should be designed to meet the transportation requirements; the transportation mode of the product includes road transportation, railway transportation, air transportation and water transportation, etc.
    (2) Appropriate protective measures, safety measures and emergency measures during transportation should be considered, such as the safety measures and emergency measures during the transportation of products such as shockproof, fireproof, ammunition products and other flammable, explosive, corrosive and radioactive products. measure.

3. **Storage design**

    (1) The storage method should be determined according to the expected use and maintenance requirements of the product and the characteristics of the technical state; the storage method includes warehouse, open air with covering, open air without covering, special storage, etc.
    (2) The storage method should be coordinated with the packaging protection level of the product.
    (3) When deciding to adopt a special storage method, various factors should be fully considered and carefully weighed.
    (4) Analysis of storage tasks shall be carried out to determine the composition, style and required space of storage facilities of each maintenance level.
    (5) The storage grade environment of the storage facilities should be determined in coordination with reference to the relevant regulations and in combination with the actual storage environment conditions.

(6) Storage facilities should have corresponding protective measures such as moisture-proof, mildew-proof, salt spray-proof, freeze-proof, fire-proof, anti-static, radiation-proof, explosion-proof, and shock-proof.

4. **Loading and unloading design**
   (1) According to the weight, size, fragility, safety requirements and site conditions of the goods to be loaded and unloaded, appropriate mechanical loading and unloading or manual loading and unloading methods should be designed.
   (2) The items to be loaded and unloaded should have hooks, hoisting, limit, prevent falling, collision, pressure loss and other marks or relevant documents and specifications to ensure the safety and reliability of loading and unloading and avoid losses caused by improper loading and unloading.

3.3.15 Reliability Design of Non-electronic Products

3.3.15.1 Overview

The various reliability design methods described in the above sections of this chapter are applicable to digital medical equipment, but in addition to electronic products, digital medical equipment also has a large number of non-electronic products, including mechanical, optical, hydraulic, electrical, etc. Its reliability problem has become more and more prominent. Due to the characteristics of non-electronic products, their reliability design methods are different from those of electronic products, and the theory and technology of design and experiment are being further improved. The non-electronic products mentioned here refer to all products (or non-electronic parts of a device) other than pure electronic products, which are characterized by a wide variety and low standardization, and the failure of such products is due to fatigue, wear, Caused by aging, corrosion and other reasons, it belongs to the consumption type failure mode, and its failure rate does not meet the assumption of constant failure rate. Therefore, it is difficult to implement quantitative reliability analysis and design.

Reliability engineering is developed gradually by studying the reliability of electronic products with electronic products as the pioneer, and has formed a set of relatively perfect theories and methods, which has made great contributions to improving the reliability of electronic products. The failure rate of electronic products basically conforms to the so-called "bath tub curve", which divides the life span of electronic products into three stages: early failure period, accidental failure period, and wear and tear failure period. In the early failure period, the failure rate of the product is monotonically decreasing; after entering the accidental failure period, the failure rate of the product tends to stabilize and is approximately constant; then after a long period of time, enter the wear and tear period, the failure rate of the product rises sharply and is soon scrapped. But the life of non-electronic products is only one stage, and the failure rate is monotonically increasing, that is, the wear and tear type failure, does not meet the "bottom of the tub" constant failure rate assumption. Therefore, most of the reliability theories, methods and standards that are generally applicable to electronic products cannot be applied to non-electronic products, especially the quantitative reliability design and analysis is difficult to implement. However, practice shows that the reliability design guidelines, failure mode, effects and criticality analysis (FMECA), fault tree analysis (FTA), and other qualitative reliability techniques and methods are not only fully applicable to non-electronic products, but are also effective.

Although domestic and foreign engineering circles have poured a lot of manpower and financial resources into the reliability quantitative analysis and design of non-electronic products, due to the limited available data (failure rate, etc.), and it is very difficult to obtain these data, therefore, So far, no universally applicable methods and standards have been formed. Although some failure rate statistical models and failure rate data books for non-electronic products have been formed, they are not universal and not enough to be used as a direct basis for predicting the reliability of non-electronic products. In this case, the engineering community generally believes that for non-electronic products, the most effective way is to find problems, sum up experience, and improve design through long-term use, so as to improve product reliability. In fact, this is the basic idea of establishing reliability design criteria. To this end, the following are recommended:

(1) From the management level, formulate corresponding specifications for the design, process, manufacturing, testing, packaging, transportation, storage, use, repair and maintenance of non-electronic products, and strengthen management and supervision to ensure that products Inherent reliability and operational reliability.
(2) From the design level, for the designated non-electronic products, the design experience and use experience of similar products can be used for reference, and on this basis, the "design specifications" and "reliability design criteria" for this product are formulated, including structural form, "Quantitative models" and "qualitative criteria" for strength, stiffness, factor of safety, raw materials, resonant frequencies, etc.
(3) Apply the "Failure Mode, Effect and Criticality Analysis (FMECA)" technology to the design of non-electronic products. FMECA is a bottom-up (from component to system) reliability analysis technology, starting from the lowest component failure, and analyzing the consequences of the failure layer by layer until the system level product. First of all, find out all possible failures of all the constituent units of the system, and analyze these failures one by one, including the failure mode, failure mechanism and the impact of the failure on the system. Then, classify the failures according to the severity of the impact, identify the "fatal" failures, and design countermeasures to prevent them. At the same time, the results of FMECA are also the basis for determining key and important parts. FMECA is a qualitative analysis method that does not require mathematical operations, is simple and easy to implement, and has remarkable effects, and is very popular among technicians. But FMECA also has its limitations,

it can only do single factor analysis. If a certain top-level failure requires several factors (bottom-level failures) to occur simultaneously, FMECA will be helpless. Therefore, it is necessary to use "Failure Tree Analysis (FTA)" as a supplement.

(4) FTA is a top-down (from system to component) reliability analysis technique. First determine the top event, which is the least expected system-level failure, and search for all the direct causes of the failure down to the bottom layer. FTA can not only find out possible hardware failures, but also find out software failures, environmental factors and human factors. FTA can analyze not only single-factor failures, but also multi-factor failures (combination of several unit failures). FTA is applicable to any stage of the system life cycle, especially the early design stage, to find out the weak links in the system as early as possible, and take effective preventive measures in the design to improve the inherent reliability of the product.

(5) FMECA is an indispensable basic work of FTA, and FTA is the development and supplement of FMECA. The joint application of the two (analyzing the "fatal failure" found by FMECA as the top event of FTA) will receive a lot of attention. Good results.

(6) When designing the mechanical structure of the product, the problem of preventing misinstallation of fittings must be carefully considered. It must be guaranteed from the design that under no circumstances can wrong or reversed fittings be installed. Similarly, the problem of preventing misinstallation of fittings cannot be left to the operator, and the "sense of responsibility" of the operator cannot be placed.

3.3.15.2 Characteristics of Reliability of Non-electronic Products

Compared with electronic products, the reliability of non-electronic products has the following characteristics:

(1) The failure of non-electronic products is mainly wear-and-tear failure (such as fatigue, aging, wear, corrosion, strength degradation, etc.), while the failure of electronic products is mainly caused by accidental factors.

(2) The failure rate of wear-and-tear failure increases with time, so the change of the failure rate of non-electronic products with time is generally not a constant value.

(3) There are many failure modes of non-electronic products, and even the same part has multiple important failure modes. The failure modes of non-electronic products can generally be divided into the following types:

- Damaged failure modes: such as fracture, excessive deformation, plastic deformation, cracks, etc.;
- Degradation failure modes: such as aging, corrosion, wear, etc.;
- Loose failure mode: such as looseness, desoldering, etc.;

- Improper failure mode: such as improper clearance, improper stroke, improper pressure, etc.;
- Blockage or leakage failure mode: such as blockage, oil leakage, air leakage, etc.;
- Functional failure mode: such as unstable performance, performance degradation, abnormal function, etc.

(4) Most of the components of non-electronic products are non-standard, and their failure statistics are very scattered, which makes it difficult to count failure data.
(5) Different failure modes of non-electronic products are often correlated, and failure mode correlation needs to be considered in reliability analysis.

3.3.15.3 Characteristics of Reliability Design of Non-electronic Products

The reliability design of non-electronic products is different from the design method of electronic products. The reliability design of non-electronic products has the following basic characteristics:

1. **Taking stress and strength as random variables at the starting point**

Recognize that the stress and material strength of the parts are not constant, but random variables, with discrete nature, mathematically must be described by the distribution function, which is due to the variability and statistical nature of the load, strength, structural dimensions, working conditions, etc.

2. **Apply probability and statistical methods to analysis**
3. **Quantitatively answer the failure probability and reliability of the product**

First of all, it is admitted that the designed product has a certain failure probability, but it cannot exceed the allowable value specified in the technical file. And it can quantitatively give the failure rate and reliability of the designed product.

4. **A variety of reliability indicators are available**

The reliability design of non-electronic products requires selecting different and most suitable reliability indicators according to the specific conditions of different products, such as failure rate, reliability, Mean Time Between Failures (MTBF), maintenance degree, and effectiveness. Reliability indicators and evaluation methods should be selected at the beginning of the design stage.

5. **Emphasize the leading role of design on product reliability**

Emphasize that the reliability of the product is fundamentally determined by the design, and the design determines the inherent reliability of the product. If the design is not proper, the product will be unreliable no matter how good the manufacturing process is and how high the management level is. Give a part enough inherent reliability in its design, and the part will be inherently reliable.

6. **Environmental factors must be considered**

Environmental conditions such as high temperature, low temperature, shock, vibration, humidity, salt spray, corrosion, sand and dust, wear and tear have a great influence on stress, which in turn has a great influence on reliability. Studies have shown that the tails of the stress distribution have a much greater impact on reliability than the tails of the strength distribution, so quality control of the environment will bring much greater benefits than quality control of the strength.

7. **Maintainability must be considered**

For products whose reliability index is based on availability, such as construction machinery, no matter how good the inherent reliability of product design is, maintainability must be considered, otherwise it is impossible to maintain a high availability of the product. Therefore, from the beginning of the design, it is necessary to link the inherent reliability and the service reliability as an overall consideration, and analyze whether it is better to improve the maintainability or improve the reliability in order to achieve the specified effectiveness of the equipment or system.

8. **From a holistic, systematic point of view**

Consider the design issues from the point of view of the whole, system and ergonomics, and pay more attention to the total cost of the product in the whole life cycle rather than just the purchase cost.

9. **Recognize the need for reliability growth during design and afterwards**

During the initial design, development, and testing of a product, its reliability is often improved. This improvement is usually due to changes in some factors. For example, after a failure occurs, the analysis of the cause of the failure provides information to improve reliability, and the accumulation of experience in the design and development process will also improve the design and manufacturing process. Product reliability. Therefore, if the reliability of the product is regularly evaluated in the initial stages of product design, development, testing, and manufacturing, it will be found that the reliability characteristics will gradually increase and the reliability will be improved. This phenomenon is called "reliability". increase". GB The definition of reliability growth in 3187 is: as the product design, development, and production stages are gradually carried out, the reliability characteristics of the product are gradually improved. Reliability growth tends to saturate when the reliability level approaches the inherent reliability of the design. These forecasts and reports of reliability growth give an indication of progress towards reliability goals.

3.3.15.4 Main Contents of Reliability Design of Non-electronic Products

The main contents of the reliability design of non-electronic products are as follows:

(1) Study the failure physics and failure model of the product;
(2) Determine the reliability index and grade of the product;
(3) Reasonable allocation of product reliability indicators;
(4) Carry out reliability design for parts based on the specified reliability index.

3.3.15.5 Methods and Steps of Reliability Design for Non-electronic Products

Since complex and expensive parts and systems have high requirements for reliability, it is necessary to ensure that the specified target reliability is designed into the parts and thus into the system. Therefore, the reliability design methods and steps of non-electronic products are as follows:

(1) Put forward the design task and specify detailed indicators including technical, performance and reliability indicators.
(2) Determine the relevant design variables and parameters. These variables should have an impact on the design outcome, be independent of each other, and be measurable before, after and during the experiment.
(3) Carry out Failure Mode, Effect and Criticality Analysis (FMECA).
(4) Determine the independence of the failure modes of the parts. If the properties of one failure mode are affected by another failure mode, the stress and strength under the affected failure mode shall be corrected so that the calculated reliability of each failure mode is independent of each other.
(5) Criteria for determining the failure mode. There are many possible failure modes of non-electronic parts, such as: material yield, fracture, fatigue, excessive deformation, pressure bar instability, corrosion, wear, creep, excessive noise, excessive amplitude, etc. Commonly used criteria are: maximum normal stress, maximum shear stress, maximum deformation energy, maximum strain energy, maximum strain, maximum deformation, deformation energy under fatigue, maximum total strain under fatigue, maximum allowable corrosion amount, maximum allowable Amount of wear, maximum allowable amplitude, maximum allowable creep, etc.
(6) Determine the stress function and the stress distribution under each failure mode.
(7) Determine the strength calculation formula and the strength distribution under each failure mode.
(8) Determine the reliability associated with the stress distribution and strength distribution for each fatal failure mode.
(9) Determine the overall reliability of the part considering all failure modes simultaneously.
(10) Determine the confidence level of part reliability. Reliability is for parts, and confidence is for sample test results.
(11) Calculate the reliability of all key components in the system according to the above steps.
(12) Perform failure tree analysis (FTA) on the system.
(13) Calculate the reliability of the subsystem and the whole system.
(14) If necessary, the content of the entire design can be optimized.

3.4 Implementation and Application of Reliability Design Criteria

3.4.1 *Purpose of Going Forward*

The reliability design criteria for digital medical equipment is a basic quality management document. The "direct purpose" of establishing and implementing the reliability design criteria is to improve the design quality, while the "ultimate purpose" is to improve the quality of products. As a directive document, reliability design criteria must be conscientiously implemented. In the design, the designers are required to compare and implement each item one by one, and each item should have a clear design measure. Therefore, it has the following realistic and long-term significance:

1. **Regulate the design behavior of designers**

Reliability design criteria can provide a specific and operable "guideline" for the qualitative design of reliability, so that designers have rules to follow. Therefore, the design behavior of designers can be regulated by implementing reliability design criteria.

2. **Avoid low-level design mistakes**

The inherent reliability of a product is an inherent inherent attribute of the product, which is endowed by design and guaranteed by manufacturing and management, but the design process plays a decisive role. When designers are designing products, if they can seriously implement the guidelines, they can avoid some negligence or mistakes (low-level mistakes) that should not happen, thereby improving the design quality and truly putting the phrase "reliability is designed" into practice. to the point. Therefore, implementing reliability design criteria in the design process is an important means to improve the inherent reliability of products.

3. **To check the quality of the design**

Product reliability and performance are both product quality indicators. Generally speaking, performance indicators can be tested with instruments and meters, but the confirmation of reliability indicators is much more difficult. Implementing reliability design criteria can help solve this problem. After the design work is completed, the quality department shall organize a one-by-one inspection of the implementation of the criteria, and submit a "Reliability Design Criteria Compliance Verification Report". Although it is not possible to quantitatively confirm whether the reliability of the product meets the standard, it is possible to know qualitatively whether the reliability of the designed product is high or low.

4. **Provide a basis for design review**

During the product design review, the "Criteria Compliance Verification Report" should be submitted to the review expert group for review. This is not only a further confirmation of the quality of the design, but also a recognition of the quality of the work of the inspection team, avoiding the formality of the inspection work.

5. **Facilitate continuous growth in reliability**

The design of digital diagnosis and treatment equipment has passed the "guideline compliance verification" and design review, which does not mean the end of the work. With the deepening of the product development process, the breakthrough of key technologies, and the implementation of failure zeroing measures, etc., it may lead to design changes. In the process of design changes, new technologies, new processes, new materials, new components, etc. are often used. All these improvement measures should be supplemented to the original guidelines and implemented one by one. This process has to be carried out until the product life cycle end of Therefore, the process of supplementing, revising and re-implementing the standards is also the process of increasing product reliability.

6. **Conducive to the inheritance of knowledge**

In the long-term engineering practice, scientific and technical personnel (not just limited to designers) have a lot of experience, lessons and experience, which are scattered in their personal notepads or in their minds. These intangible things are actually a part of the enterprise's very valuable and extremely valuable knowledge wealth. It would be a pity if no one cares about it and let it go away. By establishing and implementing reliability design criteria, these scattered and intangible knowledge wealth can be collected, summarized and improved to make it a criterion, which can not only guide the current product design, but also benefit the inheritance of knowledge and the development of newcomers. nourish. Now that knowledge can be passed on and newcomers can be cultivated, the "sustainable development" of the enterprise is also reasonable.

3.4.2 Implementation

The main body of implementation and application of reliability design criteria for digital medical equipment should be designers, including hardware designers, structural designers, software designers, etc. During the design process of digital medical equipment, designers should implement the reliability design criteria specified in Sect. 3.3 into the design work one by one, and the circuit, drawing reviewers and quality specialists should also refer to the corresponding reliability when carrying out the review work. design guidelines.

The implementation process of reliability design criteria is shown in Fig. 3.15.

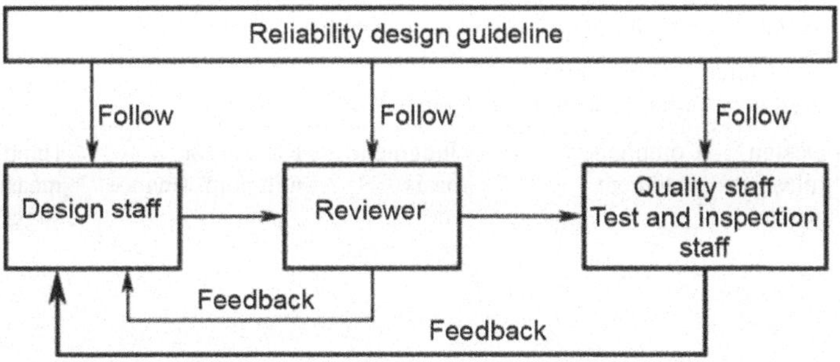

Fig. 3.15 Implementation process of reliability design criteria

3.5 Checking and Rectification of Reliability Design Criteria

3.5.1 Overview

After completing the design of each stage of digital medical equipment, the designer should write a compliance verification report for implementing the reliability design criteria, and the report should list the design measures taken to meet the requirements of each criterion.

Compliance check of reliability design criteria is an important reliability work. Through the compliance check of the design criteria, it is helpful to discover the hidden dangers of reliability in the product design, and can provide support for improving the reliability level of the product. Its requirements are:

1. During the development process, the reliability design guidelines should be analyzed to determine whether the product reliability design meets the requirements of the design guidelines, and to identify the existing problems and take improvement measures as early as possible.
2. For the results of the analysis/evaluation of the implementation of the design guidelines, prepare and submit a compliance check report of the reliability design guidelines and submit it to the project leader for approval as one of the reliability evaluation materials. If no technical measures are taken for individual clauses, the reasons shall be fully explained and the approval of the highest technical person in charge of the research and development unit shall be obtained.
3. The reliability design guidelines compliance check team should be responsible for completing the compliance check of the reliability design guidelines.

Reliability design guidelines compliance verification methods can be divided into qualitative analysis of compliance and compliance scoring methods.

Table 3.27 Reliability design criteria compliance checklist

Model: Product Name: Product number:
Reliability Designer: Auditors: Total Page: Page No

Serial number	Design rules article	Compliance statement		Judgment basis (design measures)	Reason for non-conformance	Handling measures and suggestions
		yes	no			
-	-	-	-	-	-	-
-	-	-	-	-	-	-

3.5.2 *Qualitative Analysis Method for Compliance*

Table 3.27 is for the compliance checklist of reliability design criteria.

Use Table 3.24 to check each design criterion. For the "conforming" clauses, tick "√" in the "yes" column of "conformity", and fill in the "judgment basis"; for the "non-conforming" clauses, in Tick "√" in the "No" column of "Is it compliant", and fill in the "Reasons for Non-Conformity Items" and "Treatment Measures and Suggestions".

3.5.3 *Compliance Scoring Method*

When conducting the compliance inspection of reliability design criteria, relevant experts can be invited to participate in the evaluation, and it is recommended to adopt the weighted scoring method. The principle is: for each reliability design criterion, determine its basic score according to its implementation; then multiply it by the weighting coefficient to get the score of each criterion; the total score of the product reliability design criterion is equal to the weighted score of each design criterion average value.

1. **Weighting principle**

The impact on reliability is considered by assigning different weights to each design criterion. According to the relative importance of each criterion to the reliability, the weights from 1 to 10 are respectively determined. The general principles are:

(1) For critical criteria that meet reliability requirements, the weighting coefficient is specified to be 8–10.
(2) For important but not critical design criteria that meet the reliability requirements, the weighting coefficient is specified to be 4–7.
(3) It is beneficial to reliability, but for unimportant design criteria that meet reliability requirements, the weighting coefficient is specified to be 1–3.

2. **Reliability compliance score value requirements**

The developer shall determine the minimum required value for compliance evaluation of reliability design criteria. Due to the wide range of evaluation objects, it is impossible to recommend a single "most reasonable" minimum requirement value. After the weighting coefficients of the reliability design criteria of specific products are determined, the final score of 100 indicates that the reliability design criteria have been fully integrated into the design. The goal should be to ensure that the design can meet the specified reliability design criteria 100%. For specific instruments or equipment, this goal should be adjusted according to the actual situation and possibility, and 100 points cannot be required. It usually takes a negotiation process to finally determine the minimum required value of the reliability design criterion compliance score, which is often not only due to the limitation of design technology, but also considers the cost, schedule, and impact on other professional projects. The minimum required score is generally 85 to 95 points.

3. **Weighted scoring step**

    1. Based on the reliability design criteria, establish the reliability design criteria compliance scoring table, the format is shown in Table 3.28.
    2. Determine the weighting coefficient of each criterion W_i, and its range is $1 \leq W_i \leq 10$, and fill it in the scoring table.
    3. Determine the scoring method adopted, with a score of 0 to 100, of which 100 means that the reliability criteria are fully implemented (meeting the requirements of the criteria), and 0 means that the reliability design is not considered.
    4. Analyze and count the applicable objects of each design criterion according to the design data N_t, and fill in the scoring table.
    5. Analyze and determine the object tree that meets the criteria requirements of each design criterion N_0, and fill in the scoring table.
    6. Calculate the scores of each design criterion according to the scoring method S_i, the specific method is as follows:

Scores for each reliability design criterion: $S_i = \frac{N_0}{N_t} \times 100.$. For items that can only be answered "Yes (in compliance with the design criteria)" or "No (in compliance with the design criteria)", when answering "Yes",; when answering "No" $S_i = 100$, $S_i = 0$.

7. Calculate the overall reliability design criteria compliance score of the product

$$S_T = \sum_{i=1}^{n} W_i S_i \Big/ \sum_{i=1}^{n} W_i$$

In the formula:

S_T—Product reliability design criteria compliance score;

n—Number of entries of reliability design criteria.

4. **Compliance inspection report**

Table 3.28 Reliability design criteria compliance scoring form

Product name					Total page	Page no
Serial number	Design Guidelines entry	Weighting coefficient W_i	Applicable objects of design criteria N_t	Meet design guidelines number of objects N_0	Score $S_i = \frac{N_0}{N_t} \times 100$	Weighted score $S_{wi} = W_i S_i$
1						
2						
3						
…						
Reliability design criteria compliance score		$S_T = \sum S_{wi} / \sum W_i = XX$				
			Compliance checker:		Date:	

After completing the compliance inspection of each item of the reliability design criteria, a compliance inspection report of the reliability design criteria should be prepared, the main contents of which include:

(1) Product function and design description.
(2) Instructions for compliance inspection.
(3) Conformity inspection conclusion (including main problems and suggestions for improvement).
(4) Members of the compliance inspection team and their signatures.

5. **Precautions**

1. The R&D unit should formulate corresponding product reliability design criteria based on product characteristics.
2. The reliability design criteria should fully absorb the mature experience and failure lessons of similar product design at home and abroad.
3. The reliability design criteria should be gradually improved, that is, to increase the effective clauses and remove invalid clauses according to the product development situation, so as to improve the applicability of the criteria.
4. The content of reliability design criteria should be operable and easy for designers to implement.
5. The reliability design criteria should pay attention to the coordination and mutual echo with the maintainability, testability, safety and supportability design criteria.
6. Selection principle of reliability design criteria for electronic products: Electronic products are characterized by electronic components as the main working components and electrical signals as the main control parameters. In each technical classification of the above-mentioned reliability design

criteria, there are criteria clauses applicable to electronic products. Therefore, relevant items can be selected from the above-mentioned reliability design criteria to form reliability design criteria for electronic products.

7. Principles for selection of reliability design criteria for non-electronic products: non-electronic products generally refer to all non-electronic products. The lack of reliability data and other characteristics have great difficulties in reliability design. In the reliability design criteria of technology classification, derating design and electromagnetic compatibility design are not suitable for the reliability design of non-electronic products, and there are optional items in other categories. In addition, for the typical failure modes of non-electronic products, anti-fatigue design, anti-wear design, anti-corrosion design, anti-fracture design, anti-leakage design, and anti-loosening design criteria should also be formulated.
8. Pay attention to collecting and accumulating information items of reliability design criteria, and establish an information database to provide support for reliability design.

3.5.4 Rectification of Reliability Design

After completing the compliance verification of the reliability design criteria, the inspectors of the reliability design criteria of digital medical equipment should output a list of non-conformities, analyze the non-conformities, explain the reasons for the non-conformities, and put forward reliability improvement suggestions in a timely manner. Designers need to rectify non-conforming items according to the reliability design criteria, further optimize the product system structure, adopt new materials, new technologies and new processes, improve the quality level of various components and parts used in products, and increase redundant designs. Adjust its safety factor and derating factor, improve thermal design and operating environment conditions, and improve product reliability through the above measures.

The reliability design rectification process is shown in Fig. 3.16.

3.6 FAQs About Reliability Design Implementation

Product reliability is designed, produced, and managed. According to the failure statistics of a certain manufacturers digital diagnosis and treatment equipment, 50% of the failures are caused by the design, 40% of the failures are caused by the process, and the other 10% of the failures are caused by the material. It can be seen that the design and process of the product have a great influence on the reliability of the product. Product reliability design is a key link in the process of product reliability. It determines whether the product can meet the reliability requirements, and provides the basis for the follow-up process (maintenance, support, etc.), and also affects the

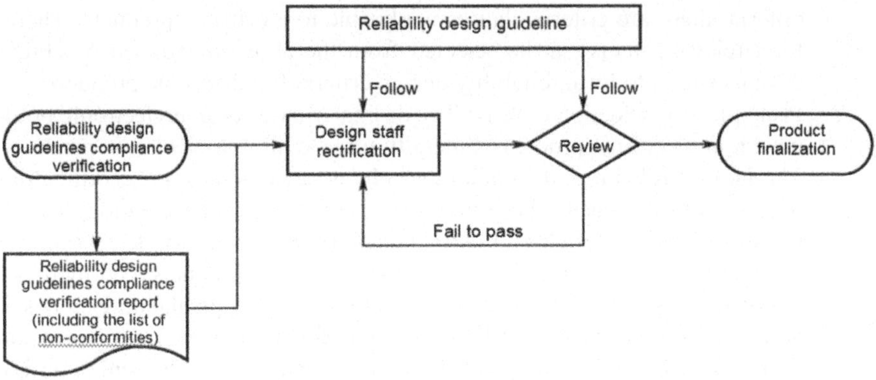

Fig. 3.16 Rectification process of reliability design

product quality provided to customers. Whether it meets the requirements of the market and obtains customer satisfaction. However, many enterprises have many problems in the implementation of product reliability design analysis, mainly as follows:

(1) Defining reliability requirements is the driving force for implementing reliability design, and establishing reliability design criteria is the foundation for realizing systematization and specialization of reliability design. Putting forward clear and qualitative reliability requirements or even quantitative reliability index requirements is the basis for promoting the reliability design of the project team; most designs without reliability requirements can only be empirical and scattered designs that rely on personal professionalism and consideration; on the basis of clarifying the reliability requirements, the requirements and verification elements of the reliability design criteria can be further clarified, so that the reliability design can be promoted to specialization and systematization.
(2) The reliability design and analysis of the product is not clearly divided in each stage of the project life cycle, or its management and review arrangements are ignored. Reliability design and analysis must be included in the product design and manufacturing process, but companies often do not formulate and implement product reliability assurance programs, do not follow the principle of prevention first and early control, and fail to implement product reliability well Standard terms for design and analysis.
(3) The review method of product reliability design and analysis is improper, or the problem is not identified in the verification and confirmation activities of product design and development, or the necessary improvement measures are not proposed for the problem. The main manifestations are: the enterprise cannot strictly carry out the reliability review, and cannot insist on carrying out the reliability review in stages; the review work lacks professionalism and the support of external experts.

(4) Engineers in charge of hardware and software design lack reliability design concepts, cannot take the initiative to implement reliability design methods into design work, or do not implement them properly, and completely ignore or even have no knowledge of reliability design principles.
(5) Design engineers pay too much attention to product performance indicators and ignore the reliability level. They always feel that things should be made first and then reliability. Practice has proved that technical design and reliability design are concurrent projects, which should not only be considered, but also can greatly shorten the practice of future mill engineering. While pursuing high performance and multiple functions (making the product more complex), design engineers choose a balance point in the game of performance and reliability, which not only meets the performance requirements of customers, but also ensures the reliability level of the product, avoiding future The huge workload, technical manpower consumption and economic loss caused by a large number of unreliable products after the product is launched.
(6) On the basis of the design, good materials (components, raw materials, structural parts, shelf products, etc.) should also be selected. For example, for the sake of economy, components with lower reliability levels are selected, which reduces the overall reliability level of the product, and may even bring economic losses far greater than the savings in material costs.
(7) Reliability work requires the collaborative work of a team, but in the actual development process, it is often mistaken for the work of reliability engineers, which will lead to design engineers not cooperating with the work requirements put forward by reliability engineers. Execution, which ultimately leads to the inability to implement reliability requirements into product design and manufacturing.
(8) There are no perfect and fully applicable reliability design criteria, and do not expect to obtain a perfect book of product reliability design criteria from outside. The real and most practical design criteria are the summarization of failure cases and lessons learned in the product's own R&D process. We should pay attention to summarization and induction in our daily work, and gradually form design guidelines with our own characteristics.
(9) Reliability design criteria should be implemented rather than formulated. Don't spend a lot of time formulating the criteria and spending little time on implementing the criteria. Reliability design criteria will be experienced in the implementation and verification, and will be continuously improved. As long as it is continuously implemented and verified, and continuously modified and improved, the reliability design criteria will become more and more applicable as time goes by.

3.7 Summary

This chapter elaborates on the development, implementation and verification of the reliability design guidelines for digital medical equipment, and summarizes a set of reliability design methods based on the evaluation of reliability design guidelines compliance. The reliability design guidelines are obtained by summarizing and refining the successful experiences and failed lessons accumulated by designers in long-term engineering practice. The reliability design guideline should be a mandatory document, and the clauses in it are the qualitative reliability requirements that must be implemented one by one when the product design is carried out. When the design work is completed, the project manager or reliability engineer will check the implementation of the guidelines in the design process according to the guidelines. By developing and implementing the reliability design guidelines, the "design quality" and "manufacturing quality" are improved, and the ultimate goal is to improve product reliability.

Chapter 4
Failure Model Analysis Method of Digital Diagnosis and Treatment Equipment

4.1 Overview of Failure Model Analysis Method

Failure model was proposed in the "13th Five-year-plan" special guidelines for digital diagnosis and treatment. Therefore, this chapter summarizes the technologies related to failure model to provide a reference method for supporting the failure model analysis. Technologies related to failure model mainly include fault tree modeling and analysis, reliability modeling and prediction technology, failure mode, effect and criticality analysis (FMECA), failure mode and failure model of mechanical parts and electronic components, failure distribution model and statistical analysis. Each technology is briefly introduced as follows:

(1) Fault tree modeling and analysis: taking the undesired product failure event or catastrophic criticality event as the top event, we find out the necessary and sufficient direct causes of the failure event (also called bottom event, including hardware, software, environment, human factors, etc.) layer by layer through the failure cause-effect logic analysis from top to bottom in strict accordance with the hierarchy, draw a fault tree, and finally find out all possible causes and combinations of causes leading to the top event, and use the basic failure rate data of each bottom event to calculate the probability of occurrence of the top event and the importance of the bottom event. Fault tree modeling and analysis establishes a tree structure model of the fault tree, and the probability of the top event can be calculated by using the probability theory method and the basic data of the occurrence probability of the basic event, which includes the qualitative fault tree model and the quantitative top event occurrence probability model. The fault tree modeling and analysis are particularly suitable for analyzing the unexpected fault consequence events of the whole diagnosis and treatment equipment and the core components thereof, and can find out all the factors of the unexpected fault consequence events, provide reference for taking preventive and remedial measures, and improve the safety and effectiveness of the diagnosis and treatment equipment.

X. Li et al., *Reliability Engineering Technology of Digital Diagnosis and Treatment Equipment*, https://doi.org/10.1007/978-981-99-5522-0_4

(2) Reliability modeling and prediction: taking a tier of digital medical equipment as the object, to decompose its composition into basic units, establish the reliability model of the tier, and use the reliability data of its basic units to predict the failure rate of the tier under the given conditions. Reliability modeling and prediction is a bottom-up, local-to-whole process that uses the known failure rate of a lower-level composition to extrapolate the failure rate of its higher-level product through a failure model. Reliability modeling and anticipation contains a qualitative reliability block diagram model and a quantitative failure rate calculation mathematical model, which is especially suitable for the design phase to assess whether the level product meets the specified failure rate or the assigned reliability index requirements, and to provide reference for the comparative demonstration, preference and optimization of design solutions.
(3) Failure mode, effect and criticality analysis: it is a generalized analysis method that analyzes all possible failure modes of a product and their possible effects, and classifies each failure mode according to the severity of its effects and its probability of occurrence Failure mode, effect and criticality analysis is a bottom-up inductive analysis method that helps to understand all possible potential problems of the product and take targeted preventive measures. Failure mode, effect and criticality analysis includes the failure mode of basic component unit, the impact of failure on the products of the upper three levels, and the qualitative criticality or quantitative criticality of failure, so as to take preventive, remedial and verification measures for the failure unit with large failure impact and great criticality and its corresponding failure mode.
(4) Failure mode and failure physical model: failure mode refers to the form, shape and phenomenon of product failure, which is the external macroscopic expression of product failure. Failure mechanism refers to the physical, chemical or other reasons and processes that cause the failure of components and materials. The failure of mechanical parts and components is often caused by physical and chemical reactions. The failure mechanism and failure physical model can provide important help for the study of product life and the design and implementation of accelerated test.
(5) Failure distribution model and statistical analysis: a function of the cumulative failure probability distribution is used to express the failure distribution pattern of the product in the process of use. The failure distribution function and its parameters can be fitted by using the item and fault information, and the conformity of the selected failure distribution can be confirmed. The cumulative failure probability can be predicted by using the failure distribution function, and the failure distribution law of the item can be found out and the reliability can be predicted. The failure distribution model and statistical analysis can provide a means to analyze the historical service data of products and find out the distribution law of product life. The commonly used failure distribution models include exponential distribution, Weibull distribution, Lognormal distribution, etc.

4.2 Fault Tree Modeling and Analysis

4.2.1 *Overview of Fault Tree Modeling and Analysis*

Fault Tree Analysis (FTA) is to find out the necessary and sufficient direct causes of the fault event (also called bottom event, including hardware, software, environment, human and other factors) by using the unwanted product failure event or catastrophic criticality event as the top event and finding out the necessary and sufficient direct causes of the failure event layer by layer through a strict top-to-bottom failure cause-effect logic analysis. etc.), draw a fault tree, and finally find out all possible causes and combinations of causes leading to the top event, and the probability of occurrence of the top event and the importance of the bottom event can be calculated by using the basic failure rate data of each bottom event.

Using the fault tree modeling and analysis can quickly and effectively grasp the possible major consequences and high frequency of fault causes, prevent major accidents and reduce the probability of high frequency fault. It also greatly simplifies the reliability of the workload and improves the analysis effect and efficiency.

Generally, the repairable product corresponds to the concept of failure, and the irreparable product corresponds to the concept of failure. The technical principles and methods are the same. In addition, as the process of fault tree analysis usually needs to be modeled first and then analyzed, it is uniformly called fault tree modeling and analysis.

This chapter mainly introduces the principles, methods, implementation procedures and relevant precautions of fault tree modeling and analysis. In the development, production and using stage of digital diagnosis and treatment equipment, the fault tree modeling and analysis technology can be used to prevent major consequences of events, find the reasons related to the top event, and formulate troubleshooting manuals and programs for support.

4.2.2 *Key Points of Work Items*

(1) In order to ensure the timeliness of the analysis work, fault tree analysis should be carried out at the early stage of product development, and fault tree analysis reviews should be conducted before major field tests, and supplemented, modified, iterated and improved at each development stage to reflect changes in product technology status and processes, adopting the method of improvement while building the "tree";
(2) In the design process, the principle of "The one who designs takes the responsibility of analysis" is implemented. And experienced design, production and use personnel are invited to participate in the tree building work to ensure the correctness of the logical relationship of the fault tree;

(3) In case of failure, the "tree" shall be built by the person in charge of the accident, and relevant personnel shall assist;
(4) In the fault tree analysis, it is assumed that the bottom events are independent from each other;
(5) The fault tree of complex products should be modularly decomposed and simplified;
(6) The product design improvement measures formulated by the fault tree analysis, must be implemented in the drawings and relevant technical documents, to ensure that the analysis results in a timely manner to implement the product design;
(7) In engineering practice, for large or complex products, CAD software should be used to assist in fault tree analysis as much as possible to improve efficiency and save manpower.

4.2.3 Definition of Fault Tree Analysis

4.2.3.1 Fault Tree

(1) The fault tree is a logic diagram used to indicate which components of a product have faults or external events, or a combination of them, that will cause a given fault to occur in the product. FTA is a special kind of inverted tree logic causality diagram. The elements of the diagram are events and logic gates. The input event of the logic gate is the "cause" of the output event, and the output event is the "effect" of the input event; events are used to describe the status of system and meta-component failures, and logic gates link events together to represent the logical relationships between events. If the bottom event of a fault tree describes one state, and its inverse event also describes a single state, it is called a two-state fault tree.
(2) If the bottom event of a fault tree describes one state, and its inverse event includes two or more incompatible states, it is called a multi-state fault tree.

4.2.3.2 Fault Tree Analysis

Fault Tree Analysis (FTA) is an analysis technique that determines various possible combinations of product failure causes and their probability of occurrence by analyzing the hardware, software, environmental, and human factors that may cause product failures in a system, drawing a fault tree graph according to rules, and calculating it based on a mathematical model. Fault tree analysis takes an undesired product failure event (or catastrophic product criticality), i.e., the top event, as the target of the analysis, and finds out the necessary and sufficient direct causes of the failure event layer by layer through a strict top-down failure cause-effect logic analysis, using deductive reasoning, and finally finds out all the causes and combinations of causes that lead to the top event and calculates their probability of occurrence, and then seeks to reduce its probability of occurrence through design improvement and implementation of effective failure detection, maintenance and other measures, and gives suggestions for product improvement. Fault tree analysis can analyze the effect of a combination of multiple fault factors on the product.

4.2.3.3 Fault Tree Analysis Events and Symbols

See Table 4.1 for common events and their symbols of fault tree.

1. **Bottom Event**

A Bottom Event is a cause event in a fault tree that causes only other events. It is located at the bottom of the fault tree in question and is always an input event rather than an output event of a logic gate.

2. **Result Event**

Table 4.1 Common events and symbols of fault tree

Symbol		Note:
Bottom Event	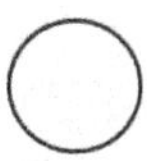	Basic Event Components under the condition of the design of the operation of the random fault events, in general, its fault distribution is known, can only be used as the input of the logic gate and not as the output; Solid line circle indicate product faults , dotted line circle indicate human faults.
Bottom Event	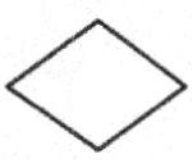	Undeveloped Event Refers to the omission of events, generally used to represent those that may occur, but the probability value is small, or for the system does not need further analysis of the failure event. They can be neglected in qualitative and quantitative analysis
Result Event	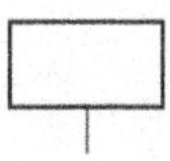	Top Event The final outcome event of interest in a fault tree analysis. Unwanted failure events that have significant impact on the technical performance, economy, reliability and safety of the system, and the top event can be determined by FMECA analysis; it is located at the top of the fault tree and is always the output event of the logic gate in the fault tree under discussion rather than the input event
	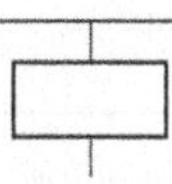	Intermediate Event The resulting event between the bottom and top events. It is the output event of a logic gate and the input event of another logic gate at the same time
Special Events	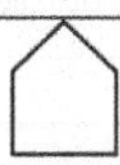	Switch Event Special events that have occurred or will occur
	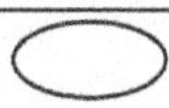	Conditional Event Special event describing the specific limitations of the logic gate's functioning

A Resultant Event is an event that is caused by another event or a combination of events in a fault tree analysis. It is at the output of a logic gate. Result events are divided into top events and intermediate events.

3. **Special Events**

Special Event refers to the fault tree analysis need special symbols to indicate its particularity or attention to the event. Special events are divided into switch events and condition events.

4.2.3.4 Fault Tree Analysis, Logic Gates and Symbols

The logic gates and their symbols commonly used in the fault tree are as follows, see Table 4.2 for details.

1. **AND Gate**

Bi (I = 1, 2, … n) for the input of the gate event, A for the output of the gate event, Bi occurs at the same time, A must occur, this logical relationship is called time. The logical expression is:

$$A = B_1 \cup B_2 \cup \ldots \cup B_n$$

2. **OR Gate**

Bi (i = 1,2, … n) in at least one event occurs, A occurs, this logical relationship is called the event and. The logical expression is:

$$A = B_1 \cup B_2 \cup \ldots \cup B_n$$

Table 4.2 Common logic gates and their symbols in fault tree

Symbol		Symbol		Symbol	
AND Gate	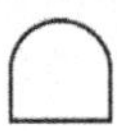	OR Gate	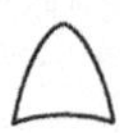	NOT Gate	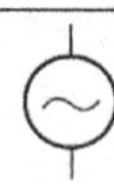
Sequential AND	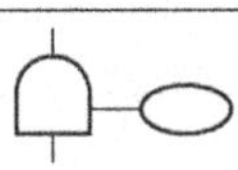	Forbidden Gate	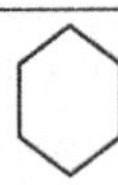	Exclusive OR Gate	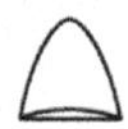
Voting Gate	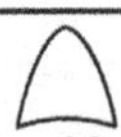 m:0:0	Priority-AND Gate	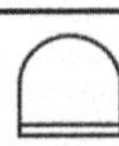	/	/

3. NOT Gate

Output event A is the inverse of input event B. In the fault tree, the NOT Gate is seldom used, because the inverse event of the original event can be used to describe.

4. Sequential AND

Output event A occurs only if sequence event B occurs according to the specified "sequence condition."

5. Inhibit Gate

The occurrence of input event B causes output event A to occur only when the "inhibit condition" occurs.

6. Exclusive-OR Gate

The occurrence of either of input event 1, 2 can cause output event A to occur, but input events 1, 2 cannot occur simultaneously. The logical expression is:

$$A = (B|_1 \cap B_2) \cup (B_1 \cap B_2)$$

7. Voting Gate

if at least *r* of that n input occurs, the output event A occurs;

8. Priority-AND Gate

A and B are base events or intermediate events or sub-fault trees. When A and B occur at the same time or A before B, C will happen.

9. Spare Gate

An output event occurs when the number of spare parts is less than the number required. Transfer symbols include the same transfer symbol and similar transfer symbol, as shown in Table 4.3.

Table 4.3 Identical and similar transition symbols

Symbol		Note:
Identical Transfer Symbol	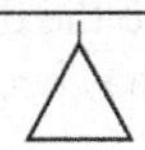	Located at the bottom of the fault tree, indicating that some branches of tree A are elsewhere
	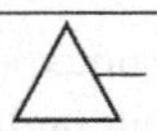	At the top of the fault tree, indicating that tree A is a subtree of a fault tree drawn in another section
Similar Transfer Symbol	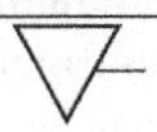	Located at the bottom of the fault tree, indicating that similar parts of the tree branch in another place, the bottom event with a different event number
	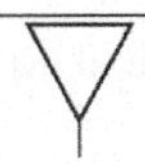	At the top of the fault tree, indicating that tree A is a subtree of a similar fault tree drawn elsewhere

(1) Identical Transfer Symbol

Represents a transfer of the same failure event. in order to reduce that repeated work and simplify the fault tree, this kind of transition symbol is generally use. Add the corresponding label respectively from somewhere into, or go to somewhere, can also be used for fault tree page.

(2) Similar Transfer Symbol

Indicates a transition where the fault event structure is similar but the event number is different. In order to simplify the fault tree and reduce the repeated work, this kind of transition symbol is generally used. Add the corresponding label respectively from somewhere into, or go to somewhere, can also be used for fault tree page.

4.2.3.5 Cut Set and Minimal Cut Set

(1) Cut Set

Cut Set is a set of bottom events in a fault tree. When these bottom events occur simultaneously, the top event must occur.

(2) Minimal Cut Set

Minimal Cut Set is a cut set in which the number of bottom events cannot be reduced further, i.e., the set of bottom events remaining after removing one bottom event from the minimal cut set is not a cut set. A minimal cut set represents a fault mode of the system, and finding all minimal cut sets of the fault tree is the task of qualitative analysis of the fault tree.

4.2.4 General Requirements for Fault Tree Analysis

4.2.4.1 Purpose of the Fault Tree Analysis

The objectives of the FTA are as follows:

(1) From the perspective of safety, it can be used to compare the design of various digital diagnosis and treatment equipment; Or a design has been determined to assess whether safety requirements are met;
(2) As for the reliability test of digital medical device, the unexpected fatal event caused by the combination of a plurality of non-fatal fault event may be found through the FTA, and corresponding improvement measures are taken accordingly;
(3) To provide the basis for the development of digital medical equipment use and maintenance procedures;

(4) For those who have never been involved in the design, use and maintenance of digital medical equipment, the fault tree provides them with a visual management, a "guide" for use and maintenance, or a "clue list" for finding faults.

4.2.4.2 Timing of Fault Tree Analysis

Fault tree analysis is applicable to the development, production and use stages of digital medical equipment: as an analysis tool to identify potential design problems, fault tree analysis can be applied to various design stages of new or improved products, including the specific content of the design is not very complete early design stages. This early work should be expanded upon as information on the system design and its components becomes available. A fault tree can also identify potential problems that may arise from a product's physical design, environmental or service stresses, manufacturing process defects, and from operating or maintenance processes.

(1) Do fault tree analysis at the same time of product design to find weak links in reliability and safety, so as to take improvement measures to improve reliability;
(2) During the development process, each sub-system and each component of the digital diagnosis and treatment equipment forms its own fault tree analysis report, such as the bogie fault tree analysis report, etc. Sub-components and components can also form their own special fault tree analysis report; According to the characteristics of various models, different types of fault tree analysis reports are formed;
(3) After a major failure or accident occurs during operation or testing, use fault tree analysis to find the cause of the major failure or accident, and provide support for "returning to zero". A fault tree analysis can be reported on its own or as part of a fault zeroing report.

4.2.4.3 Fault Tree Analysis Categories

Fault tree analysis includes qualitative analysis and quantitative analysis.

Qualitative analysis is the most basic task of failure tree analysis, which aims to find the cause events and combinations of cause events that lead to the occurrence of the top event, i.e., to identify the set of all failure modes that lead to the occurrence of the top event; to help analysts identify potential failures and discover design weaknesses in order to improve the design; and also to guide fault diagnosis and improve use and maintenance programs. Qualitative analysis can identify the entire minimum set of cuts in the failure tree, and the minimum set of cuts can be analyzed to identify weaknesses and develop improvement measures accordingly. The quantitative analysis is based on the qualitative analysis and uses the reliability data of the bottom event to quantitatively calculate the failure tree, to obtain the probability of occurrence of the top event, the probability of occurrence of each minimum cut set and the importance of the minimum cut set and the bottom event, to find the weak links, and to prioritize the improvement measures according to the results of the importance analysis. Weaknesses are identified and improvement measures are prioritized based on the results of the importance analysis. The failure tree analysis is mainly based on qualitative analysis in the proposal stage and the initial prototype stage, and a combination of qualitative and quantitative analysis is used as much as possible in the test and finalization stages.

4.2.4.4 Relationship Between FTA, FMEA and ETA

Fault tree analysis is closely related to Failure Mode and Effects Analysis (FMEA). FMEA is basically a single factor analysis method, which only considers the impact of a certain failure mode, without considering the combined impact of several failure modes. Through FMEA, the key failure mode that affects safety and mission success can be found out, and the fault tree can be established for multi-factor analysis to find out the combination of various failure modes and provide a basis for improving the design. That is to say, FMEA is the basis of fault tree analysis. In general, single-factor FMEA is performed first, and the failure mode with high severity or criticality is found, which is regarded as the top event, and a fault tree is established to perform multi-factor fault tree analysis.

Event Tree Analysis (ETA) starts from an initial cause event and analyzes all possible consequence events caused by the state combination of subsequent events in time sequence, while fault tree analysis starts from an undesired consequence When an event starts, analyze the cause event or combination of cause events that caused the consequence event according to a certain logical relationship. Due to the different emphases between these two methods, when analyzing the security and reliability of complex systems, the two methods of event tree analysis and fault tree analysis can be combined and applied to give full play to the respective advantages of the two methods. Advantages to find out the cause of system failure more effectively. When to combine these two methods:

- It is easier to construct sequences of events than to construct relationships between causes;
- The resulting fault tree may be very large;
- Often there will be separate teams doing different parts of the analysis.

When the above conditions exist, the potential undesired event between function and technology can be analyzed first, and this event can be used as the top event of fault tree analysis and the input event of event tree analysis.

4.2.5 Detailed Work Requirements for Fault Tree Analysis

The main working steps of fault tree analysis are shown in Fig. 4.1.

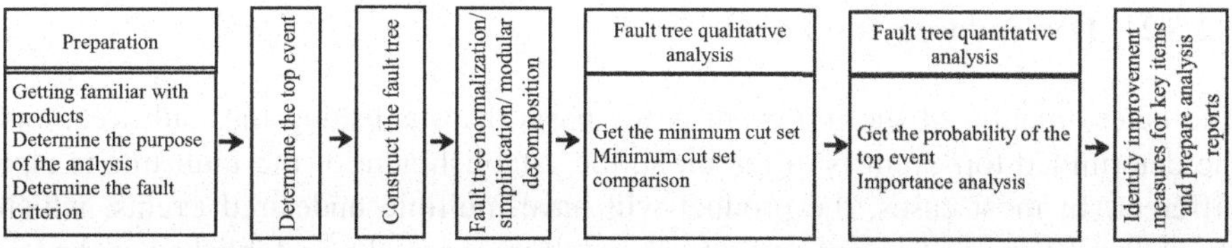

Fig. 4.1 Main working steps of fault tree analysis

4.2.5.1 Preparations for Fault Tree Analysis

1. **Product familiarization work**

Familiar with product design instructions, design drawings (such as schematic diagrams, structural diagrams, flow charts), test methods for each assembly level, test requirements for each assembly level and other relevant materials (operating procedures, maintenance procedures), and thoroughly grasp product design intent, structure, functions, boundaries and environmental conditions; when analyzing the fault tree of digital medical equipment, attention should be paid to understand the relationship between the interfaces of each subsystem and each component.

Identify the influence of human factors and software on the product, identify the various possible state modes of the system, analyze the mutual transformation between these modes, and draw the product state mode and transition diagram if necessary to help clarify the relationship between normal or faulty products relationship; in the fault tree analysis, the different working modes of the product in various states such as ground test, operation, and shutdown should be analyzed to find out the relationship between them.

Before a fault tree analysis, it is best to conduct an FMEA to help identify top events and subsequent events at all levels. According to the complexity of each component, if necessary, a product system reliability block diagram should be drawn to help correctly form the top structure of the fault tree and realize early modularization of the fault tree, reducing the scale of the tree.

2. **Determine the purpose of the analysis**

Analysts should clarify the purpose of fault tree analysis based on task requirements and product understanding. For the same product, if the analysis purposes are different, the established fault trees are also different.

3. **Determining failure criteria**

According to the product function and performance requirements, determine the failure criterion of the product. Only when the failure criterion is accurate, can we identify what is the failure, so as to determine the necessary and sufficient cause of the failure.

4.2.5.2 Determining Top Events

The determination of the top event is the basis of establishing the fault tree, and the determined top event is different, so the establishment of the fault tree is also different. In most cases, the product will have multiple undesired events, which should be determined one by one, and the fault tree should be established as the top event and analyzed separately; moreover, the product will have multiple working modes, and the top event should be analyzed separately in each working mode. The way to determine the top event is as follows:

(1) Carry out fault tree analysis during the design process, and generally select and determine the top event from failures that significantly affect product technical performance, economy, reliability and safety;
(2) If FMECA has been carried out before the fault tree analysis, the top event can be determined from the system failure modes with severity I and II;
(3) After a major failure or accident occurs, such an event can be taken as the top event. The definite top event must be strictly defined, otherwise the built fault tree will not achieve the expected purpose.

4.2.5.3 Establishment of Fault Tree

After the top event is determined, the basic rules and methods for building a fault tree should be followed, and the logical reasoning relationship between the failure events should be expressed by using the special event and logic gate symbols for the fault tree, and the required fault tree should be constructed.

1. **Basic rules for fault tree analysis**

   (1) Clearly establish the boundary conditions of the tree

   The boundary of the fault tree should be consistent with the boundary of the system in order to avoid omissions and repetitions. According to the boundary conditions, it is clear where the fault tree needs to be built. Usually the boundary conditions include the following aspects:
   (1) Determine the top event;
   (2) Determine the initial conditions, which are compatible with the top event. For any component with more than one working state, its working state shall be specified as the initial condition;
   (3) Events that are not allowed by regulations refer to events that are not allowed to occur when the tree is built.

(2) Simplify system configuration

Simplified system composition can consider the following aspects:

(1) Make necessary reasonable assumptions about the system, such as ignoring human faults, ignoring some equipment or wiring failures, making conservative assumptions about some equipment, etc.

(2) For complex systems, on the basis of FMEA, the unimportant parts of the top event can be discarded to simplify the system, and then the tree can be built

(3) Strictly define failure events

Failure events must be strictly defined, otherwise the built fault tree will be incorrect. As for the result event, it should be expressed as "what is the failure" and "under what circumstances" as needed. For example, "the pressure tank bursts when the pump starts" "the light bulb does not light when the switch is turned on".

(4) Trees should be built step by step from top to bottom

The construction should be carried out step by step from top to bottom, and any input to the next logic gate should not be performed until all necessary and sufficient direct inputs of the same logic gate are not listed. For a huge fault tree, there may be many inputs at each level, and each input may still be a huge sub-tree. Therefore, building trees step by step can avoid omissions.

(5) Direct gate-to-gate connection when building a tree is not allowed

Direct gate-to-gate connection without passing through the result event is now allowed when building a tree. The output events of each gate should be clearly defined. The main purpose is to prevent the builder from developing the subtree without defining the intermediate events in words, and secondly, the gate-to-gate connection fault tree makes it difficult for the reviewer to judge whether it is right or wrong.

(6) Concrete the abstract description of the event

In order to drive the fault tree down, it is necessary to gradually replace the more abstract indirect events with more concrete direct events, so that it is also possible to form "event-event" strings without any logic gates when building the tree, which should also be defined one by one and written in long boxes.

(7) Dealing with common cause events and mutually exclusive events

A common failure cause can cause different component failures or even different system failures. Common-cause failure events are referred to as common-cause events. For common cause events present in the fault tree, the same event label must be used. Events that cannot occur at the same time are mutually exclusive events. For the events and subtrees at the input end of the AND Gate, attention should be paid to whether there are mutually exclusive events. If there are, XOR Gate transformation should be used to process them.

2 **Fault tree establishment process**

Figure 4.2 shows the process of establishing a fault tree. The specific instructions are as follows:

(1) Take the top event as the output event, analyze and establish all the direct cause events that lead to the top event as the next-level input events, establish the logic gate relationship between these input events and output events, and draw the output events and input events Fault tree diagram between events;
(2) By analogy, expand these next-level events as output events, and stop until all input events are bottom events, so far the initial fault tree is established;
(3) Establish definitions and expression symbols for the events in the fault tree, use symbols to replace the event text description in the fault tree, use transfer symbols to simplify the fault tree, and realize the standardized expression of the fault tree.

Write the determined top event in the top rectangle. Put all the necessary and sufficient direct causes of the top event in the corresponding event symbols, draw the second row, and then use appropriate logic gates to connect the top event and these direct cause events according to their logical relationship in the actual system. In this way, follow the tree building rules and develop step by step until all the lowest row of causal events are bottom events, and the fault tree of the given top event is built by deductive method.

4.2.5.4 Normalization, Simplification and Modularization of Fault Trees

In order to reduce the workload of analysis, it is necessary to standardize, simplify and decompose the established fault tree.

1. **Normalization of fault trees**

of transforming the constructed fault tree into a fault tree containing only basic events, result events, and three logic gates of "and", "or" and "not" is called the normalization of fault tree.

(1) Handling rules for special events

   (1) Handling rules for undiscovered events: According to their importance and completeness of data, they can be treated as basic events or deleted. Important undiscovered events with complete data are treated as basic events; unimportant undiscovered events with incomplete data can be deleted; other situations are determined by the analysts according to the actual project.
   (2) The principle of handling switch events: treat switch events as basic events.
   (3) Processing principle of conditional events: Conditional events are always associated with special gates and processed according to the equivalent transformation rules of special gates.

(2) Equivalent transformation rules for special gates

The equivalent transformation rules of special doors are shown in Table 4.4.

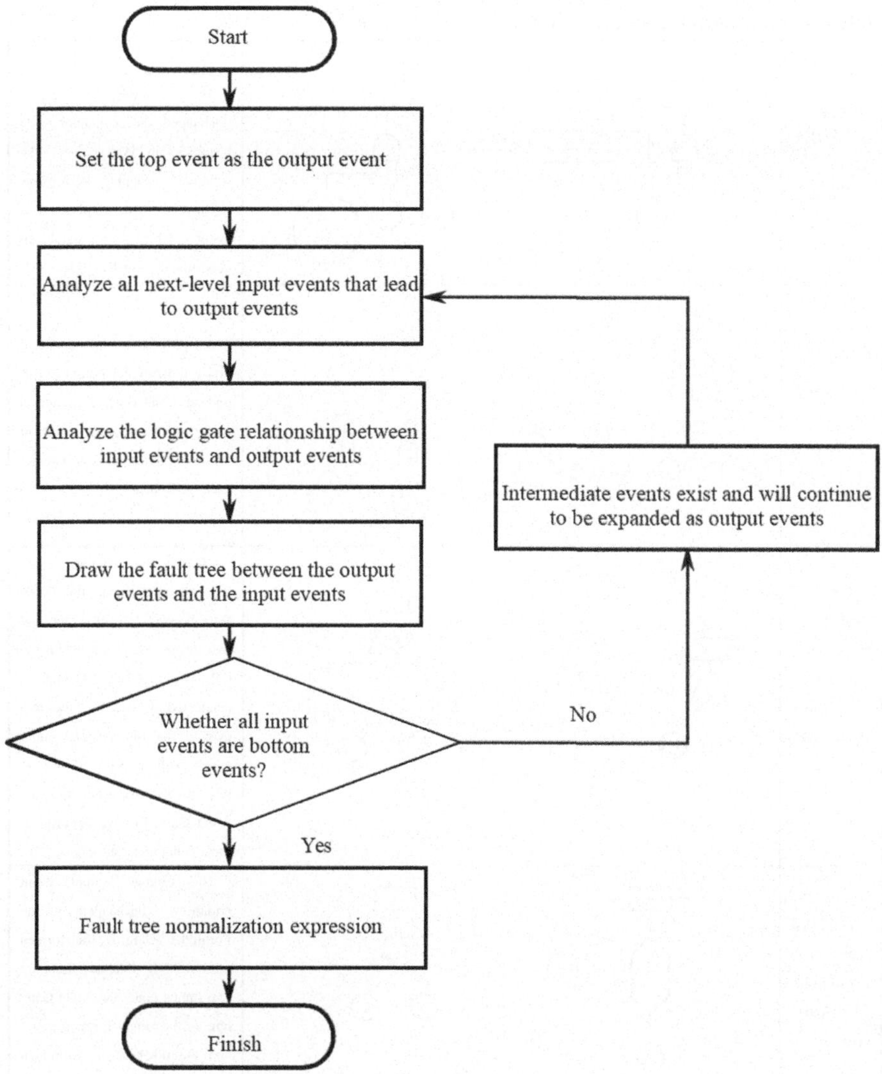

Fig. 4.2 The establishment process of fault tree

2. **Simplification of fault trees**

The simplification of fault tree is not a necessary step of fault tree analysis, and it will not affect the results of qualitative and quantitative analysis later. However, simplifying the fault tree as much as possible is an effective measure to reduce the size of the fault tree and thus reduce the workload.

(1) Use the same transfer symbol to represent the same subtree, and use similar transfer symbols to represent similar subtrees;

Table 4.4 Equivalent transformation rules for special gates

Special door	Icon	Note
Sequential AND Gate is transformed into AND Gate	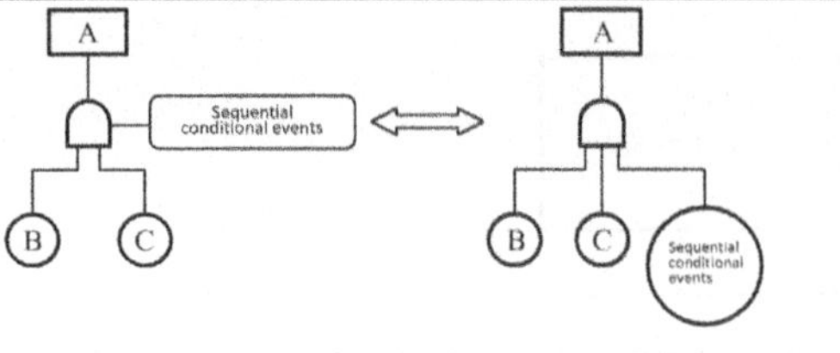	The output remains unchanged, the Sequential AND becomes an AND Gate, the original input remains unchanged, and a new input event is added — sequential conditional event X
The Voting Gate is transformed into a combination of OR Gate and Gate	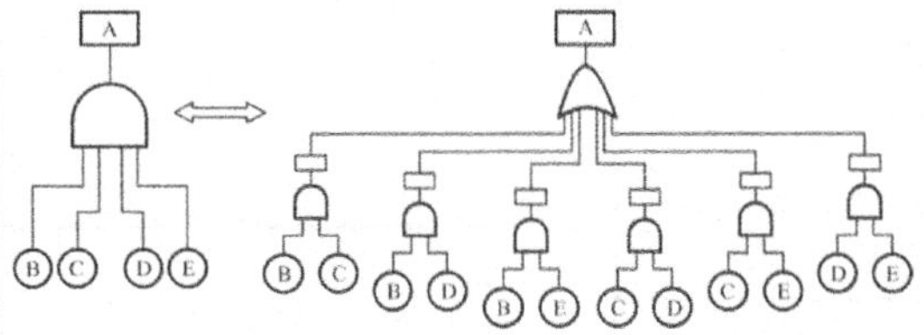	An OR Gate is connected under the original output event, and an AND Gate is connected under each input event, and there are *r* original input events under each AND Gate
The XOR Gate is transformed into a combination of OR Gate, NOT Gate and AND Gate	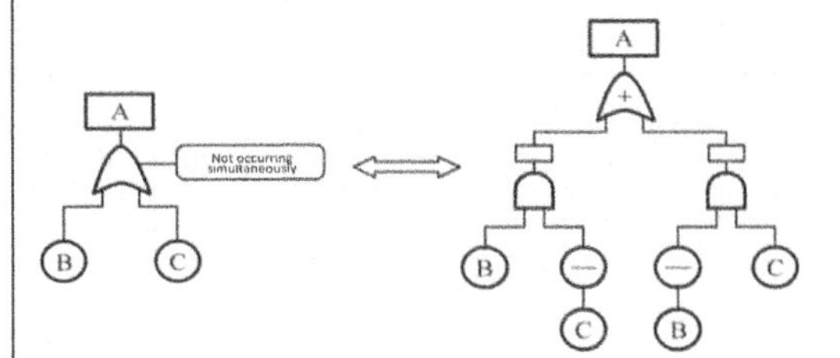	The original output event remains unchanged, the XOR Gate becomes an OR Gate, and two events are connected to the OR Gate, and an AND Gate is connected to each of the two events, and an original input event and a NOT Gate are respectively connected to each AND Gate. Receive an original input event under the gate
Forbidden Gate is transformed into AND Gate	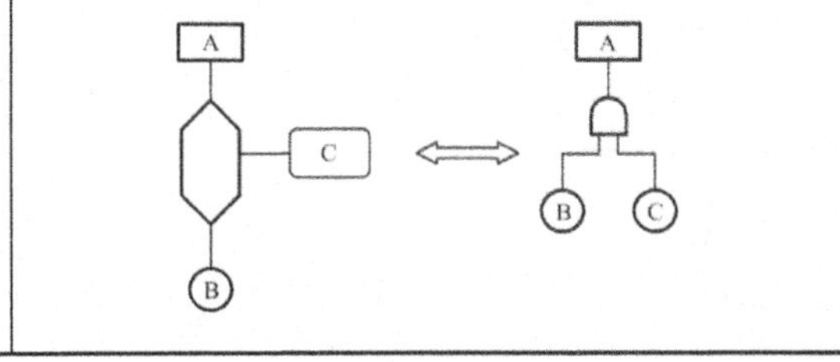	The original output event remains unchanged, the Forbidden Gate is transformed into an AND Gate, and there are two inputs under the AND Gate, one is the original input event, and the other is the forbidden condition event

(2) Remove obvious logical redundant events and obvious logical redundant gates.

According to the set (event) operation rule, the basic principle of the simplified fault tree can be obtained as follows. See Table 4.5 for the basic principle of fault tree set (event) operation, and see Table 4.6 for Boolean algebra simplification rules.

3. **Modular decomposition of fault trees**

The modular decomposition of the fault tree is not a necessary step in the fault tree analysis, and it will not affect the results of the subsequent qualitative and quantitative

Table 4.5 Basic principle of fault tree set (event) operation

Name	Mathematics symbol	Engineering symbol
Dee Morgan's theorem	$\overline{(X \cap Y)} = \overline{X} \cup \overline{Y}$ $\overline{(X \cup Y)} = \overline{X} \cap \overline{Y}$	$\overline{(X \cdot Y)} = \overline{X} + \overline{Y}$ $\overline{(X + Y)} = \overline{X} \cdot \overline{Y}$
Operation with Φ and Ω	T_J (junction temperature) $= T_A + 30\,°C$ (intergated circuit))	$\Phi \cdot X = \Phi \cup \Phi + X = X$ $\Omega \cdot X = X \cup \Omega + X = \Omega$ $\overline{\Phi} = \Omega, \quad \overline{\Omega} = \Phi$
Common relation	$X \cup (\overline{X} \cap Y) = X \cup Y$ $\overline{X} \cap (X \cup \overline{Y}) = \overline{X} \cap \overline{Y} = \overline{(X \cup Y)}$	$X + \overline{X} \cdot Y = X + Y$ $\overline{X} \cdot (X + \overline{Y}) = \overline{X} \cdot \overline{Y} = \overline{(X + Y)}$

Table 4.6 Boolean algebra simplification rules

Name	Mathematics symbol	Engineering symbol
Commutative law	$X \cap Y = Y \cap X$	$X \cdot Y = Y \cdot X$
	$X \cup Y = Y \cup X$	$X + Y = Y + X$
Associative law	$X \cup (Y \cap Z) = (X \cap Y) \cap Z$	$X \cdot (Y \cdot Z) = (X \cdot Y) \cdot Z$
	$X \cup (Y \cup Z) = (X \cap Y) \cup Z$	$X + (Y + Z) = (X + Y) + Z$
Distributive law	$X \cap (Y \cup Z) = (X \cap Y) \cup (X \cap Z)$	$X \cdot (Y \cdot Z) = X \cdot Y + X \cdot Z$
	$X \cup (Y \cap Z) = (X \cup Y) \cap (X \cup Z)$	$X + Y \cdot Z = (X + Y) \cdot (X + Z)$
Idempotent law	$X \cap X = X$	$X \cdot X = X$
	$X \cup X = X$	$X + X = X$
Absorption law	$X \cap (X \cup Y) = X$	$X \cdot (X + Y) = X$
	$X \cup (X \cap Y) = X$	$X + (X \cdot Y) = X$
Complementarity	$X \cap \overline{X} = \Phi$	$X \cdot \overline{X} = \Phi$
	$X \cup \overline{X} = \Omega = 1$	$X + \overline{X} = \Omega = 1$

analysis. However, modular decomposition of the fault tree as much as possible is an effective measure to reduce the size of the fault tree and thus reduce the workload of analysis. The modular decomposition of the fault tree proceeds in the following steps:

(1) According to the definition of the module and the largest module, find out the largest possible module in the fault tree. If computer-aided software is available, it is convenient to find all the largest modules of the fault tree;
(2) Each module can perform quantitative calculation and qualitative analysis independently;
(3) Each module is replaced by an equivalent dummy bottom event to reduce the size of the original fault tree;
(4) After the qualitative analysis and quantitative calculation of the fault tree, the relationship between the top event and each module can be converted into the relationship between the top event and the bottom event according to actual needs.

4.2.5.5 Qualitative Analysis of the Fault Tree

The purpose of qualitative fault tree analysis is to find the causal event or combination of causal events that lead to the occurrence of the top event, that is, to identify all failure mode sets that lead to the occurrence of the top event, to determine the cut set and minimum cut set of the fault tree, and to perform the minimum cut set and bottom cut set. The comparative analysis of events determines the more important bottom events from a qualitative point of view, helps analysts discover potential faults, exposes weak links in the design, so as to improve the design, and can also be used to guide fault diagnosis and improve use and maintenance programs.

1. **The role of the minimum cut set**

A minimum cut set represents a failure mode of the system, and the task of qualitative fault tree analysis is to find all the minimum cut sets of the fault tree. The role of the minimum cut set is mainly reflected in two aspects:

(1) Prevent failure. If the design can ensure that at least one bottom event in each minimum cut set does not occur (the probability of occurrence is extremely low), then the top event does not occur. Therefore, finding the minimum cut set is of great significance to reduce the risk of potential failure of complex systems and improve system design. Starting from the state of ensuring the normal operation of the system, for a system failure mode, it is only necessary to avoid the occurrence of any one of the bottom events to eliminate the corresponding failure mode.
(2) System fault diagnosis and maintenance. When performing fault diagnosis, if a component is found to be faulty and repaired, the system can restore its function, but its reliability level cannot be restored. Because from the concept of the minimum cut set, it can be seen that the system fails only when all the components in the minimum cut set fail, and as long as any component is repaired, the system can resume its function, but at this time, there may still be other components in the same minimum cut set. If the failed component is not repaired, the probability of the system failing again is high. Therefore, during system fault diagnosis and maintenance, other component faults in the same cut set should be traced and all repaired, so that the system reliability and safety design level can be restored.

2. **The method of finding the minimum cut set**

After completing the tree building and normalizing the fault tree, it is necessary to calculate the minimum cut set of the fault tree. Uplink method and downlink method are commonly used to calculate the minimum cut set. For complex fault trees, fault tree analysis software tools are commonly used to find the minimum cut set. See Table 4.7 for the steps of the ascending method and descending method to solve the minimum cut set of the fault tree.

4.2.5.6 Quantitative Analysis of Fault Tree

The purpose of quantitative fault tree analysis is to:

(1) Use the occurrence probability of the bottom event to calculate the occurrence probability of the top event to determine the reliability of the system;
(2) Determine the occurrence probability of each minimum cut set in order to improve the design and improve the reliability and security level of the system.

Table 4.7 Steps for solving the minimum cut set of the fault tree by the upward method and the downward method

Project	Upward method	Downward method
Features	Starting from the bottom event, search for the event set step by step from bottom to top, and finally obtain the minimum cut set of the fault tree	Starting from the top event, search for event sets step by step from top to bottom, and finally obtain the minimum cut set of the fault tree
Step	(1) Determine all bottom events; (2) The logic gate corresponding to the bottom event of the analysis; (3) The input event of the logic gate is represented by the event operation relationship ("AND Gate" is represented by a Boolean set; "OR Gate" is represented by a Boolean sum); (4) Iterate upwards according to step (3) until the top event of the fault tree; (5) Simplify the obtained Boolean equation with Boolean operation rules; (6) Finally, the simplest formula for representing the top event by the sum of bottom event products is obtained; (7) In the simplest formula, the "product " item of each bottom event represents a minimum cut set of the fault tree, and all the " product " items are all the minimum cut sets of the fault tree	(1) Determine the top event; (2) Analyze all corresponding logic gates of the top event; (3) Expand the top event into the input event of the logic gate (the input events connected with the "AND Gate" are listed in the same row; the input events connected with the "OR Gate" occupy a row respectively); (4) According to step (3), each intermediate event is expanded downward according to the same rules until all events are bottom events; (5) Each row in the last column of the table is a cut set of the fault tree; (6) Through the comparison between cut sets, use the rules of Boolean algebra to merge and eliminate elements, and finally get all the minimum cut sets of the fault tree

The quantitative analysis process of the fault tree mainly includes assumption analysis, top event probability, calculation method of top event occurrence probability, and importance analysis.

1. **What-if analysis**

    (1) The bottom events in the fault tree are independent of each other. This independence is mainly judged from the perspective of engineering practice. If some bottom events are not independent of each other, there will be a large error in the calculation according to the assumption of statistical independence, and it should be corrected;
    (2) Each bottom event or top event has two states of occurrence and non-occurrence;
    (3) The fault distribution of the bottom event is exponential distribution. Otherwise, it is difficult to obtain accurate results analytically.

2. **Top event probability**

The occurrence probability of the top event can be solved by the minimum cut set. In engineering, CAD software should be used to assist calculations as much as possible to ensure calculation efficiency and accuracy.

3. **The calculation method of top event occurrence probability**

In most cases, the bottom event may appear repeatedly in several minimum cut sets, that is, the minimum cut sets are intersected. At this time, the accurate calculation of the top event probability must use the probability formula of compatible events, and in engineering In practice, precise calculation is not necessary, and the following method of approximate calculation of top event occurrence probability can usually meet engineering needs.

$$F_s = P(T) = P\left(\bigcup_{i=1}^{R} K_i\right) = \sum_{i=1}^{R} P(K_i) \tag{4.1}$$

In the formula:

$P(T)$ Top event probability;
$P(K_i)$ The probability of occurrence of the i-th minimum cut set;
R The minimum number of cut sets.

4. **Importance analysis**

The contribution of the bottom event to the occurrence of the top event is called the importance of the event. Importance is a function of product structure, life distribution of components, and time. Components in the fault tree can have multiple failure modes, and each failure mode corresponds to a basic event. The importance of a component is equal to the sum of the importance of the basic events it contains. The purpose of importance analysis is to improve and perfect product design, determine the parts of the product that need to be tested, and formulate a checklist for product fault diagnosis. Importance analysis includes probability importance, structure importance and key importance etc. The physical meaning of probability importance is: the degree to which the bottom event causes the probability of the top event to change. The physical meaning of structural importance is: the critical degree of the purely physical position of the bottom event in the system has nothing to do with the failure probability itself, and can be used in the design to determine whether the physical composition of the system meets the requirements. The physical meaning of the key importance degree: Considering the relative failure rate and probability importance of the bottom event at the same time, it reflects the nature that it is more difficult to improve a more reliable bottom event than a less reliable bottom event.

(1) Probability importance

The definition of probability importance: the degree to which the change in the occurrence probability of the i-th bottom event causes the change in the occurrence probability of the top event.

Its mathematical expression is:

$$\Delta g_i(t) = \frac{\partial F_S(t)}{\partial F_i(t)} \tag{4.2}$$

In the formula:

$\Delta g_i(t)$ It is the probabilistic importance of the *i-th component*;
$F_S(t)$ System unreliability function;
$F_i(t)$ Component unreliability function.

It can be seen from the definition that the significance of the probability importance is: the degree to which the change of the unreliability of the ith component causes the change of the system unreliability.

(2) Structural importance

The definition of structural importance: the importance of the position of the bottom event i in the system. Its mathematical expression is:

$$I_i^{\varphi} = \frac{1}{2^{n-1}} n_i^{\varphi} \tag{4.3}$$

$$n_i^{\varphi} = \sum_{i=1}^{2^{n-1}} [\varphi(1_i, X) - \varphi(0_i, X)] \tag{4.4}$$

$[\varphi(1_i, X) - \varphi(0_i, X)]$ is the system structure functional change when the *i-th* component changes from normal state (0) to fault state (1), and at this time, other components remain unchanged.

The bottom event i of the system changes from a normal state (0) to a fault state (1), and when other components remain unchanged, the system may have the following four states:

(1) From the status of the bottom event i being normal and the top event being normal to the bottom event i being faulty, the top event is also faulty, that is, the state of the top event has changed, and the change value is 1;
(2) From the state of bottom event i normal and top event normal to bottom event i failure, top event is still normal, that is, the state of top event has not changed, and the change value is 0;
(3) The state of the bottom event i is normal, the state of the top event failure is changed to the state of the bottom event i failure, and the top event is still faulty, that is, the state of the top event has not changed, and the change value is 0;
(4) The state of the bottom event i is normal and the top event is faulty becomes the state of the bottom event i fault and the top event is normal, that is, the state of the top event has changed, and the change value is -1. Since the study is a monotonically correlated system (that is, the state change direction of the components in the system is always consistent with the state change direction of the system), the last case is not considered.

(3) Key importance

The definition of key importance: the relative change rate of the occurrence probability of the top event caused by the relative change of the occurrence probability of the *i*th bottom event. The mathematical expression is:

$$I_i^{\mathrm{CR}}(t) = \frac{F_i(t)}{F_S(t)} \cdot \Delta g_i(t) \tag{4.5}$$

In the formula:

$F_S(t)$ system unreliability function;
$F_i(t)$ the unreliability function of the i-th component;
$\Delta g_i(t)$ The probability importance of the i-th component.

4.2.5.7 Fault Tree Analysis Report

The main contents of the fault tree analysis report are:

1. **Foreword**

The purpose and timing of preparing the fault tree analysis report shall be stated. The timing refers to the development stage of the analysis, and the purpose mainly refers to the analysis task, the scope involved and so on.

2. **Product description**

It mainly includes the functional principle, composition interface, boundary definition, operation state and working condition description of the product, etc.

3. **Basic assumption**

In order for the analysis to be practical, several basic assumptions should be made. Such as ground launch status or air launch status, etc.

4. **Definition and criteria of failure**

Give a clear meaning of the fault, and analyze which state the product is in is a fault.

5. **Definition and criterion of top event**

For the events that the product does not want to happen, define them as top events one by one and analyze them separately. On the basis of FMEA, it is best to select one of the failure modes from the system failure modes whose failure severity is Class I and II to be determined as the top event.

6. **Fault tree construction**

It is not necessary to give a detailed tree building process, but there must be a complete fault tree.

7. **Normalization, simplification and modular decomposition of fault trees**

Normalization of the fault tree is essential, and simplification and modular decomposition may be considered as appropriate.

8. **Qualitative analysis of fault trees**

Determine the minimum cut set of the fault tree, and analyze the minimum cut set.

9. **Quantitative analysis of fault tree**

It mainly includes the calculation of the occurrence probability of the fault tree top event and the analysis of the importance.

10. **Conclusions and recommendations of fault tree analysis**

According to the results of qualitative and quantitative analysis, the weak link of the design is given, and corresponding improvement suggestions are put forward.

11. **Appendix**

The attachments may include necessary charts and explanatory materials not given in the previous part; other product information that needs to be supplemented; importance ranking table, etc.

4.3 Reliability Modeling and Prediction

4.3.1 Overview

The failure rate is the ratio of the number of failures of a batch of products within a certain period of time to the total working time. The failure rate is proportional to the frequency of failures when the product is used. The failure rate is an important indicator to measure the reliability of a product. Modeling and prediction is a method used to estimate whether a digital medical device meets specified reliability requirements.

This section mainly introduces the principles and methods of reliability modeling and prediction, its implementation procedures and related precautions. In the development stage of digital medical equipment, reliability modeling and prediction technology can be used to establish a product reliability model, predict the basic failure rate and task failure rate of the product, and help designers understand the reliability level of the design scheme in the design stage. It is used to compare different design schemes and judge whether the design scheme meets the specified reliability index requirements.

4.3.2 Reliability Prediction Standard and Introduction

4.3.2.1 GJB/Z 299C-2006 Standard Introduction

The full name of GJB/Z 299C-2006 standard is *Electronic Equipment Reliability Prediction Manual.* This standard provides data and methods for reliability prediction of electronic equipment and systems. This standard introduces component stress analysis prediction method and component count reliability prediction method, which are applicable to electronic components working under normal working conditions. The component stress analysis prediction method is applicable to the equipment development stage where the product has a detailed component list and the components are determined to withstand stress; the component count reliability prediction method is applicable to the preliminary design stage of product development.

The general process of electronic equipment reliability prediction is as follows:

(1) First divide the reliability prediction units, and then establish the system reliability model. It is expected that the units are relatively independent in circuit function, and their reliability models are generally series structures.
(2) Calculate the non-operating failure rate of components. For those who adopt the reliability prediction method of component stress analysis, calculate the working failure rate according to the working reliability model provided in Chap. 5 of the GJB/Z 299C-2006 standard; The general failure rate in Chap. 6 of the standard is multiplied by the general quality factor to obtain the usual value of the failure rate of a certain type of components.
(3) Add the expected failure rate of various components in the unit to obtain the expected failure rate of the unit.
(4) According to the reliability model of the equipment and system, predict the reliability indicators such as the mean time between failures of the equipment and system step by step.

Since this standard is a national military standard, it is quite authoritative in the field of reliability prediction, and many enterprise manufacturers adopt this standard when doing reliability prediction. However, since the standard was released in 2006, the data survey in the standard was based on the level of components in the early twenty-first century. At that time, the production process of components was relatively immature and the failure rate was relatively high. After nearly two decades of development of domestic components, the production process has been continuously matured, the raw materials of the components have been continuously optimized, the reliability of the components has been continuously improved, and the failure rate of the components is lower than before. If the data on the GJB 299C-2006 standard is still When predicting the reliability of newly developed products, there may be a problem that the basic failure rate of components is relatively high, resulting in poor reliability prediction results for electronic equipment.

4.3.2.2 Introduction to GJB/Z 108A-2006 Standard

The full name of the GJB/Z 108A-2006 standard is *Reliability Prediction Manual for Non-Working Conditions of Electronic Equipment*. This standard provides basic data and methods for non-working state reliability prediction of electronic equipment and systems. This standard mainly introduces the component non-working detailed prediction method and the component non-working count reliability prediction method. The component non-working detailed prediction method is applicable to the equipment development stage where the product has a detailed component list. Counting reliability prediction method is suitable for the preliminary design stage of product development.

The general process of predicting the reliability of non-working components is as follows:

(1) First divide the reliability prediction units, and then establish the system reliability model. The divided predictive units are relatively independent in terms of circuit function, and their reliability models are generally in series structure;
(2) Calculate the non-operating failure rate of components. For those who adopt the "Detailed Prediction Method of Non-operating Reliability of Components", calculate their non-operating failure rate according to the non-operating reliability prediction model provided in Chap. 5 of this standard, then the non-working failure rate of a certain type of component is obtained by multiplying the non-working general failure rate in Chap. 6 of the standard by the non-working quality coefficient;
(3) Add the non-operating failure rate of various components in the expected unit to obtain the expected non-operating failure rate of the unit;
(4) According to the reliability model of the equipment and system, predict the non-working state reliability of the equipment and system step by step.

4.3.2.3 Introduction to GB/T 7289-2017 Standard

The full name of the GB/T 7289-2017 standard is Standard Conditions for the Reliability Failure Rate of Electrical Components and the Stress Model for Failure Rate Conversion. Using this standard is equivalent to adopting IEC 61709-2011 Electric Components Reliability Reference Conditions for Failure Rates and Stress Models for Conversion standards. This national standard stipulates how to use failure rate data to predict the reliability of electronic components in electronic equipment. However, this standard does not provide the basic failure rate of components. The stress model converts the failure rate of one working condition into the failure rate of another working condition, which enriches the usage scenarios of reliability prediction. The author believes that there is a certain risk in doing this kind of conversion in the reliability prediction. For example, although some digital medical equipment is applied on a ship or a car, instead of being applied on a fixed and good ground, the equipment cabin where the digital medical equipment is located Corresponding environmental protection design has been done inside, such as shock absorption, moisture-proof, etc. The actual environmental impact of components is close to the fixed and good ground, which will cause the situation that the use scene does not match the actual environment, resulting in a deviation in the conversion of failure rate. Therefore, readers are advised to conduct analysis in combination with the actual use of components when using this standard for failure rate conversion, and do not directly apply the failure rate conversion stress model in the standard easily.

4.3.2.4 Introduction to GB/T 37963-2019 Standard

The full name of the GB/T 37963-2019 standard is *Electronic Equipment Reliability Prediction Model and Data Manual*. This standard is compiled with reference to the International Electrotechnical Commission IEC TR 62380-2004 standard, but the data of the two standards are not completely equivalent. This standard gives the prediction model, impact factor characterization and related data of common component types, and is suitable for reliability prediction in the field of civil industry. Under the assumption of a constant failure rate of components, the failure rate of non-redundant equipment can be obtained by accumulating the failure rate of components. When the type of components, use environment and stress conditions are relatively clear, the estimated model provided by this standard can be used The failure rate of each component is calculated by stress analysis method. If the use of environmental stress is not clear, the product failure rate can be estimated according to the counting prediction method provided in this standard, but the accuracy of the result of the counting method is relatively low.

4.3.3 Modeling and Prediction Assumptions

4.3.3.1 Assumptions for Reliability Modeling

The assumptions for reliability modeling are as follows:

- The system and its constituent units only have two states of failure and normal, and there is no third state;
- All inputs of the system are within the specified range, that is, the system failure caused by input errors is not considered;
- When performing reliability modeling, simple structural parts in the system may not be considered;
- When there is sufficient evidence to show that the reliability level of a certain product is very high, the product may not be considered in system reliability modeling;
- When software reliability is not included in the system reliability model, it should be assumed that the entire software is completely reliable;

- When human reliability is not included in the system reliability model, it should be assumed that the human is completely reliable and there are no interaction problems between the human and the system.

4.3.3.2 Assumptions for Reliability Prediction

The assumptions for reliability prediction are as follows:

- Unless otherwise specified, the failure distribution of the product uses an exponential distribution;
- Unless otherwise specified, the expected product failures are independent of each other;
- Basic reliability is expected using failure rate and mean time between failures as the expected parameters (the two are reciprocally related in an exponential distribution), and mission reliability is expected using mission reliability as the expected parameter;
- The target of reliability prediction should be the specified value in the mature period, and the predicted value should generally not be lower than 1.25 times the specified value in the mature period.

4.3.4 Reliability Modeling Steps

4.3.4.1 Task Analysis

Reliability models can be divided into basic reliability models and task reliability models. Generally, when establishing the basic reliability model of the system, the system is regarded as a full series model of each component.

When establishing a task reliability model, it is necessary to clarify what the task to be analyzed is, and for the task to be analyzed, which functions of the system are involved, which functions are necessary, and which functions are unnecessary. And form the fault criterion of the system. All software and hardware failures involved in all necessary functions affecting the completion of system tasks shall be counted as failure events.

The mission of the system can generally be derived from the life profile and mission profile. The life profile and task profile describe the timing, duration, operating modes and environmental conditions of all events and environments that the product may experience.

4.3.4.2 Functional Analysis

The purpose of product function analysis is to distinguish the functional relationship among the units that make up the product. These functional relationships mainly include functional hierarchical relationship, functional interface relationship, working mode and working sequence of each unit.

The function of the product is realized by the functions of each unit that makes up the product. Through the process of functional decomposition from top to bottom, the functional hierarchy of the product can be obtained.

In the process of product function decomposition, the interface relationship between lower-level functions should be further clarified, that is, the input and output of each function should be clarified.

When a product can complete a specific function in multiple ways, it has a working mode of replacement (complete replacement or partial replacement). In addition, in order to ensure the correct realization of product functions, the product may also have fault detection, fault isolation, etc. It is very important to distinguish these working modes for the correct establishment of product reliability models.

During the entire process of completing the task, the product works in a certain sequence. Some products may work continuously for a long time, and some products may work intermittently for a short time, or work in a certain way during a certain period of time. Worked another way at another time. Distinguishing the working sequence of the product is also the basis for correctly establishing the reliability model.

The functional logic relationship of the product can be described by a functional block diagram or a functional flow chart.

4.3.4.3 Fault Definition

An event or condition in which a product or a part of a product cannot or will not perform its intended function, known as a failure. For a specific product, it should be combined with its function to give the product failure criterion, that is, the failure criterion. The failure criterion is the limit value for judging whether the product constitutes a failure, and should generally be determined according to each specified performance parameter and allowable limit of the product. The failure criterion of the basic failure rate refers to the failure caused by the product itself that needs to be repaired. The failure criterion of the task failure rate refers to the failures that affect the completion of the product task. For example, the fault discrimination criteria for digital medical equipment are:

- Failures caused by non-human (including software and hardware) within the service life are counted as associated failures that affect the basic failure rate;
- In the task profile, any failure that cannot complete the specified task is counted as an associated failure that affects the task.

4.3.4.4 Establishment of Reliability Block Diagram

After the above-mentioned relevant analysis, the interdependence between all units of the product when performing tasks should be expressed from the perspective of reliability through a concise and intuitive method, which is to establish a reliability block diagram. The reliability block diagram is used to describe the reliability (or fault) logical relationship between the units that make up the product, and is generally expressed by the reliability block diagram model. Each box in the block diagram represents a functional unit related to product reliability. Both the basic reliability model and the task reliability model can be represented by a reliability block diagram.

The basic reliability model is a reliability model used to estimate the maintenance and support requirements caused by the failure of products and their constituent units. After any unit in the system (including the reserve unit) fails, it needs to be repaired or replaced, which will generate maintenance and guarantee requirements, so it can be regarded as a model for measuring maintenance manpower and use guarantee costs. The basic reliability model is a full series model, even if there are redundant units, it should be treated as series. Therefore, the higher the failure rate of each unit in the digital medical equipment system, the higher the basic failure rate of the system.

The mission reliability model is a reliability model used to estimate the probability of a product completing a specified function during the execution of a mission, describe the predetermined function of each unit of the product during the mission completion process, and measure the effectiveness of the work. Obviously, the lower the failure rate of units required to complete tasks in the digital medical equipment system, the lower the system task failure rate. Different mission profiles correspond to different mission reliability models, and the mission reliability models must establish their own models for the mission profiles.

4.3.4.5 Establishment of Mathematical Model of Failure Rate

The reliability block diagram shows the logical relationship between the failure rate of the product and its units, and the mathematical model of the failure rate shows the quantitative relationship between the failure rate of the product and its units, which requires the established reliability block diagram, establish corresponding mathematical models. The functional relationship between the failure rate of each unit and the system failure rate is expressed by mathematical formula, and the reliability prediction is based on this.

4.3.4.6 Determining the task time model

The model accounts for events and conditions related to specific use cases of the system, such as during the use of a certain type of digital medical equipment, some parts of the system are not always working. Therefore, it must be corrected when establishing a mathematical model, that is, it needs to be corrected with the duty factor of the system. The duty factor refers to the ratio of the working time of the subsystem to the working time of the system. Generally, it can be corrected as follows.

Assuming that the failure rate of the subsystem (the life obeys the exponential distribution) is negligible when it is not working, that is:

$$R(t) = \exp(-\lambda \times t \times d) \tag{4.6}$$

In the formula:

$R(t)$ The reliability of the subsystem;
λ Failure rate of subsystem (1/h);
t The working time of the system (h);
d Duty factor, $d = S/F$.

4.3.5 *Typical Reliability Models*

Typical reliability models are divided into reserve models and non- reserve models, and reserve reliability models are divided into working reserve models and non-operating reserve models according to whether the reserve unit and the working unit work at the same time. A typical classification of reliability models is shown in Fig. 4.3.

4.3.5.1 Series Model

Failure of any one of all the constituent units of the system will lead to the failure of the whole system. Such a system is called a series system. The series model is one of the most commonly used and simplest models.

The reliability block diagram of the series model is shown in Fig. 4.4, and its mathematical model is:

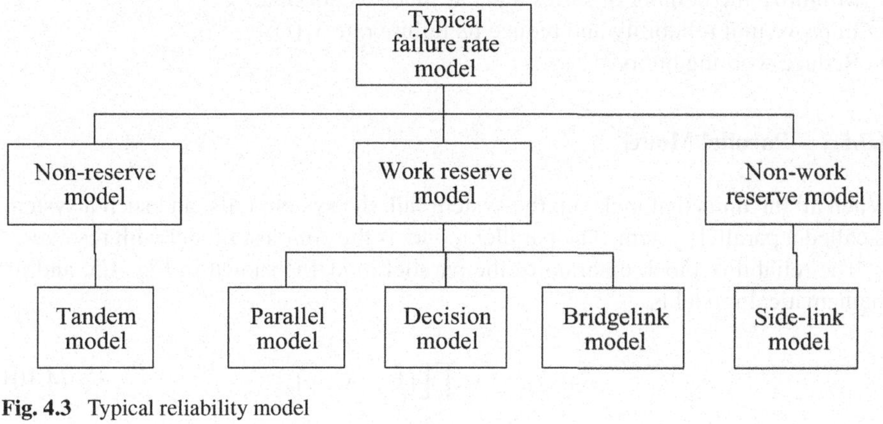

Fig. 4.3 Typical reliability model

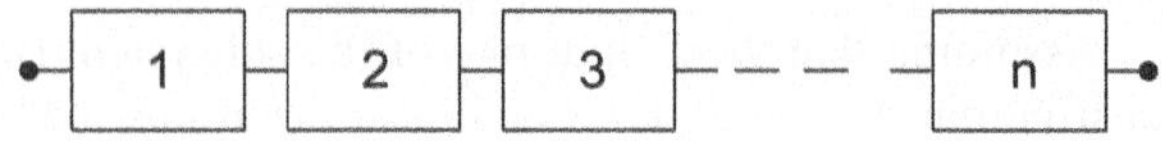

Fig. 4.4 Reliability block diagram of the series model

$$R_s(t) = \prod_{i=1}^{n} R_i(t) = \prod_{i=1}^{n} \mathrm{e}^{-\int_0^t \lambda_i(t)\,\mathrm{d}t} \tag{4.7}$$

In the formula:

$R_s(t)$ The reliability of the system;
$R_i(t)$ The unit reliability;
$\lambda_i(t)$ The failure rate of the unit;
n the number of units that make up the system.

When the life distribution of each unit is exponential distribution, the life of the system also obeys the exponential distribution, and the failure rate of the system λ_s λ_i is the sum of unit failure rates:

$$\lambda_s = -\frac{\ln(R_s(t))}{t} = -\sum_{i=1}^{n} \frac{\ln(R_i(t))}{t} = \sum_{i=1}^{n} \lambda_i \tag{4.8}$$

The Mean Time Between Failure (MTBF) of the system:

$$\mathrm{MTBF} = \frac{1}{\lambda_s} = \frac{1}{\sum_{i=1}^{n} \lambda_i} \tag{4.9}$$

from formula (4.7) that the reliability of the system is the product of the reliability of each unit, the more units, the smaller the system reliability. From the design point of view, in order to improve the reliability of the series system, the following three aspects can be considered:

- Minimize the number of series units as much as possible;
- Improve unit reliability and reduce its failure rate $\lambda_i(t)$;
- Reduce working hours t.

4.3.5.2 Parallel Model

When all the units that make up the system fail, the system fails, and such a system is called a parallel system. The parallel model is the simplest model with reserves.

The reliability block diagram of the parallel model is shown in Fig. 4.5, and its mathematical model is:

$$R_S(t) = 1 - \prod_{i=1}^{n} [1 - R_i(t)] \tag{4.10}$$

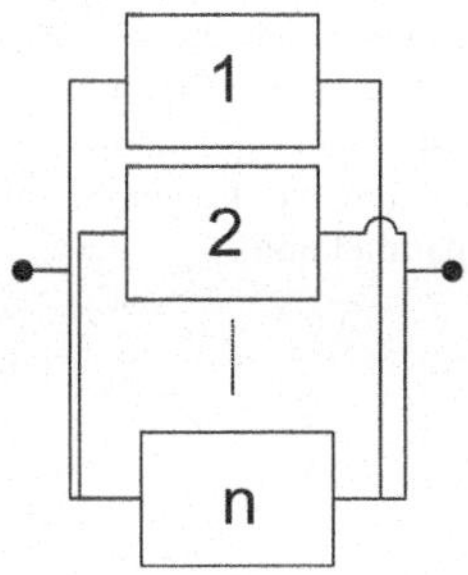

Fig. 4.5 Reliability block diagram of the parallel model

In the formula:

$R_s(t)$ The reliability of the system;
$R_i(t)$ The unit reliability;
n The number of units that make up the system.

When the life distribution of each unit of the system is exponential distribution, for the most commonly used two-unit parallel system, there is

$$R_s(t) = e^{-\lambda_1 t} + e^{-\lambda_2 t} - e^{-(\lambda_1+\lambda_2)t} \quad (4.11)$$

The Mean Time Between Critical Failures (MTBCFS) of the system is:

$$T_{\mathrm{BCF}_s} = \int_0^{\infty} R_s(t)\mathrm{d}t = \frac{1}{\lambda_1} + \frac{1}{\lambda_2} - \frac{1}{\lambda_1+\lambda_2} \quad (4.12)$$

Although the unit failure rate λ_1, λ_2 is constant, the failure rate of the parallel system $\lambda_s(t)$ is no longer constant. The failure rate curve of the parallel model is shown in Fig. 4.6.

When the lifetime distribution of each unit in the system is an exponential distribution, for n a parallel system of units with the same distribution, we have

$$R_s(t) = 1 - (1 - e^{-\lambda t})^n \quad (4.13)$$

$$T_{\mathrm{BCF}_s} = \int_0^{\infty} R_s(t)\mathrm{d}t = \frac{1}{\lambda} + \frac{1}{2\lambda} + \cdots + \frac{1}{n\lambda} \quad (4.14)$$

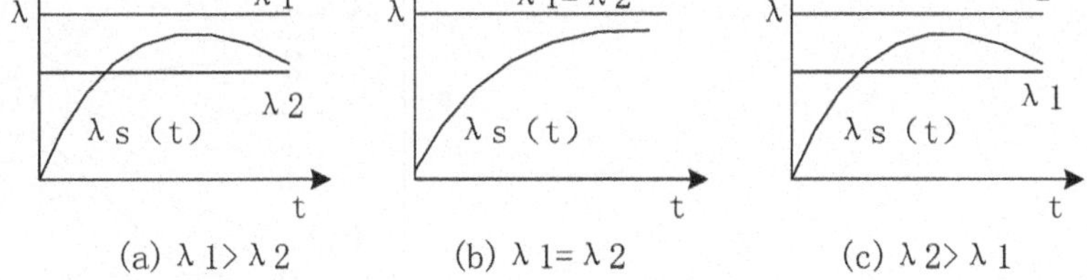

Fig. 4.6 Parallel model failure rate curve

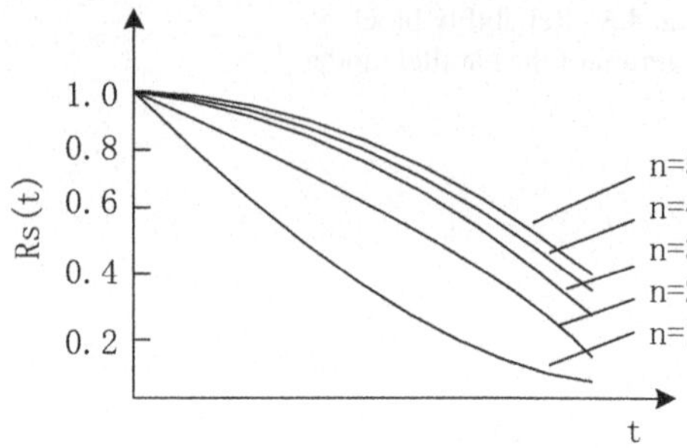

Fig. 4.7 The relationship between the reliability function of the parallel system and the number of parallel units

The relationship between the reliability function of the parallel system and the number of parallel units is shown in Fig. 4.7. It can be seen from the figure that compared with the non-reserve single unit, the reliability of the system is significantly improved, especially when $n = 2$ the reliability is improved more significantly. When there are too many units connected in parallel, the reliability improvement speed is greatly slowed down.

4.3.5.3 Decision *(n, r)* Model

N voting system consisting of units and a voting device. When the voting device is normal, the number of normal units is not less than $r(1 \le r \le n)$ and the system will not fail. Such a system is called $r/n(G)$ voting system. It is a form of work reserve model.

$r/n(G)$ system's reliability block diagram of the system is shown in Fig. 4.8.

$r/n(G)$ system's mathematical model of the system:

$$R_s(t) = R_m \sum_{i=r}^{n} C_n^i R(t)^i (1 - R(t))^{n-i} \tag{4.15}$$

In the formula:

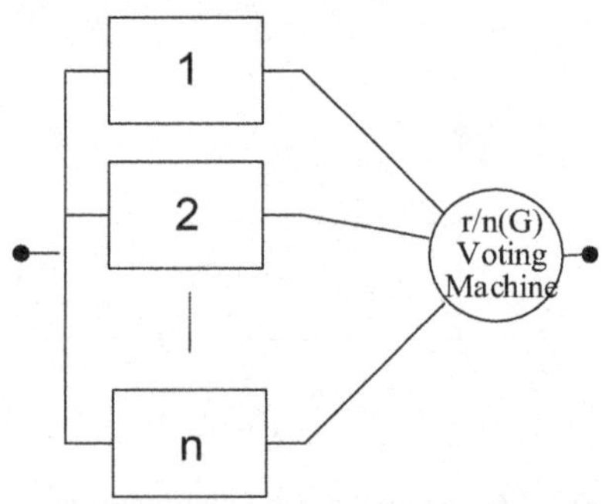

Fig. 4.8 *r*/*n* (G) System's reliability block diagram

$R_s(t)$ The reliability of the system;
$R(t)$ The reliability of system components (each unit is the same);
R_m The reliability of the voting device;

the exponential distribution of $r/n(G)$ the failure rate, the reliability λ of the system:

$$R_s(t) = R_m \sum_{i=r}^{n} C_n^i e^{-i\lambda t}(1 - e^{-\lambda t})^{n-i} \tag{4.16}$$

When the reliability of the voting machine is 1, the task time T_{BCF_S} between fatal failures of the system is:

$$T_{\mathrm{BCF}_s} = \int_0^\infty R_s(t)\mathrm{d}t = \sum_{i=r}^{n} \frac{1}{i\lambda} \tag{4.17}$$

In $r/n(G)$ system, the system is normal when n must be an odd number (let is $2k+1$) and the number of normal units of the system must be greater than or equal to $k+1$ that of the system. Such a system is called a majority voting system. A majority voting system is $r/n(G)$ a special case of the system. The two-out-of-three system is a commonly used majority voting system, and the reliability block diagram of the 2/3 system is shown in Fig. 4.9. When the reliability of the voting machine is 1 and the failure rate of the constituent units is constant λ, the mathematical model is:

$$R_s(t) = 3e^{-2\lambda t} - 2e^{-3\lambda t} \tag{4.18}$$

$$T_{\mathrm{BCF}_s} = \frac{5}{6\lambda} \tag{4.19}$$

When the reliability of the voting machine is 1:
$r = 1$, $1/n(G)$ is a parallel system,

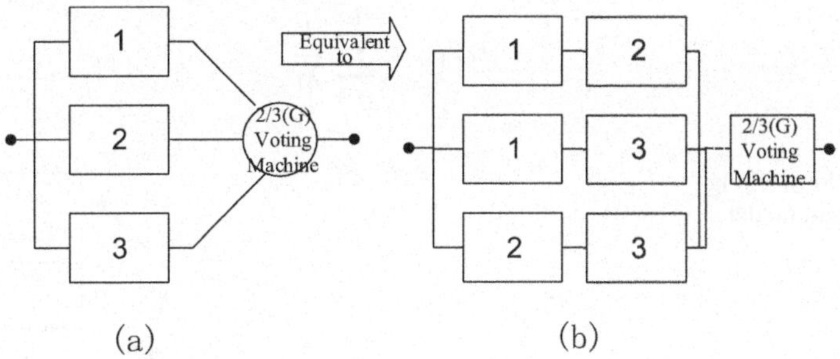

Fig. 4.9 2/3 System reliability block diagram

$$R_s(t) = 1 - (1 - R(t))^n \tag{4.20}$$

$r = n$, $n/n(G)$ is a series system

$$R_s(t) = R(t)^n \tag{4.21}$$

$r/n(G)$ system's MTBCFS of the system is smaller than that of the parallel system and larger than that of the series system.

4.3.5.4 Parallel Model

Only one of the n units that make up the system works. When the working unit fails, it is transferred to another unit to continue working through the conversion device. The system fails until all units fail. It is called a non-working reserve system, also known as a bypass system.

Non-working reserve system model is shown in Fig. 4.10.

The reliability mathematical model of the non-working reserve system is as follows:

(1) Assuming that the reliability of the conversion device is 1, the system T_{BCF_s} is equal to the sum of each unit T_{BCF_i}:

$$T_{\mathrm{BCF}_S} = \sum_{i=1}^{n} T_{\mathrm{BCF}_i} \tag{4.22}$$

In the formula:

T_{BCF_s} The Mean Time Between Critical Failures of the system;
T_{BCF_i} The Mean Time Between Critical Failures of the unit;
n The number of units that make up the system.

(2) When the life of each unit of the system obeys the exponential distribution:

$$T_{\mathrm{BCF}_S} = \sum_{i=1}^{n} \frac{1}{\lambda_i} \tag{4.23}$$

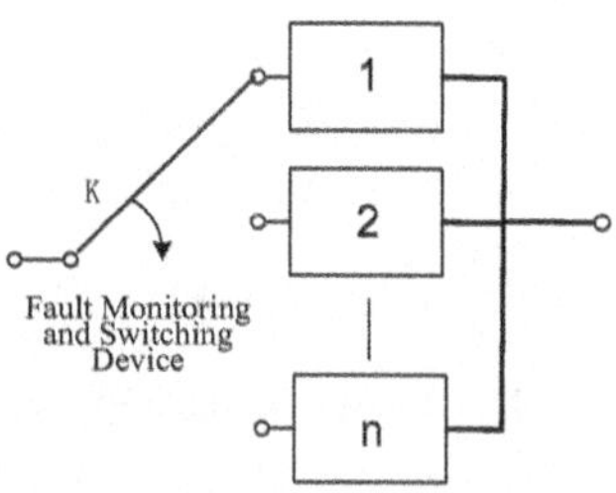

Fig. 4.10 Not working reserve system model

In the formula:

T_{BCF_s} The Mean Time Between Critical Failures of the system;
λ_i The failure rate of the unit;
n The number of units that make up the system.

(3) When all units of the system are the same:

$$T_{BCF_S} = \frac{n}{\lambda} \tag{4.24}$$

$$R_s(t) = e^{-\lambda t}\left[1 + \lambda t + \frac{(\lambda t)^2}{2!} + \cdots + \frac{(\lambda t)^{n-1}}{(n-1)!}\right] \tag{4.25}$$

For a non-operating reserve system consisting of two different units commonly used ($n = 2, \lambda_1 \neq \lambda_2$):

$$R_s(t) = \frac{\lambda_2}{\lambda_2 - \lambda_1} e^{-\lambda_1 t} + \frac{\lambda_1}{\lambda_1 - \lambda_2} e^{-\lambda_2 t} \tag{4.26}$$

$$T_{BCF_s} = \frac{1}{\lambda_1} + \frac{1}{\lambda_2} \tag{4.27}$$

(4) Assuming that the reliability of the conversion device is constant R_D, the two units are the same and the service life obeys the exponential distribution of the failure rate λ, the reliability of the system is:

$$R_s(t) = e^{-\lambda t}(1 + R_D \lambda t) \tag{4.28}$$

(5) For two different units, the failure rates are λ_1, λ_2:

$$R_s(t) = e^{-\lambda_1 t} + R_D \frac{\lambda_1}{\lambda_1 - \lambda_2}(e^{-\lambda_2 t} - e^{-\lambda_1 t}) \tag{4.29}$$

$$T_{BCF_s} = \frac{1}{\lambda_1} + R_D \frac{1}{\lambda_2} \tag{4.30}$$

The advantage of the non-working reserve system is that it can greatly improve the reliability of the system. Its disadvantages are: ① The complexity of the system is increased due to the addition of fault monitoring and switching devices; ② The reliability of the fault monitoring and switching devices is required to be very high. Otherwise the benefits of stockpiling would be severely diminished.

4.3.5.5 Bridging Model

The realization of some redundant forms or alternative working modes of the system does not adopt the parallel, voting or side connection model, but a bridging form. Therefore, in the logical description of the reliability model, a logical relationship like a bridge structure in the circuit appears. The functional block diagram and reliability block diagram of the bridge model system are shown in Fig. 4.11. The establishment of its mathematical model is relatively complicated, and a general expression cannot be established. Let's deepen the understanding of the bridging model by analyzing a specific case.

A certain system consists of five parts A, B, C, D, and E. Under the condition of normal power supply, any one of equipment B and D can work normally to complete the task. When switch E is open, generator A supplies power to device B, and generator C supplies power to device D. If generator A fails, isolate generator A and close one-way switch E, and generator C supplies power to equipment B and D. If the generator C fails, the switch E does not work, and the equipment D cannot work.

It can be seen from the model in the figure that the units in the reliability block diagram in the bridging model have a flow direction (reflected by the connection direction), which reflects the flow relationship between system functions. In the typical model presented earlier, the reliability box is undirected, that is, bidirectional. The units in the reliability block diagram can be undirected units or directed units, which are used to represent different process logic relationships.

We use a simple method to establish the reliability mathematical model of this example. By observing and analyzing the reliability block diagram in Fig. 4.11b, we can know that when units A and B, units C and D, or units B, C and E are all normal, the system functions normally. The mathematical model of system reliability is:

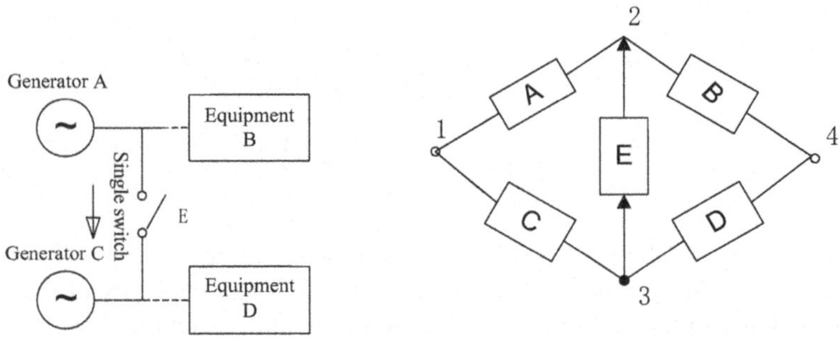

(a) Function Block Diagram (b) Reliability Block Diagram

Fig. 4.11 Functional block diagram and reliability block diagram of the bridge model system

$$
\begin{aligned}
R_s(t) = {} & R_A(t)R_B(t) + R_C(t)R_D(t) + R_B(t)R_C(t)R_E(t) \\
& - R_A(t)R_B(t)R_C(t)R_D(t) - R_A(t)R_B(t)R_C(t)R_E(t) - R_B(t)R_C(t)R_D(t)R_E(t) \\
& + R_A(t)R_B(t)R_C(t)R_D(t)R_E(t)
\end{aligned}
\tag{4.31}
$$

4.3.6 Reliability Prediction Method

The reliability prediction should be deepened with the progress of the research and development work, and different methods are generally selected in three stages. See Table 4.8 for the selection of prediction methods at different development stages.

According to product characteristics and information status, different reliability prediction methods can be selected. For a large and complex complete machine, the component-based reliability modeling and prediction method can avoid the basic modeling problem of a large number of components, and can also reduce the workload of complete machine reliability modeling and prediction. For newly developed components, the counting method and stress analysis method based on the basic failure rate of components can solve the problem of missing information on newly developed components. For improved products, using the similar product method, through comparative analysis, the reliability prediction can be completed simply and quickly.

Table 4.8 Selection of prediction methods in different development stages

Development stage		Design	Initial design	Detailed design	Scope of application
Prediction method	Similar product law	√	√	√	Non-electrical products, improved modified products with similar product data
	Expert Scoring	/	√	√	Non-electrical products, newly developed products, improved and modified products without similar product data
	Component counting	√	√	/	Electronic product
	Stress analysis	/	√	√	Electronic product

4.3.6.1 Component Counting Method

1. **Method description**

In the preliminary design stage, the working state reliability of electronic components is estimated using the component counting method. The type and quantity of all components, the quality level of components and the working environment of the equipment shall be given in the estimation report according to Table 4.9. The domestic components are estimated according to the data and methods provided in GJB/Z 299C-2006; the imported components are estimated according to the section 4 method in MIL-HDBK-217F (Notice 2).

2. **Example of component counting method**

A certain digital diagnosis and treatment equipment consists of 4 adjustment diodes, 2 synthetic resistors, and 4 mica capacitors, all of which are made in China, and the quality level is B_1. The working environment of the equipment is a laboratory. Calculate the basic failure rate for the device.calculation steps:

(1) For domestic devices, use GJB/Z 299C-2006 for prediction;
(2) Determine the working environment category of the equipment: G_B;
(3) Determine the types of components: adjusting diodes, synthetic resistors, and mica capacitors;
(4) Determine the quality grade of components, all of which are B_1;
(5) Check Tables 6.19, 6.21, and 6.22 in GJB/Z 299C-2006 to determine the general failure rate of components:

Adjustment diode: $\lambda_{G1} = 0.077\ (10^{-6}/\mathrm{h})$

Synthetic resistor: $\lambda_{G2} = 0.0028\ (10^{-6}/\mathrm{h})$

Mica capacitor: $\lambda_{G3} = 0.0061\ (10^{-6}/\mathrm{h})$

(6) Check Tables 6.3 and 6.4 in GJB/Z 299C-2006 to determine the quality factor of components:

Adjustment diode: $\pi_{Q1} = 0.5$

Synthetic Resistor: $\pi_{Q2} = 0.6$

Mica capacitor: $\pi_{Q3} = 0.5$

Table 4.9 Predicted example of component counting method

Serial number	Component category	Quantity N	Quality level	Quality factor πQ	Environment category	λG (10^{-6}/h)	$N\lambda G$ (10^{-6}/h)	Note

(7) Determine the number of components:

Adjustment diode: $N_1 = 4$;

Synthetic resistor: $N_2 = 2$;

Mica capacitor: $N_3 = 4$;

(8) Calculate the basic failure rate of the equipment:

$$\begin{aligned}\lambda_{\text{device}} &= N_1\lambda_{G1}\pi_{Q1} + N_2\lambda_{G2}\pi_{Q2} + N_3\lambda_{G3}\pi_{Q3} \\ &= 4 \times 0.077 \times 0.5 + 2 \times 0.0028 \times 0.6 + 4 \times 0.0061 \times 0.5 \\ &= 0.16956\left(10^{-6}/\text{h}\right)\end{aligned}$$

$$\text{MTBF}_{\text{device}} = 1/\lambda_{\text{device}} = 5897617.36(\text{h}) \tag{4.32}$$

See Table 4.9 for an example of component counting method prediction.

4.3.6.2 Component Stress Analysis Method

1. **Method description**

In the detailed design stage of digital diagnosis and treatment equipment, the component stress analysis method is used to predict the failure rate of components in working state. The failure rate of domestic components is predicted according to the data and methods provided in GJB/Z 299C-2006; the failure rate of imported components is predicted according to the data and methods provided in MIL-HDBK-217F. Pay attention to the following requirements when making estimates.

(1) Entry requirements

In order to ensure the credibility of the forecast, the quantity, category, model, quality grade, and main parameters of all components and parts should be given in the forecast report according to Table 4.10.

(2) Integrity requirements

The forecast report should have complete forecast steps and processes, and explain each step in detail. For each type of component, its predicted model is listed, and the value of each coefficient, component failure rate, unit reliability prediction results, etc. are listed according to Table 4.10.

(3) Selection of estimated data

The data of domestic or foreign components should be used for prediction according to the actual situation of digital medical equipment. It cannot be divorced from the actual situation, and all of them should be estimated according to imported components, and it should not appear that imported components are used in electronic

Table 4.10 Prediction table example of component stress analysis method

Serial number	Components serial number	Components model	Components category	Quantity N	Quality grade	Each π coefficient	λb (10^{-6}/h)	Work failure rate (10^{-6}/h)		Note
								λp	$N\lambda p$	

equipment, but all of them are based on domestic components. Forecast situation. The selection of components shall be stated in the forecast report.

(4) Selection of expected temperature

When predicting, the case temperature or junction temperature of the components should be evaluated according to the expected environment where the digital medical equipment is installed and used. The determination of the temperature should be analyzed in the forecast report.

When thermal analysis data is lacking, according to the engineering experience of digital medical equipment, the following formula can be used to calculate the junction temperature of components:

$$T_J\,(\text{junction temperature}) = T_A + 20\,^\circ\text{C}\ (diode)) \tag{4.33}$$

$$T_J\,(\text{junction temperature}) = T_A + 30\,^\circ\text{C}\ (transistor)) \tag{4.34}$$

$$T_J\,(\text{junction temperature}) = T_A + 30\,^\circ\text{C}\ (\text{intergated circuit})) \tag{4.35}$$

Among them, T_A is the ambient temperature where the components work.

(5) Selection of derating factor

The design of digital diagnosis and treatment equipment should strictly follow the derating guidelines issued by the overall design unit for derating. Special circumstances beyond the scope of derating guidelines should be approved by the technical director of the equipment manufacturer, and such situations should be reported in the forecast report. Be explained.

(6) Selection of quality coefficient

The quality factor should be correctly selected according to the quality grade of the selected components. For domestic components, according to the actual selected quality grade, select the corresponding quality grade coefficient from GJB/Z 299C-2006. For imported components, according to the actual selected quality grade, from MIL-HDBK-217F *MIL ITARY* Select the corresponding quality grade coefficient in *HANDBOOK RELIABILITY PREDICTION OF ELECTRONIC EQUIPMENT.*

(7) Selection of environmental categories and coefficients

According to the daily use environment of digital diagnosis and treatment equipment, when selecting the environmental factor, select according to the environmental classification in Table 4.3-1 of GJB/Z 299C-2006. The commonly used use environment of digital diagnosis and treatment equipment is as follows:

(1) When the digital diagnosis and treatment equipment is used in a good environment on the ground that can maintain normal climate conditions and the

mechanical stress is close to zero, and in a laboratory or hospital with good maintenance conditions (such as temperature and humidity control), the environment category should be selected as a good ground ($G_{B)}$;

(2) When the digital diagnosis and treatment equipment is used in an ordinary building or on a fixed rack with good ventilation, and is in an environment less affected by vibration and shock, such as the environment where ordinary household appliances are located, the environment category is selected as general ground fixation ($G_{F1)}$;

(3) When the digital diagnosis and treatment equipment is used in a relatively stable moving state, and the use environment is affected by vibration and shock, such as on an ambulance or other driving vehicles, the environment category should be selected as smooth ground movement ($G_{M1)}$.

(8) Other requirements

For the components that cannot be found in the cited standards but are used in the actual design, according to the actual situation of the components, refer to and quote other documents, or refer to the situation of similar components, and give the failure rate after analysis and correction data, such situations should be detailed in the forecast report.

2. **Example of component stress analysis method**

(1) Digital circuit

The digital circuit 54LS00 is a domestic device, the quality level is B $_1$, and the environmental category is G_B. Calculate the failure rate of the device.
calculation steps:

(1) For domestic devices, use GJB/Z 299C-2006 for prediction;
(2) 54LS00 is a bipolar digital circuit, check the Table 5.2.2–1 of GJB/Z 299C-2006, the reliability model is:

$$\lambda_P = \pi_Q[C_1\pi_T\pi_V + (C_2 + C_3)\pi_E]\pi_L \tag{4.36}$$

(3) The quality level of the device is B $_1$, check the Table 5.2.2–3 of GJB/Z 299C-2006, and get the quality factor $\pi_Q = 0.5$;
(4) The digital diagnosis and treatment equipment is used in the laboratory, the environmental category is GB, check the Table 5.2.2–2 of GJB/Z 299C-2006, and the environmental coefficient π E = 1.0 can be obtained;
(5) Check Table 5.2.2–4 of GJB/Z 299C-2006. Combined with the fact that the chip meets the response standard and has been produced stably, the maturity coefficient π L = 1.0 can be obtained;
(6) Ambient temperature TA = 41 °C, TJ = TA + 30 = 71 °C, check the Table 5.2.2–6 of GJB/Z 299C-2006, get the temperature coefficient πT = 0.87;

(7) There are four gates in 54LS00, check the Table 5.2.2–17 of GJB/Z 299C-2006, take the number of circuit gates 50 and below, and get the circuit complexity failure rate C1 = 0.1227, C2 = 0.0100;
(8) 54LS00 is a 14-pin dual in-line package (DIP-14), check the Table 5.2.2–31 of GJB/Z 299C-2006, and get the package complexity C3 = 0.0558;
(9) Check Table 5.2.2–14 of GJB/Z 299C-2006, the circuit is a non-CMOS circuit, and the voltage stress coefficient π V = 1.0;
(10) Calculate the working failure rate of the device:

$$\begin{aligned}\lambda_P &= \pi_Q[C_1\pi_T\pi_V + (C_2 + C_3)\pi_E]\pi_L \\ &= 0.5 \times [0.1227 \times 0.87 \times 1.0 + (0.01 + 0.0558) \times 1.0] \times 1.0 \\ &= 0.0862745(10^{-6}/\text{h})\end{aligned}$$

(2) Semiconductor discrete devices

A low-frequency plastic-encapsulated switching diode in the United States has a quality grade of special military grade and an environmental category of G_B. Calculate the failure rate of the device.

Calculation steps:

(1) For foreign devices, use MIL-HDBK-217F (Notice 2);

"Basic Failure Rate Table" of MIL-HDBK-217F, and the reliability model is:

$$\lambda_p = \lambda_b\pi_T\pi_s\pi_c\pi_Q\pi_E \tag{4.37}$$

(2) For switching diodes, check 6.1 of MIL-HDBK-217F, and get the basic failure rate $\lambda_b = 0.0010$;
(3) Ambient temperature $T_A = 50$ °C, $T_J = T_A + 20 = 70$ °C, check the "Temperature Coefficient" table in section 6.1 of MIL-HDBK-217F, and get the temperature coefficient $\pi_T = 3.9$;
(4) The application state of the device is a switching diode, and the conduction voltage is 0.33 V. Check the "Application Coefficient" table in Sect. 6.1 of MIL-HDBK-217F, and the application coefficient $\pi_s = 0.11$
(5) The device is encapsulated in plastic, corresponding to the quality level of plastic. Checking Sect. 6.1 "quality factor" table in MIL-HDBK-217F, it can be got that the quality factor $\pi_Q = 8.0$.
(6) The connection construction factor of the device is a non-metallic connection inside. Check the "Connection Construction" table in Sect. 6.1 of MIL-HDBK-217F, and the quality factor $\pi_c = 2.0$;

The environmental category is G_B, check the "Environmental Coefficient" table in Sect. .1 of MIL-HDBK-217F, and get the environmental coefficient π_E = 1.0;
(7) Calculate the working failure rate of the device:

$$
\begin{aligned}
\lambda_p &= \lambda_b \pi_T \pi_s \pi_c \pi_Q \pi_E \\
&= 0.001 \times 3.9 \times 0.11 \times 8.0 \times 2.0 \times 1.0 \\
&= 0.006864 \times 10^{-6}/\text{h}
\end{aligned}
$$

(3) Passive components

For a domestic metal film resistor, the quality grade is B_1, and the environmental category is G_B. Calculate the working failure rate of the device.

Calculation steps:

(1) For domestic devices, use GJB/Z 299C-2006 for estimation.
(2) Metal film resistors, check GJB/Z 299C-2006, the general resistor reliability model is:

$$
\lambda_p = \lambda_b \pi_E \pi_Q \pi_R \tag{4.38}
$$

(3) The rated temperature of the resistor is 125 °C, the rated power is 0.5W, and the actual power used is 0.3 W, so the electrical stress ratio S is 0.6, and the shell temperature of the device is 40 °C. Check GJB/Z 299C-2006 for 5.5.2-1, the basic failure rate $\lambda_b = 0.0045$;
(4) The environmental category is G_B, check the Table 5.5.2-2 of GJB/Z 299C-2006, and get the environmental coefficient $\pi_E = 1$;
(5) The quality level of the device is B_1, check the Table 5.5.2-3 of GJB/Z 299C-2006, and get the quality factor $\pi_Q = 0.6$;
(6) The resistance value of the resistor is 300 kohms, check the Table 5.5.2-4 of GJB/Z 299C-2006, and the resistance coefficient $\pi_R = 1.6$;
(7) Calculate the working failure rate of the device:

$$
\begin{aligned}
\lambda_p &= \lambda_b \pi_E \pi_Q \pi_R \\
&= 0.0045 \times 1 \times 0.6 \times 1.6 \\
&= 0.00432 \times 10^{-6}/\text{h}
\end{aligned}
$$

component stress analysis method prediction table.

4.3.6.3 Similar Products Method

1. **Method description**

The similar product method is to use the reliability data of existing mature products similar to the product to estimate the reliability of the product. The reliability data of mature products mainly come from field statistics and laboratory test results.

The similarity factors considered by the similar product law generally include:

- The similarity of product structure and function;
- The similarity of design;

- The similarity of materials and manufacturing processes;
- The similarity of service profiles (assurance, usage and environmental conditions).

2. **Estimated procedure for similar products method**

(1) Identify similar products

Considering the aforementioned similar factors, select the product that is most similar to the new product and has reliability data.

(2) Analyze the impact of similar factors on reliability

Analyze the impact of various factors considered on product reliability, analyze the design differences between new products and old products and the impact of these differences on reliability.

(3) Reliability prediction of new products

According to the aforementioned analysis, determine the ratio *k of the reliability value* (failure rate, reliability, etc.) of the new product and the old product. Of course, these ratios should be evaluated by experienced experts. Finally, the reliability of the new product is predicted based on the ratio.

$$\lambda_{\mathrm{N}} = \lambda_{\mathrm{O}} \times k \tag{4.39}$$

(4) Example of similar products method

For example, for a photon stimulated emission loss compound microscope, its reliability index is known $\lambda_{\mathrm{O}} = 126.87 \times 10^{-6}$, and the failure rate of each module before upgrading is shown in Table 4.11.

In order to improve the width of field of view and camera precision of this type of microscope, two improvement measures have been taken for this compound microscope:

- The photon imaging laser is upgraded to a two-photon imaging laser;
- The hardware structure of the electronic control system remains unchanged, and only the software function is optimized.

Table 4.11 Failure rate of each module before upgrade

Serial number	Module	Failure rate ($\times 10^{-6}$/h)
1	Photonic imaging lasers	32.64
2	Scanning imaging module	18.72
3	Fluorescence imaging module	22.53
4	CMOS camera	38.79
5	Electronic control system	14.19

Table 4.12 (Product name) example of prediction table for similar products

Serial number	Unit name	Similar product name	Similarity coefficient $k\ i$	Similar product failure rate	Unit failure rate $\lambda\ i$ ($\times 10^{-6}$/h)

It is estimated that the new microscope is very similar to the original microscope, the difference is that the photon imaging laser is upgraded to a two-photon laser. Compared with the single-photon laser, the new two-photon laser has higher step energy and higher reliability. High, but there is no statistical data on the failure rate of new products. According to the expert score, the reliability ratio k is 0.96, and the failure rate of the new two-photon imaging laser can be predicted:

$$\lambda_{SN} = \lambda_{SO} \times k = 0.96 \times 32.64 \times 10^{-6} = 31.3344 \times 10^{-6} \tag{4.40}$$

Then the reliability index of the new two-photon microscope can be obtained $\lambda_N = 125.5644 \times 10^{-6}$, and the (product name) similar product method prediction table is shown in Table 4.12.

4.3.6.4 Scoring Prediction Method

1. **Method description**

Experienced designers or experts score several factors that affect reliability, such as unit complexity, technical level, working hours, and environmental conditions, and conduct a comprehensive analysis of the scores to obtain the relative reliability ratio of each unit product. A product with known reliability data is used as a benchmark to predict the reliability of other products. When applying this method, this book stipulates that the time factor is based on the working time of the digital medical equipment system, that is, the predicted unit λ is based on the working time of the system.

2. **Scoring factor**

Factors usually considered in the scoring prediction method are: complexity, technical level, working hours and environmental conditions. In engineering practice, the scoring factors can be increased or decreased according to the characteristics of the product.

3. **Scoring principle**

We use the expected parameter of product failure rate to illustrate the scoring principle. The scoring principles are as follows:

- The scores of various factors range from 1 to 10, with higher scores indicating poorer reliability.

- Complexity: it is based on the number of components that make up the unit and the ease of their assembly to assess the simplest rating of 1 point, the most complex rating of 10 points.
- Technical level: Evaluated according to the maturity of the current technical level of the unit, with 10 points for the lowest level and 1 point for the highest level.
- Working time: Evaluated according to the working time of the unit, the premise is to take the working time of the system as the time reference. When the system is working, the unit that works all the time is rated as 10 points, and the unit that works for the shortest time is rated as 1 point.
- Environmental conditions: Evaluated according to the environment in which the unit is located, 10 points for the unit that will withstand extremely harsh and severe environmental conditions during the working process, and 1 point for the best environmental conditions.

4. **Scoring**

Experienced designers or experts are invited to rate several factors that affect reliability, such as unit complexity, technical level, working time and environmental conditions, and the number of raters is at least 5. First, the raters score each product according to the scoring principle, and then the person in charge of reliability prediction synthesizes the scores of each product by each rater, that is, the 4 factor scores of each product are the average of the scores of each rater. value.

5. **Scoring reliability prediction**

Knowing the failure rate of a certain unit λ^*, the failure rate of other units is:λ_i

$$\lambda_i = \lambda^* \cdot C_i \tag{4.41}$$

In the formula:

i = 1, 2, ..., nThe number of units;
C_i Scoring coefficient for the i-th unit.

$$C_i = \omega_i / \omega^* \tag{4.42}$$

In the formula:

ω_i The score of the i-th unit;
ω^* The failure rate λ^* is the number of scores for the unit.

$$\omega_i = \prod_{j=1}^{4} r_{ij} \tag{4.43}$$

In the formula:

Table 4.13 Calculation of the failure rate of a radiotherapy system

Serial number	Unit name	Complexity r_{i1}	Techinque level r_{i2}	Operating hours r_{i3}	Environmental conditions r_{i4}	Scores for each unit ω_i	Grading coefficient for each unit $C_i = \omega_i/\omega^*$	Unit failure rate λ i ($\times 10^{-6}$/h)
1	A 1	5	6	5	5	750	0.3	85.4
2	A 2	7	6	10	2	840	0.336	95.6
3	A 3	10	10	5	5	(ω^*) 2500	1.0	(λ^*) 284.5
4	A 4	8	8	5	7	2240	0.896	254.9
5	A 5	4	2	10	8	640	0.256	72.8
6	A 6	6	5	5	5	750	0.3	85.4

Table 4.14 (Product name) score prediction table

Serial number	Unit name	Complexity r_{i1}	Techinque level r_{i2}	Operating hours r_{i3}	Environmental conditions r_{i4}	Unit score ω_i	Unit grading factor $C_i = \omega_i/\omega*$	Unit failure rate λ i ($\times 10^{-6}$/h)

r_{ij} The score of the first i unit and the first factor j;
$j = 1$ Complexity;
$j = 2$ Technical level;
$j = 3$ Working hours;
$j = 4$ Environmental condition.

6. **Scoring example**

A radiotherapy system consists of six sub-systems, A_1 to A_6.. It is known that the failure rate of A_3 is 284.5×10^{-6}/h, that is, $\lambda^* = 284.5 \times 10^{-6}$/h, and the failure rate of other subsystems can be obtained by using the scoring method. The general calculation can be done using tables, see Tables 4.13 and 4.14.

4.3.7 Reliability Prediction Steps

1. **Estimated unit failure rate value**

The reliability prediction of the system is a bottom-up system synthesis process from the local to the whole and from the small to the large. Therefore, the basic failure rate of the system and the failure rate value of the unit in the task reliability model (unit refers to the smallest level product when reliability is predicted, which can be components or equipment, or subsystems or systems) should be estimated first. That is, according to the development stage and characteristics of the product, choose the appropriate prediction method to calculate the failure rate value of each product.

2. **The estimated failure rate of the system**

After obtaining the failure rate value of each product (box) in the reliability block diagram, the failure rate value can be calculated according to the failure rate mathematical model of the system.

3. **Comparison with failure rate requirements or assigned values for the system**

For systems and products that have proposed failure rate requirements, the reliability prediction value must be compared with the failure rate requirement value (specified value) or assigned value (specified value) to judge whether the design meets the failure rate requirement.

4. **Identify weak links affecting system reliability**

Arrange the expected reliability values of the products that make up the system from low to high, and the products that are ranked first are the weak links in reliability, and design improvement measures must be taken until the re-estimated results meet the requirements.

4.3.8 System Reliability Prediction Requirements

System reliability prediction is based on the predicted value of each unit that makes up the system, and according to the system reliability model, the basic failure rate and task failure rate of the system are predicted. For the use of previous systems or finished products (without any improvement/modification), and the purchased shelf products are no longer predicted for reliability, their previous statistical values or reliability indicators are directly used.

4.3.8.1 Basic Reliability Prediction

The basic reliability model is a series model, assuming that the system components are independent of each other, then:

$$\begin{aligned} R_S(t_s) &= R_1(t_1) \cdot R_2(t_2) \cdot \cdots \cdot R_n(t_n) \\ \text{MTBF} &= \int_0^{\infty} R_S(t_S)\,\mathrm{d}t_S \end{aligned} \tag{4.44}$$

$$\overline{\lambda_S} = 1/\text{MTBF} \tag{4.45}$$

In the formula:

$R_S(t_s)$ System reliability;
$R_i(t_i)$ The reliability of the i-th unit;
t_s System working time (h);
t_i The working time of the i-th unit (h);
$\overline{\lambda_S}$ System average failure rate (1/h).

If the life of each unit obeys the exponential distribution, and it is $d_i = t_i/t_S$ assumed that the failure rate of the product is zero when it is not working, then

$$\begin{aligned} R_S(t_s) &= e^{-\lambda_1 t_1} \cdot e^{-\lambda_i t_i} \cdots e^{-\lambda_n t_n} \\ &= e^{-(\lambda_1 d_1 + \lambda_2 d_2 + \cdots + \lambda_n d_n)t_s} \\ &= e^{-\sum_{i=1}^{n} \lambda_i \cdot d_i t_s} \end{aligned} \tag{4.46}$$

In the formula:

λ_i Failure rate of the i-th unit (1/h);
d_i The duty cycle of the i-th cell.

Since each unit obeys the exponential distribution and is a series model, the system must also obey the exponential distribution, that is:

$$R_S(t_s) = e^{-\lambda_s t_s} = e^{-\sum_{i=1}^{n} \lambda_i \cdot d_i t_s} \tag{4.47}$$

Therefore:

$$\lambda_s = \sum_{i=1}^{n} \lambda_i d_i \tag{4.48}$$

In the formula:

λ_s System failure rate (1/h)
λ_i the failure rate of the i-th unit (1/h)

Strictly speaking, the working time of each component unit in the system is not consistent. For example, during the use of digital medical equipment, the actual working time of each unit (subcomponent) is less than the working time of the whole system.

In engineering, if the failure rate of each unit is based on the working time of the system (called the time base), that is $\lambda_i d_i = t_i/t_S = 1.0$; or the time base of the failure rate of each unit cannot be known, for simplicity, the working time of each unit in the system can be considered equal. Right now:

$$\lambda_s = \sum_{i=1}^{n} \lambda_i \tag{4.49}$$

That is to say, for the series model, the failure rate of the system is equal to the sum of the failure rates of each unit. In addition, it is worth mentioning that if the working time of some units in the system is less than the working time of the system, the predicted result according to formula (4.49) must be conservative.

The basic failure rate of digital diagnosis and treatment equipment is the prediction of the digital diagnosis and treatment equipment itself, and the calculation of the mean time between failures is shown in formula (4.48)

$$\text{MTBF} = 1/\lambda_s \tag{4.50}$$

λ_s according to formula (4.47).

4.3.8.2 System Task Reliability Prediction

When predicting mission reliability, attention should be paid to whether the previous basic reliability prediction values can be directly applied here. It should be considered that the environments of the two are different and need to be converted according to the environmental coefficient.

1. **System task reliability prediction steps**

The task reliability prediction of the system is calculated according to the task reliability block diagram method. The expected steps are as follows:

(1) Establish a task reliability block diagram of the system, and determine the working time T of the digital medical equipment system;
(2) Determine the working time t_i of each unit in the system;
(3) Calculate the operating ratio *S*/*F* of the unit:

$$(\text{S/F}) = t_i/T \tag{4.51}$$

If the MTBF of the unit is estimated based on the working time of the digital medical equipment system, its $(S/F)_i = 1.0$;

(4) Convert MTBF unit to MTBCF unit:

$$\text{MTBCF}_{\text{unit}} = \text{MTBF}_{\text{unit}}/(S/F)_i \tag{4.52}$$

(5) The reliability of the unit is:

$$R_{\text{unit}}(T) = \text{EXP}(-T/\text{MTBCF}_{\text{unit}}) \tag{4.53}$$

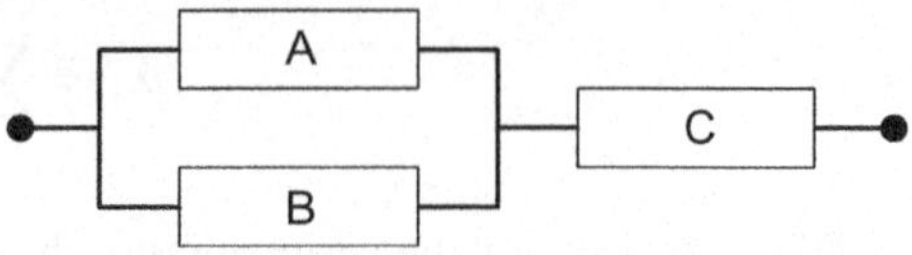

Fig. 4.12 Mission reliability model of a system

(6) Calculate the reliability of the system according to the reliability block diagram.

2. **Examples of system task reliability prediction**

The mission reliability model of a system is shown in Fig. 4.12. The MTBF of equipment A, B, and C are the same, all are 500 h, the working time is the same, all are 1 h, and *S*/*F* = 1.0. Estimated mission failure rate of the system.

Calculation process:

(1) Calculate the reliability of the unit (equipment), the MFHBF of each unit is the same, so the reliability of each unit is the same, which is:

$$R_A(T) = R_B(T) = R_C(T) = R_{unit}(T)$$
$$= \mathrm{EXP}(-T/\mathrm{MTBCF}_{unit}) = \mathrm{EXP}(-1/500) = 0.998$$

(2) The reliability of the system is:

$$R_S(T) = [1 - (1 - R_A(T))(1 - R_B(T))]R_C(T)$$
$$= \left[1 - (1 - 0.998)^2\right] \times 0.998$$
$$= 0.997996$$

4.3.9 Estimation Report

4.3.9.1 Format of the Estimation Report

The estimation report format is as follows:

(1) Overview
(2) Reference documents
(3) Reliability requirements
(4) System (product) working principle
(5) System (product) reliability model
(6) Analysis of expected results

4.3.9.2 Instructions for Preparing the Forecast Report

1. **Reliability requirements**

According to the requirements of the contract or agreement, describe the qualitative/quantitative requirements of the expected system (product) reliability, so as to compare with the expected results.

2. **System (product) working principle diagram**

Use functional block diagrams and text to briefly explain the expected system (product) composition structure and its functional relationship.

3. **System (product) reliability model**

Introduce in detail the reliability relationship among the various components of the system (product), and establish its basic reliability model and task reliability model. Simultaneously, the simplifications and assumptions in the modeling process are explained.

4. **Process estimation and its output**

Indicate the basic failure rate of the system (product), the task reliability prediction process, and the predicted final result respectively.

5. **Analysis of expected results**

The result analysis should at least include the following contents.

(1) Comparative analysis with index requirements: The system (product) reliability prediction result should be compared with 1.25 times of the reliability requirement value (maturity period), and a conclusion should be given whether the requirements are met.
(2) Weak link analysis: New products are in the process of increasing reliability from the beginning of development to the maturity stage. Regardless of whether the reliability prediction value meets the requirements, the reliability weak links should be analyzed according to the reliability prediction situation, and Take necessary design or process improvement measures for weak links (generally, the external interface should not be changed) to increase reliability. The increase measures should be analyzed and explained in detail. If the external interface must be changed, it must be changed according to the requirements of the technical agreement Handle application and approval procedures.
(3) The increase in basic failure rate cannot be achieved at the expense of task failure rate. For inherent reliability weaknesses that cannot be eliminated by design, the strict quality control measures that should be taken in manufacturing should be specified.

4.3.9.3 Precautions

The reporting unit shall specify in the contract work description:

(1) Identify alternative modeling methods;

(2) Reliability parameters and constraints (including failure criteria, etc.);
(3) life profile and mission profile;
(4) The estimated method of confirmation;
(5) Source of failure rate data;
(6) Information required for support analysis;
(7) For products designated by the reporting unit, its reliability level and related use and environment information shall be provided;
(8) Information items to be submitted.

Among them, (2), (3), and (7) are matters that must be determined.

4.4 Failure Modes, Effects and Criticality Analysis

4.4.1 Overview

Failure mode, effects and criticality analysis (Failure Mode, Effects and Criticality Analysis, FMECA) is to analyze all possible failure modes of the product and their possible impacts, and evaluate the severity and probability of occurrence of each failure mode. An inductive analysis method of classification is a bottom-up inductive analysis method, which helps to grasp all possible potential problems of the product and take targeted preventive measures.

FMECA includes design FMECA and process FMECA, and design FMECA includes hardware FMECA and software FMECA. FMECA is an important work item of product reliability analysis. It can help designers to understand potential product problems more comprehensively and clearly and take necessary improvement measures. It is also a tool for maintenance analysis, safety analysis, testability analysis and support analysis Base.

Generally, repairable products correspond to the concept of failure, and non-repairable products correspond to the concept of failure. Failure mode, Effects and Criticality Analysis is usually also called failure mode, effect and criticality analysis. Criticality analysis includes qualitative analysis (criticality) and quantitative analysis. Analysis (degree of criticality). For ease of exposition and consistency with the guidelines, it is collectively called Failure Mode, Effects, and criticality Analysis in this book.

This section mainly introduces the principles, methods, implementation procedures and related precautions of failure mode, effect and criticality analysis. In the development stage of digital medical equipment, the failure mode, impact and criticality analysis technology can be used to establish the product failure mode database, failure cause database, and preventive measure database, and take preventive and verification measures for failures with high severity levels.

4.4.2 *Work Item Highlights*

Various defects and weak links that affect product reliability should be found in product design (functional design, hardware design, software design), production (production feasibility analysis, process design, production equipment design and use) and use, in order to improve digital diagnosis and treatment. The quality and reliability level of the equipment provides the basis for improvement.

The failure mode, impact and criticality analysis is part of the design work, and the basic principle of "whoever designs, who analyzes" must be followed, and timely improvement is the basis for ensuring the effectiveness of this work.

4.4.3 *Failure Mode, Effect and Criticality Analysis Method*

This part describes the hardware FMECA and software FMECA methods of Design FMECA (D-FMECA), as well as the process FMECA method.

4.4.3.1 Function and Hardware FMECA

1. **Function and FMECA connotation**

    (1) Functional FMECA: According to each functional failure mode of the product, analyze the possible causes and effects of the functional failure mode. When using this method, output functions should be listed one by one. Generally, the product is analyzed downward from the "initial agreement level", that is, the analysis is top-down, and it can also be analyzed from any functional level of the product to any direction.

(2) Hardware FMECA: According to each hardware failure mode of the product, analyze the possible causes and effects of the hardware failure mode. Generally, the analysis is from the component level to the equipment level, that is, bottom-up analysis, and can also be analyzed from any level of product to any direction.

2. **Scope of analysis**

The functional and hardware FMECA analysis scope should cover all components on the digital medical equipment system:

- For electronic components or systems: components, boards/modules, equipment level, subsystems, systems;
- For mechanical components or systems: smallest decomposable parts and standard parts, structural details, assemblies, equipment, subsystems, systems

3. **Agreed level of analysis**

The agreed levels of analysis include: component level (infield replaceable unit), equipment level (outside replaceable unit), subsystem level, system level, and machine level.

4.4.3.2 Software FMECA

Refer to GJB/Z 1391-2006 to carry out FMECA work on each system, subsystem, software (program), module, and statement, confirm reasonable and effective corrective measures and implement them in the design in time, and provide corresponding basis for maintenance work and guarantee work.

1. **Scope and levels of analysis**

The scope of software FMECA analysis should cover the embedded software, communication software, task system software and corresponding software/hardware integrated system of the digital medical equipment system. The whole machine is analyzed sequentially.

2. **Agreed level of analysis**

The agreed levels of analysis include: module level, subroutine level, program level, software/hardware integrated system level, and complete machine level.

4.4.3.3 Process FMECA

Refer to GJB/Z 1391-2006 to carry out FMECA work on the product process, confirm reasonable and effective corrective measures and implement them in the process in time to ensure and improve product process reliability.

1. **Timing and scope of analysis**

Before the product process feasibility analysis and production tooling preparation, process FMECA work should be carried out from parts to systems. Process FMECA mainly considers the analysis of product trial production process, and may also include process FMECA of packaging, storage, transportation and other processes.

2. **Clarify the relationship between process FMECA and design**

The defects in the process FMECA cannot be overcome by changing the product design, mainly by taking effective measures in the process design and process FMEA, and the principle of " whoever designs the process, who analyzes it " should be adhered to. In the process FMECA, product design characteristics should also be fully considered, and product designers should be invited to participate in the analysis work as needed, and full exchanges of opinions between different departments should be promoted to ensure that the product meets the needs of "customers" to the greatest extent.

3. **Master the Iterative Process of Process FMECA**

Process FMECA is to prioritize the risk priority number (RPN) value of the process failure mode, and take effective improvement measures for key processes, and then track the improved RPN until the RPN value meets the acceptable level. Process FMECA is a dynamic and iterative analysis process.

4. **Accumulate experience, pay attention to information**

Like the design FMECA, the process FMECA should also accumulate information about the process failure mode, cause, severity level (S), occurrence probability level (O) and detection difficulty level (D) from similar trial production processes or procedures, and Establish a corresponding database to provide support for the effective implementation of process FMECA.

4.4.4 FMECA Work Steps

4.4.4.1 Analytical Assumptions

1 **Failure mode analysis assumptions**

The failure modes of the product should be assumed according to the function and failure criteria of the product. In order to ensure a comprehensive analysis, at least the following typical failure modes should be assumed and analyzed.

(1) Run in advance;
(2) Unable to work during the prescribed working hours;
(3) Intermittent work;
(4) Working during the stipulated unscheduled working hours;
(5) The output disappears or malfunctions during work;
(6) Decreased output or working ability;
(7) Other failure states in terms of system characteristics and work requirements or work conditions.

2. **Failure effects analysis assumptions**

Failure effects can be the consequences of dual or multiple failures. When analyzing the impact of a certain failure mode, it should be assumed that its protection device, protected part, compensation facility or redundancy/standby device also fails, and its consequences should be analyzed.

Some failures are entirely due to operator error or lightning strikes. If such a failure could have catastrophic consequences, its impact should be analyzed.

For potential failures beyond the damage tolerance, the failure modes they may develop into should be estimated and their effects analyzed.

4.4.4.2 Failure Criteria

The following failure criteria apply to reliability maintainability analysis and design, and each system should be further specified:

(1) Some functions of the digital medical equipment system are lost or will be lost;
(2) Part of the performance of the digital diagnosis and treatment equipment system is degraded or will be degraded (subject to the corresponding technical conditions);
(3) Causing disassembly, replacement or downtime for maintenance.

4.4.4.3 FMECA Work Coordination

1. **FMECA work input**

FMECA work input requirements are as follows:

(1) Overall design of the digital medical equipment system and related systems;
(2) Task profile, life profile and environmental profile of medical equipment;
(3) Functional block diagrams and reliability block diagrams of each system and equipment;
(4) Design drawings and relevant technical information;
(5) Reliability data of similar models.

2. **FMECA work output**

Requirements of FMECA are mainly in the following aspects:

(1) Determine reliability critical and important components;
(2) Reliability Centered Maintenance Analysis (RCMA);
(3) Integrated Logistics Support Analysis (ILSA);
(4) Safety analysis and evaluation;
(5) Output maintenance work and maintenance information;
(6) Formulate reliability and maintainability test plan;
(7) Improved design;
(8) Criticality matrix diagram.

3. **FMECA failure rate data sources**

   (1) When conducting criticality analysis, GJB/Z 299C-2006 should be used as the main data source for the failure rate of domestic electronic components; if there are imported electronic components, use MIL-HDBK-217F (*MIL ITARY HANDBOOK RELIABILITY PREDICTION OF ELECTRONIC EQUIPMENT*) failure rate data;
   (2) Usage information and reliability data of similar products.

4.4.5 *FMECA Detailed Work Requirements*

The hardware and software of each system of digital diagnosis and treatment equipment must undergo FMECA, and the scope of analysis covers all electronic systems of the entire digital diagnosis and treatment equipment system.

For the work of influence degree, due to the lack of domestic data at present, in the analysis of existing digital medical equipment, the failure rate of each component is mainly listed.

4.4.5.1 Function and Hardware FMECA Working Rules

According to the technical status of the product, make a list of hardware products, divide them by function, and evaluate each failure mode according to the function of the product. When analyzing, list each level of the product, and then analyze its possible failure modes and their impact. The failure effects of products at all levels are related to subsystems and system functions. This method can be analyzed from the component or component level and then extended to the system level, that is, bottom-up analysis.

The main steps of function and hardware FMECA are shown in Fig. 4.13.

1. **Function and hardware FMECA system definition**

The first step in performing functional and hardware FMECA is to define the object system to be analyzed, including:

(1) Determine the task function and working mode of the system;
(2) Determine the life profile, task profile and environmental profile of the system;
(3) Determine the task time of the system;
(4) Determine the block diagram of the system (functional block diagram, reliability block diagram).

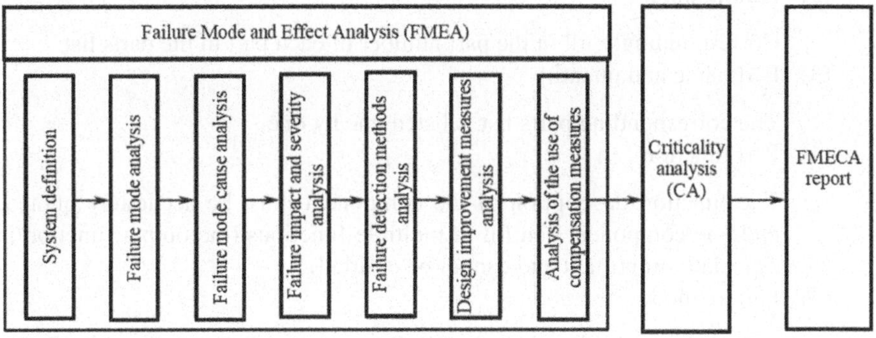

Fig. 4.13 Main steps of function and hardware FMECA

2. **Determining the agreement level**

Determine the content of the agreement level as follows:

(1) The agreed levels of hardware at all levels of digital medical equipment are divided into "whole machine-system-sub-system-replaceable unit parts (component level, board level)";
(2) The "initial agreed level" is usually a replaceable unit part;
(3) "Agreed level" refers to the products next to the upper level for list analysis. For example, when performing FMECA of a certain subsystem, fill in the name of the component (such as a certain equipment) at the agreed level, and list the analysis objects in the FMECA form. The next level of product that should be included (eg. power board, motherboard). The lowest agreed level shall be "component level or board level".

3. **Fill out the parts list**

List all widgets one level below the convention hierarchy, including:

(1) Part number, carry out accurate numbering, and assign a number to the parts with the same characteristics, same functions, and same failures;
(2) Part name;
(3) Drawing number or model;
(4) Quantity refers to the quantity of the system or equipment components including the product;
(5) Technical characteristics, detailed technical characteristics related to expected failure, such as pressure, flow, voltage, etc.;
(6) Remarks, focusing on the status in the system, relevance, combination and other qualitative technical characteristics.

4. **Hardware FMECA analysis**

(1) Invalid number

Number (Serial Number) each failure mode in the analysis Table

(2) Part number

Correspondingly fill in the part number of each part in the parts list.

(3) Part name and quantity

The corresponding parts list is listed one by one.

(4) Part function

The function description of the component must be accurately quoted, and one component can fill in multiple functions (the output function is especially important and cannot be omitted)

(5) Failure mode

Conceive and fill in all possible failure modes of the analyzed hardware (note: all, that is, complete enumeration), and the general failure modes can be considered from the following aspects:

- No function output when required;
- Loss of function (e.g. breakage);
- Malfunction (incompatibility between output and input requirements, such as shimmy, sticking, etc.);
- Degraded functionality (output outside the allowable range for stated performance, but within the driver's control limits, such as increased vibration or response time, etc.);
- Untimely function output (such as too early, too late function output). For mechanical components, failure modes should be accurately described, for example:

  (1) Damage (including: chipping, fracture, fatigue, cracks …);
  (2) Stuck (or bound, or stuck);
  (3) Degradation (including corrosion, peeling, wear …);
  (4) Disconnect, fall off;
  (5) Deformation;
  (6) Leakage;
  (7) Overheating (fire);
  (8) Explosion;
  (9) Stuck;
  (10) Toxic fumes.

(6) Cause of failure

Causes are given in relation to the assumed corresponding failure modes, and the effects of failure at adjacent and next levels of analysis should be considered. Various possible causes for the corresponding failure mode should be listed:

- Internal causes (component failure);
- For external reasons (environmental deterioration, component damage, and other external equipment/system failures), please refer to the worksheet "References for Failure Causes";
- Human errors in design, maintenance or production activities (such as dimensional errors, collisions, improper assembly, etc.) are not usually considered as causes of failure; Errors should be considered as failure causes; it must be noted that there are multiple failure causes for one failure mode. Additionally, a given cause can be the triggering event for several failure modes. Therefore, the effects and consequences of the failure mode and the cause of failure should be considered at the same time, and the possible effects should be filled in the " Failure Effect " column.

(7) Task stage

Fill in the phases of operation in which the failure may occur. If there is no specific phase, "all" should be indicated.

(8) Failure effects

Fill in the impact on the safety, task capability, performance, use and status of digital medical equipment; for each failure mode/failure cause, the failure impact on the following levels of products should be analyzed, generally divided into the following 5 parts, which should be based on It depends on the level of the analysis agreement, and the following Serial Numbers should also be used in the analysis table to distinguish the impact on different levels:

(1) Component level;
(2) Component level;
(3) Subsystem level;
(4) System level;
(5) Equipment level.

It is necessary to write out the influence or no influence on each level. If there are different influences under different working conditions, all possible reasons must be listed. If the cause of the primary failure could be a secondary failure, then that secondary failure should also be analyzed.

In addition, for hidden failures, those subordinate failures inside the system or system interface failures that will cause catastrophe or danger must find out the cause, and the dependent failures should be analyzed under the most severe conditions.

(9) Impact number

Each failure effect should be numbered according to the Serial Number. If two failure modes can cause the same effect at the system level and the digital medical equipment system level, use the same failure effect number.

(10) Design compensation guarantee measures

According to the failure effects, possible redundancy, backup modules or circuits, design tolerances, mechanical clearances, etc. should be given, and these contents should be verified and evaluated in the column of failure effects; the analysis of design assurance measures is aimed at the cause of each failure mode, Influence Proposes possible design compensation measures, which is an important link related to whether the product reliability can be effectively improved. Analysts should point out and evaluate those compensation measures that can be used to eliminate or reduce the failure effect. These compensation measures are divided into design compensation measures and operator emergency compensation measures, and maintenance work such as "part replacement" cannot be generally used as compensation measures.

(1) Design compensation measures include:

- Redundant equipment that can continue to work when the product fails;
- Safety or security devices (such as monitoring and alarm devices);

- Alternative ways of working (such as backup or auxiliary equipment);
- Design or process improvements that can eliminate or mitigate failure effects (such as optimized components, thermal design, derating design, environmental stress screening and process improvements, etc.).

(2) Compensation measures for operators:

- Special use and maintenance procedures to try to avoid or prevent the occurrence of failure;
- The most appropriate remedial action that the operator should take in the event of a failure.

(11) Detective

For each failure mode found through analysis, analyze its failure detection method in order to provide basis for system maintainability, testability design and system maintenance; failure detection methods generally include visual inspection, in-situ test and other means, such as Automatic sensing devices, sensing instruments, audio alarm devices, display alarm devices, etc.

(12) Security impact

Security severity is categorized as follows:

- CAT: Indicates catastrophic failure;
- HAZ: Indicates dangerous failure;
- MAJ: Indicates a major failure;
- MIN: Indicates slight failure;
- NSE: Indicates no security impact.

The classification of security severity corresponds to the system level of digital medical equipment. For each impact, it should be clarified whether it is a single-point failure state or a state combined with other failures.

(13) The impact of task failure rate

The impact of task failure rate corresponds to the system level of digital diagnosis and treatment equipment, and is generally divided into "affected (Y)" and "no impact (N)", and "no impact to impacted (N to Y)" can also be filled. Note in the remarks column the conditions that occur from nothing.

(14) Severity category

The category should be determined according to the following rules according to the severity of the failure impact or consequence, combined with the impact on safety and task failure rate:

(1) Category I (catastrophic failure): failure that may cause damage to digital medical equipment or even casualties;

(2) Category II (fatal failure): It will not cause damage to digital medical equipment or casualties, but may cause serious injury to personnel or serious damage to the digital medical equipment system, or failure to complete the function;
(3) Category III (critical failure): It will not cause the above consequences, but may cause minor injuries to personnel or minor damage to the digital medical equipment system;
(4) Category IV (slight failure): It will not cause the above consequences, but it will cause failure of unplanned maintenance.

(15) Failure rate

It refers to the failure rate listed for the failure mode of the product, and the main sources include:
(1) Data obtained from actual tests;
(2) Data obtained from statistical analysis;
(3) Relevant data provided by the supplier;
(4) Data obtained by analogy analysis of similar products;
(5) Data provided by standards and manuals, such as GJB/Z 299C-2006, NPRD reliability data of non-electronic components, etc.

(16) Remark column

Used to describe the following:
(1) Explanations related to other columns, such as task failure rate impact;
(2) When there is a redundancy/standby mode, the failure effect of the redundancy/standby equipment must be recorded;
(3) Basis or reasons for acceptance of Type I and Type II failure modes.

(17) Compensation measures implementation department

Mainly fill in the following contents:
(1) Design department;
(2) Manufacturing department;
(3) Purchasing department;
(4) Suppliers.

(18) Implementation of compensation measures
(1) The scope of implementation, whether all compensation measures have been implemented, and the batches of the implemented products;
(2) Description of remaining issues.

(19) Test description

Briefly describe what experiments have demonstrated the effectiveness and rationality of compensatory measures.

(20) Process inspection instructions

Briefly describe which process inspections are required for compensation measures in manufacturing to ensure.

(21) Personnel detection method

Corresponding to the failure mode, clearly describe the means by which the operator can discover the occurrence of the failure.

(22) Use repair compensation measures

After the failure occurs, the maintenance measures to be taken, such as cleaning, lubrication, in-situ adjustment, out-of-position adjustment, replacement, in-situ processing and repair, off-position processing and repair, glue injection, paint touch-up, etc.

(23) Required equipment and tools

A list of equipment and tools required for failure detection and repair, including name, model/specification and quantity.

(24) Maintenance profession and number of personnel

The specialties and number of personnel required for the detection and repair of the failure.

(25) Maintenance time

The time required for the detection and repair of the failure includes the accumulation of the following times:

- Preparation time;
- Failure identification time;
- Failure location time;
- Components-getting time;
- Failure excluding time;
- Testing time.

4.4.5.2 Software FMECA Working Rules

According to the comprehensive technical status of software/hardware products, list the products (that is, software list or program list, module list), divide by product function, and evaluate each failure mode according to function. When analyzing, list each level of the product one by one, and then analyze its possible failure modes and their impact. The failure effects of products at all levels are related to the functions of subsystems and software/hardware integrated systems. This method can be analyzed from the statement level or module level and then extended to the program level and software/hardware integrated system level, that is, bottom-up analysis.

The steps of software FMECA are similar to those of "hardware FMECA". The steps of software FMECA are shown in Fig. 4.14.

1. **Software FMECA System Definition**

The first step in performing FMECA is to define the system to be analyzed include:

(1) Determine the task function and working mode of the software system and the comprehensive relationship with the hardware system.

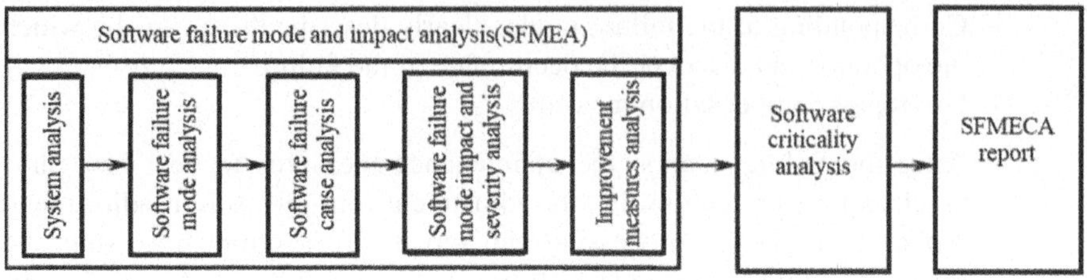

Fig. 4.14 Software FMECA steps

(2) Draw the software function flow chart. In the phase of software requirement analysis, a software requirement specification document should be formed, and the software function flow chart should be given in the document. The functional logic relationship between each software component or software unit in the software/hardware integrated system is given in the flow chart, which shows the hierarchical relationship of the software/hardware integrated system from top to bottom.
(3) Define various boundary conditions of the software.
(4) Define the software contract hierarchy. Software consists of programs, subprograms and program units.

2. **Software FMECA Forms**

(1) The software list is in the same form as the hardware FMECA parts list.
(2) The form of the analysis form is the same as that of the hardware FMECA analysis form.

3. **Software FMECA Initial Agreement Level**

It mainly includes the following contents:

(1) The agreed levels of software at all levels of digital medical equipment are divided into "whole machine—software/hardware integrated system—software (program)—subroutine—module".
(2) The "initial agreement level" is "complete digital medical equipment".
(3) "Agreed level" refers to the products immediately above the upper level for tabular analysis. For example, when performing FMECA at the software level (program level), fill in the name of the program at the agreed level, and list the analysis objects in the FMECA form. The next level of products (such as control subroutines, communication subroutines, etc.). The minimum contract level shall be "module level". The highest agreed level of the finished product should be "Software/Hardware Integrated System". The system is composed of Computer Software Configuration Item (CSCI), Hardware Technical Status Item (HWCI) and Software/Hardware Interface Specification (IRS).

In software products, it should be noted that some software modules are reused and non-developed (such as purchased or shared), and this situation should be marked in the software list. Figure 4.15 shows a software contract hierarchy diagram.

4. **Filling of the Software List**

The following contents:

(1) Software Serial Number, carry out accurate Serial Numbering, and code the same Serial Number for software with the same characteristics, same functions, and same defects;
(2) Software name;
(3) Drawing number or model;
(4) Quantity, which refers to the quantity of the system or equipment components including the software;
(5) Technical characteristics, detailed technical characteristics related to the expected failure, such as scale, control flow, data flow, boundary conditions, constraints, etc.;
(6) Remarks, emphatically explaining the status of the software in the system, relevance, combination and other qualitative technical characteristics.

5. **Software FMECA Analysis**

The filling of the software FMECA list is similar to the filling of the hardware FMECA list, and will not be elaborated here. The analysis requirements for software failure mode analysis, software failure cause analysis, software CA analysis, etc., which are different from hardware FMECA are put forward in the following.

(1) Software failure mode analysis

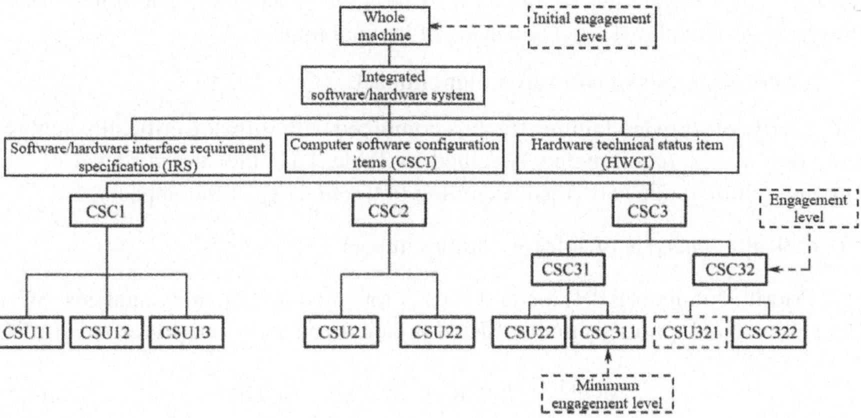

Fig. 4.15 Software agreement level diagram. *Note* CSC means Computer software component, CSU means computer software unit, CSU22 means same software unit, CSU321 means non-development software unit

Software failure modes are manifestations of software failures. The purpose of software failure mode analysis is to find out all possible failure modes for each analyzed software unit. The classification of software failure modes and their typical examples are shown in Table 4.15.

(2) Software failure cause analysis

All possible causes should be analyzed for each software failure mode. The failure of software is often caused by various defects formed in the software development process. See Table 4.16 for software failure causes according to their defect classification and typical examples.

(3) Software failure impact analysis

For each failure mode/cause of failure, the failure effects on the following levels of products shall be analyzed:

(1) Module level
(2) Subroutine level
(3) Program level
(4) System level (software/hardware system)
(5) Digital diagnosis and treatment equipment system level

Similar to hardware FMECA, it is necessary to write out the influence or no influence on each level. If there are different influences under different working conditions, all possible reasons must be listed. If the cause of the primary failure could be a secondary failure, then that secondary failure should also be analyzed.

For embedded software, the failure impact must analyze the functional impact of each software failure mode on the software/hardware integrated system. For complex software, the impact should be listed according to the above five levels; for simple software, the software/hardware can also be directly analyzed The impact of the integrated system allows direct analysis of its final impact.

(4) Severity analysis of software failure impact

The severity of software failure effects is combined with software criticality analysis. According to the requirements specified in Table 4.17, the severity level of each software failure mode is divided according to the severity of the impact.

(5) criticality analysis of software failure impact

Risk Priority Number (RPN) method is used for software criticality analysis (SCA). The software risk priority number SRPN is calculated according to formula (4.54):

$$\mathrm{SRPN} = \mathrm{SESR} \times \mathrm{SOPR} \times \mathrm{SDDR} \tag{4.54}$$

In the formula:

SESR Severity Rating for Effects of Software Failure Modes;

Table 4.15 Classification of software failure modes and their typical examples

Serial number	Category	Examples of software failure modes	
1	Common failure modes of software	(1) The runtime does not meet the requirements	
		(2) The input does not meet the requirements	
		(3) The output does not meet the requirements	
2	Detailed failure modes of software	Input failure	(1) Input not received
			(2) Wrong input received
			(3) The received data is slightly out of tolerance
			(4) The received data is moderately out of tolerance
			(5) The received data is seriously out of tolerance
			(6) Incomplete or missing parameters received
			(7) Others
		Output failure	(1) The output result is wrong
			(2) The accuracy of the output data is slightly out of tolerance
			(3) The output data accuracy is moderately out of tolerance
			(4) The accuracy of the output data is seriously out of tolerance
			(5) Incomplete or missing output parameters
			(6) The output format is wrong
			(7) The printed characters do not meet the requirements
			(8) Output typos (grammatical errors)
		Program failure	(1) The program cannot be started
			(2) Abnormal interruption during program operation
			(3) The program cannot be terminated
			(4) The program cannot exit
			(5) The program runs into an infinite loop
			(6) The operation of the program has harmful effects on other units or the environment
			(7) The program runs slightly overtime
			(8) The program runs moderately overtime

(continued)

Table 4.15 (continued)

Serial number	Category	Examples of software failure modes	
			(9) The program runs seriously timed out
			(10) Others
		Failure to meet functional and performance requirements	(1) The function/performance requirements are not met
			(2) It cannot meet the user's requirements for running time
			(3) It cannot meet the user's requirements for data processing volume
			(4) The multi-user system cannot meet the requirements of the number of users
2	Detailed failure modes of software	Other	(1) The program operation changes the system configuration requirements
			(2) The running of the program changes the data of other programs
			(3) Operating system error
			(4) Inaccurate I/O timing leads to data loss
			(5) Interface failure
			6) Human error
			(7) Hardware error
			(8) Entire system error
			(9) Unreasonable maintenance errors
			(10) Others

SOPR Software failure mode probability of occurrence rating;
SDDR Software Failure Modes Difficulty Level to Detect.

The scoring criteria are shown in Tables 4.18 and 4.19 respectively.

(6) Analysis of improvement measures

According to the cause, impact and severity level of each software failure mode, comprehensively propose targeted improvement measures.

(7) Precautions for software FMECA analysis
(1) Clarify the application focus of software FMECA in different development stages. In the stage of software requirements analysis and general design, use the functional flow chart to find out possible errors related to functions and performance in these two stages, so as to improve the requirements analysis and general design; in the detailed design and coding of software, there may

Table 4.16 Causes of software failures classified by defects and typical examples

Serial number	Software defect type	Detailed software defects	Note
1	Demand defects	(1) The formulation of software requirements is unreasonable or incorrect	
		(2) Incomplete demand	
		(3) There are logic errors	
		(4) The requirement analysis document is wrong	
2	Functional and performance defects	(1) The functions and performance specifications are wrong, or missing functions, or have redundant functions	Most prevalent and most concerned defects
		(2) The information provided to users is wrong or inaccurate	
		(3) Mishandling of abnormal situations	
3	Software structural defects	(1) Program control or control sequence is wrong	Most prevalent and most concerned defects
		(2) The processing process is wrong	
4	Data defects	(1) The data definition or data structure is wrong	Most Prevalent and most concerned defects
		(2) Data access or operation is wrong	
		(3) Variable scaling ratio or unit is incorrect	
		(4) The data range is incorrect	
		(5) Data error or loss	
5	Software implementation and coding defects	(1) Wrong coding or keys	
		(2) Violation of coding style requirements or standards	
		(3) Syntax error	
		(4) The data name is wrong	
		(5) Confusion between local variables and global variables	
6	Software/hardware interface defects	(1) The internal and external interfaces of the software are incorrect	
		(2) The relevant parts of the software are not coordinated in terms of time coordination or data throughput	
		(3) I/O timing errors lead to data loss	

Table 4.17 Scoring criteria for software failure mode effects severity rating (SESR)

Software failure impact possibility of occurrence	The extent of software failure mode effects	Rating scale
Extremely high without warning	Affect the safety of system operation, or do not comply with national security regulations, and cannot issue warnings	10
Extremely high with Warning	Affect the safety of system operation, or do not comply with national security regulations, but can issue warnings	9
Very high	Affected system loses main function and cannot operate	8
High	The system is still functional, but at a degraded level and users are unhappy	7
Medium	The system still works, but loses the convenience and comfort of use	6
Low	The system still works, but it affects the convenience and comfort of use	5
Relatively low	Slight impact	4
Very secondary	Tiny impact	3
Very minor	Minimal impact	2
None	No impact	1

Table 4.18 Scoring criteria for software failure mode occurrence probability rating (SOPR)

Software failure mode occurrence probability	Software failure mode occurrence probability P m reference range (per unit)	Rating scale
Very high (failure is almost inevitable)	$P\text{ m}\geq 5\times10^{-1}$	10
	$1\times10^{-1}\leq P\text{ m}\leq 5\times10^{-1}$	9
High (repeated failure)	$1\times10^{-2}\leq P\text{ m}\leq 1\times10^{-1}$	8
	$1\times10^{-3}\leq P\text{ m}\leq 1\times10^{-2}$	7
Moderate (occasional failure)	$1\times10^{-3}\leq P\text{ m}\leq 2\times10^{-3}$	6
	$2\times10^{-4}\leq P\text{ m}\leq 1\times10^{-3}$	5
Low (relatively few failures)	$1\times10^{-4}\leq P\text{ m}\leq 2\times10^{-4}$	4
	$2\times10^{-5}\leq P\text{ m}\leq 1\times10^{-4}$	3
Very low (nearly impossible to fail)	$1\times10^{-5}\leq P\text{ m}\leq 1\times10^{-5}$	2
	$2\times10^{-6}\leq P\text{ m}\leq 1\times10^{-5}$	1

Table 4.19 Scoring criteria for software failure mode detection probability difficulty level (SDDR)

Likelihood of software failures being detected	Software failure mode detection probability P d reference range (per unit)	Rating scale
Not sure at all	$P\text{ d}<2\times10^{-6}$ Failure cause/mechanism and failure mode may be found, or there is no such detection device at all	10
Very tiny	$P\text{ d}\approx 2\times10^{-6}$ Possibility to discover failure cause/mechanism and failure mode	9
Small	$2\times10^{-6}<P\text{ d}\leq 2\times10^{-4}$ Potential to find failure cause/mechanism and failure mode	8
Very low	$2\times10^{-4}<P\text{ d}\leq 2\times10^{-3}$ Possibility to find failure cause/mechanism and failure mode	7
Low	$2\times10-3<P\text{ d}\leq 1\times10-2$ Possibility to find failure cause/mechanism and failure mode	6
Medium	$1\times10^{-2}<P\text{ d}\leq 2\times10^{-2}$ Possible cause/mechanism of failure and failure mode found	5
Moderately high	$2\times10^{-2}<P\text{ d}\leq 5\times10^{-2}$ Possibility to find failure cause/mechanism and failure mode	4
High	$5\times10^{-2}<P\text{ d}\leq 3.3\times10^{-1}$ Failure cause/mechanism and failure mode may be found	3
Very high	$3.3\times10^{-1}<P\text{ d}$ Possibility to find failure cause/mechanism and failure mode	2
Totally sure	$P\text{ d}\approx 0$ can fully discover the failure cause/mechanism and failure mode	1

be existing and legacy functions Defects related to performance, and use the bottom-up method to verify the impact and severity of software defects, and provide information for software integration and testing;

(2) Clarify and master the main content of the basic steps of software FMECA:

- The analysis object can be a software system, subsystem, component, or a module that can be compiled separately, but the module is generally selected as the minimum analysis unit;
- Software failure modes are also the basis of software FMECA. Software is composed of several functional modules, and its failure modes include both functional failure modes and performance failure modes, but mainly functional failure modes. From this point of view, there is no essential difference between software FMECA and hardware FMECA;
- Software failure causes are caused by software defects being triggered at runtime. For hardware FMECA is to find out the potential failure of functions, and for software FMECA is to find out the key software defects under its critical calling path. Software failure is different from hardware failure. In addition to defects related to functions like hardware failure, software failure also has a defect related only to the software itself. Both defects should be corrected in the software FMECA.

4.4.5.3 Process FMECA Working Rules

1. **Purpose of Process FMECA**

The purpose of the process FMECA is to, on the premise that the product design meets the requirements, aim at the possible failure modes, causes and all the impacts on the product in each process step of the product in the production process, according to the risk priority number of the failure mode (RPN) value, formulate improvement measures for process weak links, and predict or track the effectiveness of reducing RPN value after taking improvement measures, so that RPN can reach an acceptable level, thereby improving product quality and reliability.

2. **Process FMECA Steps**

The steps of process FMECA are shown in Fig. 4.16.

3. **Process FMECA System Definition**

Like "function and hardware FMECA", process FMECA should also define the analysis object. Its content can be summarized as functional analysis, drawing "process flow table" and "parts—process relationship matrix".

Functional analysis: analyze the purpose, function, function and related requirements of the analyzed process.

Draw the "process flow table" and "parts—process relationship matrix", where the "process flow table" represents the functional requirements of the process flow related to each process. It is the preparation work of process FMECA, see Table 4.20.

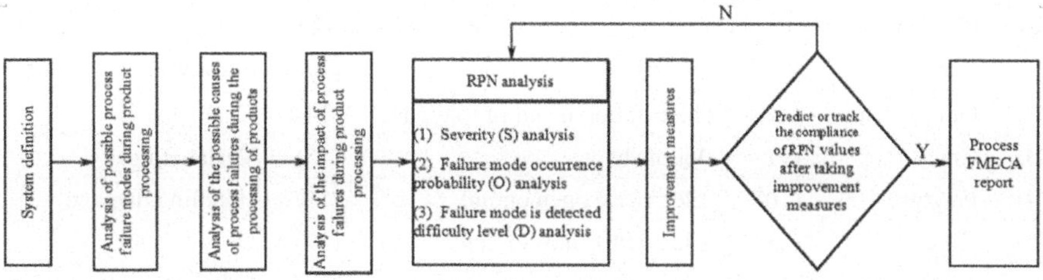

Fig. 4.16 Process FMECA steps

"Parts—process relationship matrix" indicates the relationship between part characteristics and each process of process operation. The parts-process relationship matrix is shown in Table 4.21.

4. **Process Failure Mode Analysis**

Process failure modes refer to process defects that cannot meet product processing, assembly process requirements and/or design intent. It may be the cause of a failure mode in the next (downstream) process, or it may be a consequence of a failure in a previous (upstream) process. In general, defects in product design are not considered in process FMECA. Examples (not limited) of typical process failure modes are shown in Table 4.22.

Table 4.20 Process flow sheet

Part name: production process:
Part number: department name: review: pages of pages
Name/model of equipment: analyst: approval: date of form filling:

Process flow	Enter	Output result
Process 1		
Process 2		
...		

Table 4.21 Component—process relationship matrix

Part name: production process:
Part number: department name: review: pages of pages
Name/model of equipment: analyst: approval: date of form filling:

Component Properties	Process operation			
	Process 1	Process 2	Process 3	...
Feature 1				
Feature 2				
Feature 3				
...				

Table 4.22 Examples of typical process failure modes (not limited to)

(1)	Bending	(7)	Oversize	(13)	Surface is too smooth
(2)	Out of shape	(8)	The location is out of tolerance	(14)	Unlabeled
(3)	Crack	(9)	Out of shape	(15)	Mislabeling
(4)	Fracture	(10)	(Electrical) open circuit	(16)	Handling damage
(5)	Glitch	(11)	(Electrical) short circuit	(17)	Dirty
(6)	Leakage	(12)	The surface is too rough	(18)	Leftovers

Note The failure mode should be described in physical and professional terms instead of the failure phenomenon seen

5. **Cause Analysis of Process Failure**

The process failure cause refers to why the process defect corresponding to the process failure mode occurs. Examples of typical process failure modes are shown in Table 4.23.

6. **Process Failure Impact Analysis**

The impact on the "customer" of the process defect corresponding to the process failure mode. "customer" means the next process/subsequent process, and/or end user. The impact of process failure can be divided into the next process, components and equipment.

(1) For the next process/subsequent process: the impact of process failure should be described by the characteristics of the process/process. Typical examples of the impact of process failure (for the next process /subsequent process) are shown in Table 4.24;

Table 4.23 Examples of typical process failure modes

(1)	Too much torque, too little	(11)	Tool wear
(2)	Incorrect welding current, time and voltage	(12)	Missing parts
(3)	Welding	(13)	Wrong parts
(4)	Incorrect casting gate/vent	(14)	Improper installation
(5)	Bonding is not strong	(15)	Locator wear
(6)	Incorrect heat treatment time, temperature and medium	(16)	Debris on locator
(7)	Gauge is not accurate	(17)	Broken hole
(8)	Improper lubrication	(18)	Machine settings are incorrect
(9)	The internal stress of the workpiece is too large	(19)	Incorrect programming
(10)	No lubrication	(20)	Incorrect tooling or fixtures

Table 4.24 Examples of typical process failure effects (for downstream/subsequent processes)

(1)	Unable to take out	(6)	Unable to match
(2)	Unable to drill/tap	(7)	Unable to machine the surface
(3)	Unable to match	(8)	Cause tool process wear
(4)	Unable to install	(9)	Damaged equipment
(5)	Unable to connect	(10)	Hazardous to operators

(2) For the end user: The impact of process failure should be described by the characteristics of the product. Typical examples of the impact of process failure (for the end user) are shown in Table 4.25.

7. **Risk Priority Number (RPN) Analysis**

The product of the severity level of the process failure mode (S), the probability of occurrence of the process failure mode (O) and the detection difficulty level of the process failure mode (D), namely

$$\text{RPN} = S \times O \times D \tag{4.55}$$

RPN is an evaluation of the risk level of the potential failure mode of the process, which reflects the comprehensive measurement of the possibility of the failure mode of the process and the severity of its consequences. The larger the RPN value, the more harmful the process failure mode is.

Severity level of process failure mode (S): refers to the most serious impact of a certain process failure mode in the process of product processing and assembly. See Table 4.26 for the scoring criteria of its grades.

Occurrence probability level of process failure mode (O): refers to the possibility of occurrence of a certain process failure mode. The number of levels of probability of occurrence (O) is a relatively comparative level within the scope of PFMECA, and does not represent the true probability of occurrence of process failure modes. The scoring criteria are shown in Table 4.27.

Table 4.25 Examples of typical process failure effects (for end users)

(1)	Too much noise	(9)	Unstable work performance
(2)	Excessive vibration	(10)	Excessive loss
(3)	Too much resistance	(11)	Water leakage
(4)	Laborious operation	(12)	Oil spill
(5)	Give off a nasty smell	(13)	Surface defects
(6)	Abnormal homework	(14)	Size, position, shape out of tolerance
(7)	Intermittent operation	(15)	Unplanned maintenance
(8)	Unable to work	(16)	Abandoned

Table 4.26 Scoring criteria for severity levels (S) of process failure modes

Influence level	The ultimate impact of the process failure mode (for the end user)	Final impact of process failure mode (for downstream operations/subsequent operations)	Grading scale for severity scale
Disastrous	Product damage or loss of function	Fatalities/seriously endangering the safety of workers and major environmental damage	10, 9
Serious	Product is largely non-functional/functional with reduced performance/ end user is very dissatisfied	Threat to the safety of operators, 100% of the product may be discarded/the product needs to be repaired in a specialized repair shop, and serious environmental damage	8, 7
Moderate	Product works, but performance degrades/end user is not satisfied, most cases (>75%) find product to be defective	There may be some (<100%) products that are not screened and discarded/products are repaired in special departments or off the production line and moderate environmental damage	6, 5, 4
Mild	25–50% of end users can find the product to be defective, or have no identifiable effect	Result in unscheduled product maintenance or repair	3, 2, 1

Table 4.27 Process failure mode probability (*O*) scoring criteria

Probability of failure mode occurrence	Possible failure mode probability ($P\,o$)	Level
Very high (persistent failure)	$P\,o \geq 10^{-1}$	10
	$5\times10^{-1} \leq P\,o < 10^{-1}$	9
High (frequent failure)	$2\times10^{-2} \leq P\,o < 5\times10^{-1}$	8
	$1\times10^{-2} \leq P\,o < 2\times10^{-2}$	7
Moderate (occasional glitches)	$5\times10^{-3} \leq P\,o < 1\times10^{-2}$	6
	$2\times10^{-3} \leq P\,o < 5\times10^{-3}$	5
	$1\times10^{-3} \leq P\,o < 2\times10^{-3}$	4
Low (rare failure)	$5\times10^{-4} \leq P\,o < 1\times10^{-3}$	3
	$1\times10^{-4} \leq P\,o < 5\times10^{-4}$	2
Very low (unlikely to fail)	$P\,o < 1\times10^{-4}$	1

Difficulty level of process failure mode detection (*D*): It refers to the possibility of process failure mode being detected in product processing control. The detected difficulty level (*D*) is also a relative comparison level. In order to obtain a lower detection difficulty value, product processing and assembly process control need to be continuously improved. The scoring criteria are shown in Table 4.28.

8. **Risk Priority Number (RPN) Analysis**

Table 4.28 Grading criteria for process failure mode to be detected difficulty level (*D*)

Detectability	Scoring criteria	Check method			Recommended difficulty of detection method	Grading scale for the detected difficulty level (*D*)
		A	B	C		
Almost impossible	Undetectable			√	undetectable or uncheckable	10
Very tiny	Current detection methods are almost impossible to detect			√	Detect with indirect inspection	9
Tiny	Current detection methods have only a small chance of detecting			√		8
Very small	Current detection methods have only a small chance of detecting			√		7
Small	Current detection methods can detect		√	√		6
Medium	The current detection method can basically detect the		√			5
Upper middle	Current detection methods have a greater chance of detecting	√	√			4
High	Current assays are likely to detect	√	√			3
Very high	Current testing methods will almost certainly detect	√	√			2
Affirmative	Current detection methods can certainly detect	√				1

Note Checking methods: A-use error-proof measures; B-use measuring tools to measure; C-manual inspection

An improvement measure is any process improvement measure that takes as its starting point the reduction of the severity level (*S*), the probability of occurrence level (*O*) and the difficulty of being detected level (*D*) of the process failure mode. Generally, regardless of the size of the process failure mode RPN, for projects with a severity level (*S*) of 9 or 10, measures in process design or product processing, assembly process control or preventive/improvement measures should be taken to meet the risk reduction requirements. In all cases, where the consequences of a process failure mode could be criticalityous to manufacturing/assembly personnel, preventive/improvement actions should be taken to eliminate, mitigate, control or avoid the occurrence of that process failure mode. For process failure modes that do not have improvement measures, "None" should be filled in the corresponding column of the process FMECA form.

9. **Prediction or Tracking of RPN Values**

After formulating the improvement measures, the implementation results of the improvement measures should be predicted or tracked, and the changes in the severity level (*S*) of the process failure mode, the probability level (*O*) of the process failure mode and the difficulty level (*D*) of the process failure mode being detected should be analyzed, and the corresponding RPN values should be calculated to see if they meet the requirements. When the requirements are not met, further improvement is required, and the above steps are repeated until the RPN value meets the minimum acceptable level.

10. **Process FMECA Report**

Summarize and organize the process FMECA analysis results into a technical report. Its main content includes overview, description of product processing, assembly and other processes, system definition, filling of process FMECA form, conclusions and suggestions, attached tables (such as "process flow table", "parts—process relationship matrix"), etc. The main task of implementing process FMECA is to fill in the process FMECA form (see Table 4.29). During application, the content of the table can be increased or decreased according to the actual situation.

4.4.5.4 Completion of Failure Mode List

In the FMECA report, a summary list should be filled out for failures and single-point failures with severity levels of Category I and Category II. See Table 4.30 for the list of Type I and II failure modes and Table 4.31 for the list of single point failures.

4.4.5.5 Criticality Matrix

The criticality matrix is used to determine and compare the criticality of each failure mode, and then provide a basis for determining the sequence of improvement measures.

The abscissa of the matrix is represented by the severity category, and the ordinate is represented by the product criticality C, or the failure mode occurrence probability level.

Mark the code of the product or failure mode in the corresponding position of the matrix with reference to its severity category and failure mode occurrence probability

Table 4.29 Process FMECA form

Initial engagement level: task: review:
Engagement level: analyst: approval: date of form completion:

Process name	Process function/ requirement	Failure mode	cause of issue	Failure effect			Risk Priority Number (RPN) Before Improvement			
				The impact of the next process	Component impact	Equipment impact	Severity level *S*	Occurrence probability level *O*	Detected difficulty level *D*	RPN

Initial engagement level: task: review:
Engagement level: analyst: approval: date of form completion:

Improvement measures	Responsible department	Implementation of improvement measures	Improved Risk Priority Number (RPN)				Note
			Severity level *S*	Occurrence probability level *O*	Detected difficulty level *D*	RPN	

Table 4.30 List of type I and II failure modes

Initial engagement level: task: review:
Engagement level: analyst: approval: date of form completion:

Invalidation number	Unit number	Unit name	Unit function	Failure mode	Failure effect	Impact number	Design Assurance Measures	Severity	Test Description	Process inspection	Detection method	Remark

Table 4.31 Single point of failure checklist

Initial engagement level: task: review:
Engagement level: analyst: approval: date of form completion:

Invalidation number	Unit number	Unit name	Quantity	Unit function	Failure mode	Failure effect	Impact number	Design Assurance Measures	Severity category	Compensation Measures Implementation Department	Implementation of Compensation Measures	Remark

Fig. 4.17 Example of a criticality matrix

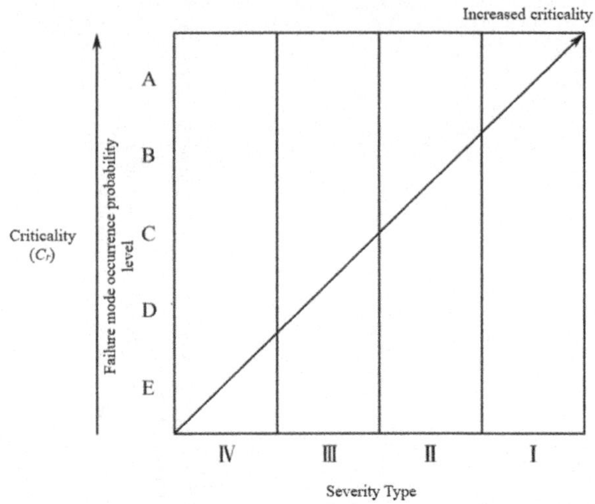

or the criticality degree of the product, so that the matrix diagram drawn in this way can show the distribution of the criticalities of each failure mode of the product.

An example of the criticality matrix is shown in Fig. 4.17. The farther the recorded failure mode distribution point is from the origin along the diagonal direction, the greater the criticality, and the need to take improvement measures as soon as possible. Drawing a good criticality matrix should be included as part of the FMECA report.

4.4.5.6 Key and Important Parts

After FMECA works, for the failure modes whose severity category in FMECA is I and II, the components with these failure modes should be classified as critical parts or important parts. Make decisions based on factors such as margin design, reliability level, concealed functions, and economics to initially determine product categories.

If the product meets one or more of the following conditions, the category can be raised or lowered on the basis of decision.

(1) Manufacturability: the process is complex and expensive;
(2) Maintainability: many maintenance man-hours and high costs;
(3) Condition of use: The component or similar component has experienced functional failures many times during its service life, and it is often in use after installation.

According to the logical decision, after the category of the component is initially determined, the product category is determined on the basis of trade-offs based on the supplementary analysis of manufacturability, maintainability and usage, combined with the following criteria for judging important parts.

(1) Criteria for judging reliability critical parts and important parts

Key Parts (Class A)

(1) The severity category is obtained through FMECA analysis. The category I with the most serious impact is aircraft crash and fatality. Components with this failure mode should be critical components.
(2) The severity category is Class II, and those that fail to cause serious personal injury, system damage, and large economic losses should also be listed as critical components.
(3) Those with high precision, high price, difficult maintenance and dependence on imports can be listed as key components.

Important Parts (Class B)

(1) The failure affecting the completion of the task, or causing the loss of the final output function should be listed as an important item.
(2) The failure affects the service life, or the failure will cause a chain reaction, which should also be listed as an important part.

(2) Output form

After the reliability critical parts and important parts are determined, they shall be part of the FMECA report, and a list of reliability critical parts and important parts shall be given.

4.5 FMECA Report

A complete FMECA report should include the following.

1. **Foreword**

Explain the purpose of implementing FMECA for a specific system, the life cycle stage of the system, and the source of the analysis task.

2. **Functional Principle of the System**

Briefly introduce the functional principle and work description of the analyzed system, specify the systems, subsystems and corresponding functions involved in this analysis, and further divide the FMECA agreement level.

3. **System Definition**

This part should include the functions or products included in the analyzed system, the failure criteria of the system, the definition of failure consequences and the corresponding severity category.

4. **Draw the Functional Block Diagram and Reliability Block Diagram of the System**

This part includes functional block diagrams and reliability block diagrams at all levels of the system and their explanations or descriptions. For a complex system, its block diagram can be used as an attachment to this analysis report instead of being included in the main text; when the system block diagram cites other design analysis reports or materials, the source of the data and reports can be directly indicated.

5. **FMECA Overview**

This section includes:

(1) Relevant descriptions of the prerequisites and basic assumptions for implementing FMECA;
(2) The source and basis of the data used in the analysis;
(3) Other relevant explanations and explanations.

6. **Conclusion and Suggestion**

This part should include the measures taken to eliminate or reduce the impact of failure, explain the single-point failure that cannot be eliminated and type I and type II failure, and suggest other possible compensation measures (such as design, process, inspection, operation, maintenance, etc.), and a description of the expected results of all actions taken.

7. **Failure Mode Effects and Criticality Analysis Form**

In the FMECA report, a summary list should be filled in respectively for the faults and single point faults with severity class I and class II. Get the list of Type I and Type II failure modes (see Table 4.32), the list of single point failures (see Table 4.33), and the list of reliability critical/important parts (see Table 4.34).

4.5.1 Failure Mode Summary Table

Through the statistics and analysis of the failure of digital medical equipment, a summary table of general failure modes of digital medical equipment is given for readers' reference. The summary table of failure modes is shown in Table 4.35.

4.6 Failure Modes and Failure Models of Mechanical Components

4.6.1 Overview

During the use of digital medical equipment, due to various reasons such as design, material, process and assembly, mechanical parts lose their specified functions and cannot continue to work, which is called failure. When the key components of

Table 4.32 List of type I and type II failure modes

Initial engagement level: task: review:
Engagement level: analyst: approval: date of form completion:

Fault	Unit	Unit name	Unit function	Failure mode	Failure effect	Impact number	Design guarantee	Severity	Test Description	Process inspection	Detection method	Remark

Table 4.33 Single point of failure checklist

Initial engagement level: task: review:
Engagement level: analyst: approval: date of form completion:

Fault number	Unit number	Unit name	Quantity	Unit function	Failure mode	Failure effect	Impact number	Design assurance measures	Severity category	Compensation measures implementation department	Implementation of compensation measures	Remark

Table 4.34 List of reliability critical/important parts

System name: task: review:
Analyst: approved: date filled:

Serial Number	Product name	Critical failure mode	Final impact	Severity category	Design improvements	Use of compensatory measures	Implementation department	Progress status	Remark

Table 4.35 Failure mode summary table

Serial number	Failure mode	Serial number	Failure mode	Serial number	Failure mode
1	General failure mode loss of function	29	No oil supply (no output)	57	Foggy
2	Unable to break	30	No air supply	58	Accumulated gas
3	Unable to get through	31	Misfire (misfire)	59	Clamp falls off
4	Unable to open	32	Not deflate	60	Screws (bolts, females), rivets fall off, degenerate, and deteriorate
5	Unable to close	33	The lights never go out	61	Ageing
6	Unable to let go	34	Tight off, not flashing	62	Serious carbon deposit
7	Short circuit	35	Not directed, not positioned	63	Dirty
8	Open circuit (open circuit)	36	Stop arm	64	Damp
9	Stuck, dead	37	Computer software failure	65	Get mouldy
10	Failure of manipulation (regulation, control)	38	Computer hardware failure	66	Rust
11	Misdirected	39	Non-working, loss of function, dysfunctional type	67	Corrosion
12	Misoperation	40	Intermittent work	68	Go bad
13	No output	41	The signal is intermittent and unstable	69	Dirty oil
14	No pressure	42	Overheat	70	Oil discoloration
15	Self unlocking	43	Large consumption of media (oil, liquid, gas, etc.)	71	Metal shavings
16	Unable to unlock	44	Parameter drift	72	Poor lubrication, other
17	Unlocked	45	Zero drift (moving)	73	Natural loss
18	No instructions	46	Out of sync	74	Unknown mode, specific failure mode for airframe and machinery, dysfunctional type

(continued)

Table 4.35 (continued)

Serial number	Failure mode	Serial number	Failure mode	Serial number	Failure mode
19	Unable to return to zero	47	Uncoordinated	75	Brake failure
20	Unable to reset	48	Poor anti-interference ability	76	Resonance
21	Unable to separate (do not throw away)	49	Leakage (liquid, gas)	77	Chatter
22	Unable to start	50	Leakage	78	Side brake
23	Unable to convert	51	Light leak	79	Hover unstable
24	No pressurization	52	Freeze	80	Vertebral instability
25	No pressure reduction	53	Oil accumulation, accumulation of water	81	Add-on bouncing
26	No cooling	54	Not sealed	82	Automatic reverse rod, drop rod
27	No heating	55	Air lock	83	Pole light
28	No power supply, power off	56	Clearance out of tolerance	84	Rod weight
85	The picture is blurry and does not fade	116	Pressure pulsation, swing	147	Desoldering
86	Did not do well	117	Rapid pressure drop	148	Welding
87	Insufficient function	118	Pressure out of tolerance	149	Fracture
88	Insufficient flexibility	119	Temperature out of tolerance	150	Crack
89	Resolution drop	120	Abnormal heating	151	Crack
90	Insulation resistance drop	121	Automatic release	152	Rupture
91	Grounding, poor grounding	122	Automatic break (off) off	153	Crack
92	Poor contact	123	Smoke (fog)	154	shaving teeth
93	Poor insulation (leakage)	124	Cable is too long or too short	155	Tooth punching (broken teeth) tooth bending
94	Very poor inspiration	125	Frequency out of tolerance	156	Trip (pull button)

(continued)

Table 4.35 (continued)

Serial number	Failure mode	Serial number	Failure mode	Serial number	Failure mode
95	Voltage out of tolerance	126	Unstable frequency	157	Bubbling
96	Current out of tolerance	127	Unstable current (swing)	158	Peeling off
97	Frequency out of tolerance	128	Unstable voltage	159	Wear and tear
98	Performance indicators are out of tolerance	129	Resistance value out of tolerance	160	Glue (glue, bond)
99	Abnormal vibration, shaking	130	The amount of amplification is out of tolerance	161	The plug (seat) is damaged
100	Abnormal swing	131	Trip switch	162	Structural interference
101	Abnormal output	132	Status switch unlimited	163	Bolt (nail), pin broken
102	Abnormal sound	133	Anti-tune	164	Spring break
103	Speed out of tolerance (abnormal)	134	Electronic-specific failure modes	165	Fixing bracket (seat) broken
104	Abnormal start	135	Screen brightness is not adjustable	166	The plug (seat) is damaged
105	Abnormal traffic	136	Damage breakdown	167	The rubber gasket (ring) is crushed
106	Manipulate anomalies	137	Fuse	168	Silver streak
107	Unusual retraction	138	Ablation	169	Broken wire exceeds the specification
108	Overload	139	Melting	170	Drop fast, burst, gap
109	Insufficient capacity	140	Burn out	171	Trachoma
110	Indicating exception	141	Out of shape	172	Wire burnt out
111	Stuck, tight, inflexible	142	Distortion	173	Contact burnout
112	Loud noise	143	Strain	174	Blown fuse
113	Big error	144	Scratch	175	Disconnected
114	Slow recovery	145	Crushed (mark)	176	Outside object injury
115	Sometimes not connected	146	Open welding	177	Damage, Damage, Loose, Off, Leaky, Blocked

(continued)

Table 4.35 (continued)

Serial number	Failure mode	Serial number	Failure mode	Serial number	Failure mode
178	Jam	192	Do not show	206	Slow orientation
179	Fall off, fly away	193	Continuous rotation	207	Abnormal interception
180	Unglue, degumming	194	Do not scan (do not search)	208	Atresia
181	Loose	195	No d istance	209	Not locked
182	Oil and gas	196	No delay	210	Mistuning
183	Not working properly	197	No self-check	211	Out of phase
184	Function failure type no signal	198	Out of tune	212	Out of tune
185	Do not track	199	No ranging	213	Self-excited
186	Unable to in touch	200	Not intercepted	214	Unstable display, reversed screen
187	Not answering	201	No video	215	Not displayed correctly
188	Not launch	202	Non-recording dysfunctional type	216	Display missing screen, drop screen
189	No self-listening	203	Weak, unclear signal	217	Short communication distance
190	Unable to alarm	204	Error indication	218	Impedance mismatch
191	No distress signal	205	Digital absence		

mechanical equipment fail, it means that the equipment is in a fault state. The failure mode of mechanical parts, that is, the external manifestation of failure, mainly manifests as wear, deformation, fracture, etc.; and the failure mechanism refers to the physical, chemical, mechanical and other changes in the failure process and the essence of the internal cause.

4.6.2 Failure Modes of Mechanical Components

4.6.2.1 Classification of Failure Modes of Mechanical Components

Under the action of one or several physical and (or) chemical factors, mechanical parts gradually change in size, shape, state or performance, and lose their intended functions in a specific form of expression. The specific form of expression referred to here is the failure model. Obviously, different physical and/or chemical processes correspond to different failure modes. The failure of mechanical parts is affected by many factors, and its failure mode is also relatively complex. Divided according to the macroscopic characteristics of the failure mode, the failure of mechanical parts can be divided into three types of failure modes: deformation failure, fracture failure and surface damage failure. On this basis, it can be further subdivided according to the failure nature and specific characteristics. Mechanical parts The failure mode classification of components is shown in Fig. 4.18.

4.6.2.2 Diagnosis of Failure Modes of Mechanical Components

Failure mode diagnosis of mechanical parts is the most important and primary work of failure analysis, which determines the direction of failure analysis to continue. The failures listed in Fig. 4.18, can often be classified as primary, secondary or even tertiary failure modes. In Fig. 4.18, fracture failure is regarded as the primary failure mode, and fatigue fracture can be regarded as the secondary failure mode. According to the level of stress, fatigue failure can be divided into three levels of fatigue failure modes: low cycle fatigue failure, high cycle fatigue failure and high and low cycle composite fatigue failure.

Generally speaking, it is not difficult to diagnose a specific failure mode, especially the diagnosis of a typical first-level failure mode. As long as a single diagnostic criterion, such as macroscopic fracture characteristics, can be obtained, the first-level failure mode The conclusion of the diagnosis. However, for the diagnosis of secondary or tertiary failure modes, it is necessary to select appropriate techniques and methods for certain quantitative analysis. For example, the diagnosis of fracture failure mode should be based on:

(1) Wreck analysis. According to the trajectory of the wreckage, the macroscopic properties of the fracture, and the deformation sequence of the fracture, etc., firstly find the initial damaged part (initiating event), and then analyze the fracture properties, crack direction, deformation, trace source, mechanical properties, and microstructure of the initial damaged part., technological process, heat treatment status, etc. are analyzed item by item and comprehensively.
(2) Stress analysis. Including the analysis and estimation of the source, nature and size of the stress, especially the analysis and calculation of the structure and stress of the initial damaged parts, the analysis of the working conditions and the environment, and a comprehensive analysis compared with the qualitative and quantitative analysis of the fracture.
(3) Failure simulation. Carry out simulation tests on the main failure models and main control parameters in the laboratory or on site, and compare and analyze the simulated failure fracture and the actual accident-causing fracture.

As another example, the secondary failure forms of wear failure include abrasive wear failure, adhesive wear failure, fatigue wear failure, oxidation wear failure, corrosion

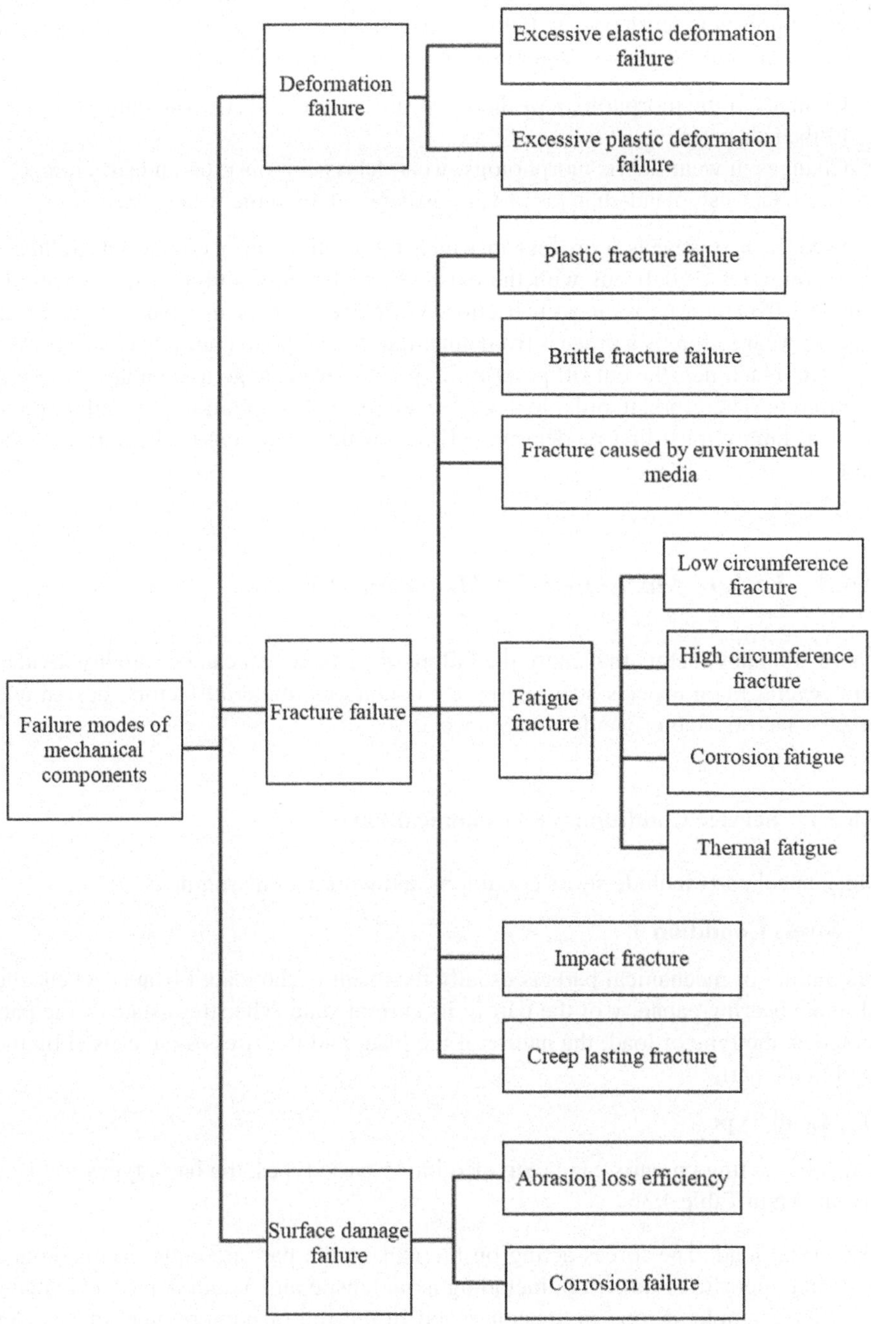

Fig. 4.18 Classification of failure modes of mechanical parts

wear failure and fretting wear failure. Each of these categories can have several tertiary wear failure modes. Diagnosis of wear failure modes is generally based on:

- Changes in the morphology of the worn surface and the structure and properties of the subsurface;
- Changes in wear debris morphology, wear debris composition and structure;
- The relationship and changes of various parameters in the wear system, etc.

However, since wear is a process in which the friction surface material gradually loses, migrates or deforms with the existence of friction, although it is generally believed that there is wear with friction, wear does not mean wear failure. From wear to wear failure is a process from quantitative change to qualitative change. For different machines, the cut-off point from quantitative change to qualitative change is different. Therefore, in order to diagnose the form of wear failure, the failure point of wear failure must first be determined specifically according to the nature of the part.

4.6.3 *Failure Mechanism of Mechanical Parts*

There are many factors that cause the failure of parts, which can be roughly divided into several main aspects such as service conditions, material factors, design and process factors, and use and maintenance.

4.6.3.1 Service Conditions of Mechanical Parts

Mechanical parts include stress conditions and working environment.

1. **Stress Condition**

The failure of mechanical parts is usually the result of the load it bears exceeds the ultimate bearing capacity of the part in its current state. The stress state of the part includes: the type of load, the nature of the load, and the stress state caused by the load in the part.

(1) **Load Type**

The loads acting on parts can be divided into 5 basic types, the basic types of loads are shown in Table 4.36.

(1) Axial load. The forces acting on the axis of the part are equal in magnitude and opposite in direction, including axial tensile and axial compressive loads. For example, a rope in tension, a rod in tension or compression, etc. Under axial load, the distribution of stress along the cross section is uniform. The relationship between the principal stress and the maximum shear stress on the part is:

Table 4.36 Basic types of loads

Serial Number	Stress distribution	Load type
1	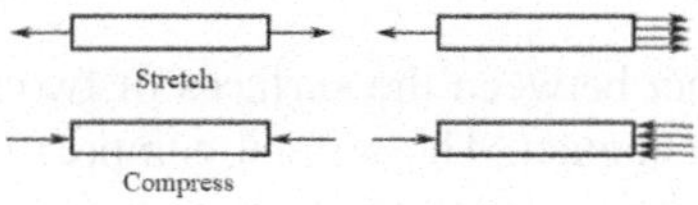	Axial load
2	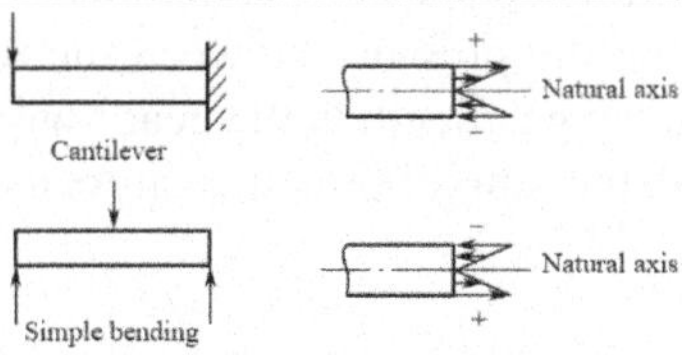	Bending load
3	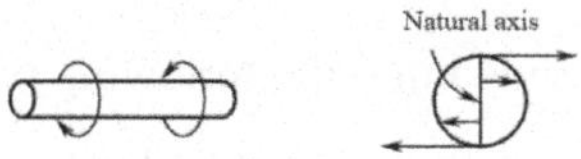	Torsional load
4	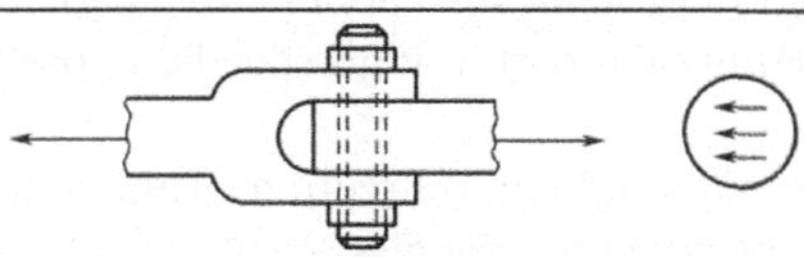	Shear load
5	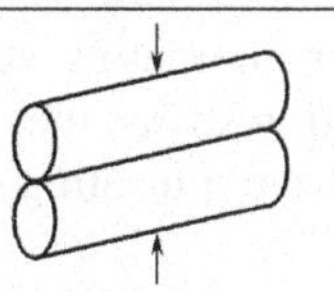	Contact load

$$\frac{\sigma}{\tau} = 2 \tag{4.56}$$

In the formula: σ is the principal stress, and τ is the maximum shear stress.

(2) Bending load. A load (and sometimes a couple) perpendicular to the axis of a part that causes the part to bend. For example, the roots of gear teeth in digital medical equipment, leaf springs of automobiles, etc., are subjected to bending loads during work. Under the action of bending load, the law of principal stress distribution on the cross section of the part is: from the maximum change of surface stress to zero stress at the neutral axis. Also, one side of the neutral axis is tensile stress, and the other side is compressive stress.

(3) Torsional load. A force couple acting in a plane perpendicular to the axis of a part, which causes the part to deform in torsion. For example, drive shafts that transmit torque, cylindrical coil springs, etc. Under the action of torsional load, the distribution law of shear stress on the cross section is: from the maximum surface to zero at the center point of the cross section (the "center point" mentioned here refers to the intersection point of the torsion central axis and the cross section).

(4) Shear load. The force that causes the relative displacement of two adjacent sections in the part. The bolt is sheared at the connection joint surface and

presses against the hole wall of the connected part. The screw is also subject to bending, but this can be ignored if the joints are tight. Under shear loading, the magnitude of the force is uniform along the cross section parallel to the maximum shear stress.

(5) Contact load. The contact between the surfaces of two parts is point contact, line contact and surface contact. The normal compressive load at the contact part after the part is loaded is called the contact load. For example, when the rolling bearing is working, the pressure between the roller and the raceway, and the pressure between the gear teeth in the gear transmission are all contact loads. Under contact load, the ratio of principal stress to maximum shear stress is indeterminate.

(2) The nature of the load

The nature of the loads can be divided into the following types:

(1) Static load. A gradual, or constant, load applied to a part.
(2) Impact load. Loads acting on a part at high speeds, impact loads often appear as energy loads
(3) Alternating load. The magnitude and direction of the load change with time, and the change can be periodic or irregular.
(4) Most machine parts work under alternating stress. Although there are many variations in the form of alternating stress, they can basically be classified into four types: symmetrical cyclic stress, pulsating cyclic stress, asymmetric cyclic stress, and random cyclic stress.

(3) Stress state

The stress state of a part refers to the stress state on each section through any point of the loaded part. Classified from different angles, the stress state of parts can be divided into unidirectional stress state, multi-directional stress state, "soft" stress state, "hard" stress state, etc.

2. **Working Environment**

Parts generally operate at room temperature and in the environment of atmospheric media, but in high temperature, low temperature or other corrosive media, many special failure types will occur.

(1) Environmental media and component failure

Environmental media include gases, liquids, liquid metals, radiation, solid abrasives, and lubricants. The failure conditions of the parts that they may cause are listed in Table 4.37 Environmental media and parts failure Table

For the accurate judgment of the failure cause of a certain part, the influence of the environmental medium must be fully considered. For example, a digital diagnostic equipment was stored in a warehouse in spring, and in autumn, it was found that the spring piece of a certain type of relay in the digital diagnostic equipment broke along the grain boundary. After failure analysis, it was determined that the stress

Table 4.37 Table of environmental media and parts failure

Medium	Possible failure
Gas: atmosphere, salt spray atmosphere, water vapor, gas-liquid two-phase flow (CO, CO_2), atmosphere containing H_2S	Oxidation, corrosion, hydrogen embrittlement, corrosion fatigue, gas-liquid flow erosion
Liquid: Cl−, OH−, NaOH, NO_{2-}, H_2S, water-solid (sand)	Corrosion, stress corrosion, corrosion fatigue, cavitation and sediment wear
Liquid metal: Hg-Cu alloy; Cd, Sn, Zn-steel, Pb-steel, Nb, K-stainless steel	Liquid brittleness, liquid metal embrittlement, Ni and Cr elements in the alloy are selectively dissolved in liquid Pb, and liquid metal corrodes
Neutron irradiation, ultraviolet irradiation	Cause material embrittlement, cause polymer material aging
Abrasives: ore, coal, rock (lubricant), slurry, aqueous solution	Combined effect of abrasive wear and corrosion wear

corrosion cracking was caused by ammonia. But no chemicals that release ammonia have ever been stored in the warehouse. Later, it was found that there was a large pile of chicken manure in the field near the south of the warehouse gate. The ammonia gas released by the chicken manure was sent into the warehouse by the south wind in spring and summer, which provided the necessary medium environment for stress corrosion and caused stress corrosion. It can be seen that if the failure analysis is not connected with the wider environment, no reliable conclusions can be drawn.

(2) Ambient temperature and component failure

The failure forms and analysis ideas of mechanical parts that may be caused by ambient temperature are listed in Fig. 4.19, the analysis ideas for failure forms of mechanical parts caused by ambient temperature.

4.6.3.2 Design, Manufacture and Component Failure

1. **Design and Part Failure**

Unreasonable design and poor design considerations are one of the important reasons for component failure. For example, the right-angled transition at the step of the shaft, too small fillet radius, sharp edges, etc. cause stress concentration, and these stress concentration points may become the origin of part damage. The cross-sectional shape of some parts is required by the part itself, such as splines, keyways, oil holes, pin holes, etc., but if the design is not thoughtful, the weakening and stress concentration of these shape features on the cross-section are not fully estimated. Or if the location is improperly arranged, it will cause early damage to the parts. Another reason is that the estimation of the working conditions of the parts is wrong, such as underestimating the possible overload in the work, resulting in insufficient bearing capacity of the designed parts.

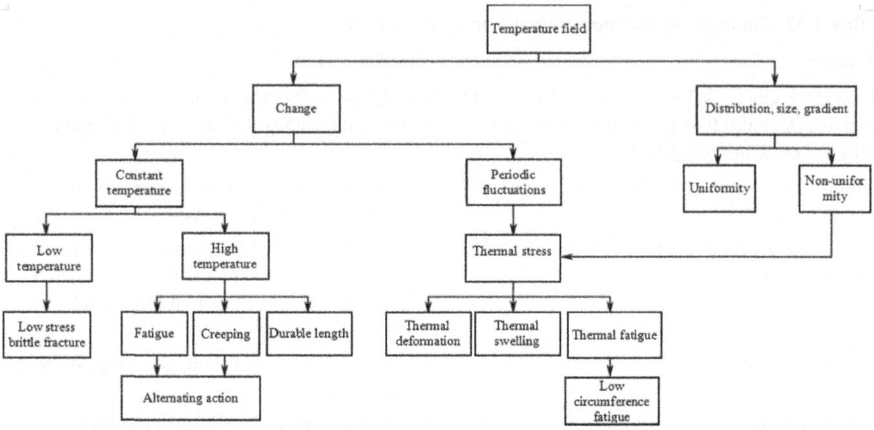

Fig. 4.19 Diagram of failure form analysis of mechanical parts caused by ambient temperature

Improper material selection is another important cause of failure. While the problem lies with the material, the responsibility lies with the designer. Most often, designers make decisions based solely on the material's general performance metrics, which simply do not reflect the material's resistance to the type of failure that occurs. Another situation is that although there is a more accurate estimate of the failure mode of the part in advance, and the corresponding performance index is proposed as the basis for material selection, due to consideration of other factors (such as economy, processing performance, etc.), different methods are used. A very suitable substitute material, thus resulting in failure.

2. **Materials, Manufacturing Processes and Part Failures**

The cause of failure of parts is also related to the intrinsic quality of the material and the quality of the mechanical manufacturing process.

(1) Metallurgical quality

The metallurgical quality of the material is an important factor for the long-term normal operation of the machine part. The metallurgical defects of the steel material, such as inclusions, pores, porosity, white spots, residual shrinkage cavities, composition segregation, etc., are the internal damage of the parts.

(2) Defects in mechanical manufacturing process

Each part is made through a series of processing techniques, no matter what kind of processing technology (casting, forging, welding, heat treatment, cutting, grinding, etc.), if the operation is not done properly, it will cause process defects and may become a part Reason for failure. Because improper manufacturing process may affect the quality of the product from the following aspects: ① Process cracks; ② High residual internal stress; ③ Poor surface quality; ④ Abnormal organizational state; ⑤ Failure to meet the required mechanical properties.

The assembly accuracy of tight fitting parts is not enough, and it will cause loosening when the machine is running, resulting in impact and noise between matching parts, thereby accelerating the failure process of parts. For example, frictional corrosion (or fretting damage, bite erosion) occurs due to slight relative movement between tight fitting parts.

4.6.3.3 Use, Maintenance and Failure of Parts

The use and maintenance status of the machine is also an aspect that must be considered in the failure analysis. The machine is overloaded during use, poorly lubricated, poorly cleaned, corroded and rusted, surface bruises, used at resonance frequencies, violation of operating procedures, accidental accidents, no regular maintenance or improper maintenance, etc., will cause early damage to parts.

For example, the analysis of 50 crankshafts of a certain engine fatigue fracture showed that 40 of them were caused by the fatigue fracture of the crankshaft after the repair, and the fillet radius of the journal was too small ($R \leq 3$ mm, design requirement $R \geq 6$ mm). Another example is the gear box of the cutter suction dredging system, which fails due to improper use, poor lubrication and poor cooling. The three gears of the gear set are all made of 12CrNi3A steel, which has been carburized and tempered at low temperature, and the carburized layer is larger than 1 mm. The gear set fails after working for 1100 h, and the failure is manifested as adhesive wear and scratches; tooth surface burns and melting; tooth top plastic deformation, tooth surface metal flows along the sliding direction, and is extruded to about 2 mm above the tooth top, and overload Folded teeth and fatigue broken teeth, etc. The inspection shows that the metallographic structure of the surface layer of the broken tooth is tempered troostite plus dispersed or intermittent network carbides, which proves that the gear has been seriously heated during the working process, and the simulation test proves that the temperature reaches 550 °C. The transmission load of this gear set is relatively high, and the working conditions are harsh, so it is a heavy-duty gear. Its failure is closely related to lubrication conditions and material strength. When the elastic fluid dynamic pressure oil film can be formed between the two gnawing teeth, the direct contact of the metal on the tooth surface can be avoided, the maximum unit pressure on the surface of the gear tooth will be greatly reduced, and the damage of the tooth surface can be significantly improved. However, the calculation according to the lubrication conditions shows that when the gears are gnawing together, an elastohydrodynamic oil film cannot be formed between the tooth surfaces, and it is in a state of boundary lubrication. The local heating of the surface layer is prone to damage such as adhesive wear, tooth surface burn and plastic flow. If this state cannot be improved in time, the damage will continue to develop and aggravate, and induce other problems, such as noise, vibration, broken teeth, etc.

The above analysis shows that improper use and maintenance is an important reason for the failure of mechanical parts.

4.6.4 *Typical Mechanical Component Life Model*

4.6.4.1 Bearing Wear Life Calculation

Bearing wear failure generally includes abrasive wear and adhesive wear. The impurity particles in the bearing will cause chiseling or plowing scratches on the surface of the raceway and the ball, causing abrasive wear; at the same time, due to the contour/peak of the raceway and the surface of the ball, the friction surface is stressed, and the local frictional heat If the surface temperature rises too high, the lubricating oil film will be broken. In severe cases, the metal on the surface layer will be partially melted, and the contact point will be stuck. The cyclic process of tearing off and re- adhesion causes adhesive wear. Abrasive wear and adhesive wear increase the clearance of the bearing, reduce the fit accuracy, and increase the noise and vibration. Therefore, the bearing radial clearance increment caused by wear is taken as the index of the bearing wear degree, the radial clearance increment is determined through the calculation of abrasive wear, and it is substituted into the adhesive wear calculation to obtain the adhesive wear life, and then from the following Calculate the wear life of the rolling bearing with the formula:

$$L_a = a_1 a_2 a_3 L_h \tag{4.57}$$

Among them, a_1 is the life correction coefficient for reliability, which can be obtained by the following formula:

$$a_1 = a\left[L_n\left({}^{100}/_{R}\right)\right]^{\frac{1}{b}} \tag{4.58}$$

Among them, R is the actual desired reliability of the bearing. For different types of bearings, the values of a, b are as follows: ball bearings, $a = 7.587$, $b = {}^{10}/_{9}$; roller bearings, $a = 4.4828$, $b = {}^{3}/_{2}$; tapered bearings, $a = 1.2063$, $b = {}^{4}/_{3}$.

a_2 is the life correction factor for materials; a_3 it is the life correction factor for operating conditions, and its value can be obtained by referring to the bearing manual.

As the amount of abrasive wear of the bearing increases, the increase in the radial clearance produces an increase in the radial clearance:

$$\Delta u_r = e_0 K_1;\ e_0 = 0.46 d^{0.67} \tag{4.59}$$

In the formula, Δu_r is the radial clearance increment; K_1 is the allowable wear factor of abrasive wear, which can be found in the bearing manual; e_0 is the wear rate related to the inner diameter of the bearing; d is the inner diameter of the bearing.

The empirical formula of adhesive wear life is established according to the test value, namely:

$$L_h = \frac{10^6}{60s_0 n}\left(\frac{\Delta u_r}{7.7K_\upsilon}\right)^{1/m} \tag{4.60}$$

In the formula, L_h is the adhesive wear life of the rolling bearing; n is the journal speed; K_υ is the volume wear degree, and its value can be obtained by checking the relevant icons in the mechanical design manual according to the product vn of the bearing outer diameter D, *the* kinematic viscosity of the lubricating oil and the bearing speed; m is an index, usually 0.1 to 0.5; s_0 it is the sliding distance per 10 ^{6} revolutions of the rolling bearing, and its value can C/P be obtained from the relevant diagram according to the bearing β and geometric parameters, $D(1+\sin\beta)$ is the standard contact angle of the bearing, C and is the rated dynamic load of the bearing, which P is The equivalent dynamic load of the bearing.

4.6.4.2 Gear Wear Life Calculation

Gear transmission is the most widely used mechanical transmission, and wear failure is the most common form of failure. About 80% of gear failures are caused by wear. According to the calculation formula of wear amount proposed by Soviet scholars, the wear life of gears is obtained. Its formula is as follows:

$$h = 2a\lambda n t z I_k \tag{4.61}$$

In the formula, λ is the sliding coefficient of the two gears, which is a measure of the relative sliding degree between the two tooth surfaces, which is equal to the ratio of the sliding velocity between the two tooth surfaces at the contact point of the gear to the tangential velocity at this point, the greater the wear, the more severe the λ wear. Generally speaking, when the pitch peripheral speed $v > 20\,\text{m/s}$, $\lambda_{\max} \leq 1.5$; $v = 2 \sim 10\,\text{m/s}$ at that time, $[e^{-\lambda t_0}]^{n-r}$. n is the speed of the gear; t is the working time of the gear; z is the number of meshing pairs of the gear under study; I_k is the wear rate, which can be obtained by looking up the table; a is the half-width of the contact area, which can be calculated according to the Hertz contact formula, namely:

$$a = 1.07\sqrt{\frac{F_n E R}{l}} \tag{4.62}$$

Among them, E is the modulus of elasticity, $E = \frac{1}{E_1} + \frac{1}{E_2}$; l is the length of the contact line; R is the comprehensive radius of curvature, $R = \frac{R_1 R_2}{R_1 + R_2}$, R_1, R_2 are the curvature radii of the large gear and the pinion respectively; F_n is the normal force of the gear teeth during meshing.

4.6.4.3 Calculation of Rubber Wear Life

There are many known wear models, among which the Archard model is the most widely recognized and applied wear model. This model points out the relationship between the wear amount and the sliding distance, load and material properties, and is applicable to various other sliding surfaces. type of wear. Its expression is as follows:

$$\hat{\lambda}\frac{\chi^2_{\alpha/2}(2r)}{2r} < \lambda < \hat{\lambda}\frac{\chi^2_{1-\alpha/2}(2r)}{2r} \tag{4.63}$$

where, V is the wear volume; F_N is the normal load, which can be calculated by Hertz contact theory or obtained by simulation when it is not directly available; is the s sliding distance; k is the wear rate $({m^2}/{N})$, which depends on the combination of materials, surface roughness, The contact temperature and other parameters of the friction pair can be obtained by looking up the Table

The wear volume per unit time can be obtained from the above formula:

$$\frac{V}{t} = kF_N\frac{s}{t} \Rightarrow V_v = kF_N v \tag{4.64}$$

where v is the sliding speed (sliding distance per unit time).

In engineering practice, v_h the wear amount represented by the wear depth is usually more practical, so the wear depth per unit time can be obtained by dividing both sides of the above formula by the nominal contact area v_h:

$$\frac{V_v}{A} = k\frac{F_N}{A}v \Rightarrow v_h = kPv \tag{4.65}$$

where, A is the nominal contact area; P is the contact stress at the contact point.

4.7 Failure Modes and Failure Models of Electronic Components

4.7.1 Overview

Electronic components refer to the basic unit that performs electrical, electronic, electromagnetic, electromechanical, and photoelectric functions in electronic circuits or electronic equipment. The basic unit can be composed of multiple parts, and usually cannot be decomposed without destruction. The failure of electronic components refers to the complete or partial loss of their functions, parameter drift, or intermittent occurrence of the above conditions. The understanding of the failure of electronic components must start with the failure mode, failure cause and failure mechanism.

Failure mode refers to the form, form and phenomenon of product failure, and is the external macroscopic manifestation of product failure. The failure modes of electronic components of the same category are also different. This chapter refers to GJB/Z 299C-2006 "Electronic Equipment Reliability Prediction Manual" to give the failure modes of the main categories of electronic components.

The failure causes of electronic components can be divided into external factors and internal factors from the way of introduction. External factors are environmental factors, electrical stress, mechanical stress, and improper use of human components. In this chapter, by analyzing the influence of external stresses such as different environmental stresses and electrical stresses on electronic components, an accelerated model of components under typical stress is given to describe the reliability characteristics of failure modes (such as average life, characteristic life, failure rate, etc.) and the accelerated stress level, providing reference for readers to carry out accelerated life tests; while internal factors are a series of physical and chemical changes in the materials and structures of electronic components, such as The change of atoms, molecules, and ions is the inherent nature of failure, and we usually call this internal cause the failure mechanism.

the failure physical models corresponding to the failure mechanisms of common electronic components, revealing the root cause of failure, failure time and stress conditions It provides reference for readers to select existing and study new failure physical models based on the characteristics of digital medical equipment products.

4.7.2 Failure Modes of Main Electronic Components

Failure physics is a discipline that studies the internal causes and mechanisms of product failure under various stresses, also known as reliability physics. In the past and even at present, failure mechanism analysis is an important part of failure physics work; however, to find out the failure development law and make quantitative predictions, a failure physics model must be established. With the in-depth development of reliability technology, failure physics models have been used in recent years highly anticipated.

This section sorts out the failure physical models corresponding to the common machine and component-level failure mechanisms, reveals the root cause of failure and the change law of failure time and stress conditions, and selects existing and Research new failure physics model to provide reference.

4.7.2.1 Primary Failure Modes of Resistors

According to the failure mode statistics of components and components in GJB/Z 299C-2006 "Electronic Equipment Reliability Prediction Manual", we can know that for fixed resistors, the main failure models are open circuit, electrical parameter drift, etc.; common resistor open circuit The reason is that when the voltage across the

Table 4.38 Common main failure modes and failure mechanisms of resistors

Resistor category	Failure mode	Failure mechanism
Thin film resistor	Open circuit	The ceramic core matrix is broken; the resistance film is broken; the lead wire is broken; the welding is bad
	Short circuit	Corona discharge
	Resistance drift	The thickness of the resistive film is uneven, and there is contamination between the resistive films
Thick film resistors	Open circuit	Terminal electrode damage; surface electrode corrosion; electric burnout; ceramic substrate fracture
	Resistance drift	Silver ion migration
Wirewound resistors	Open circuit	Winding disconnection; current corrosion; weak lead bonding; poor welding
	Resistance drift	Resistor wire aging
Potentiometer	Open circuit	Broken wire; burnt resistance band; brushes fall off
	Poor contact	Mechanical damage; aging of contact parts; poor welding
	Electrical parameter drift	Resistive material

resistor rises above the rated voltage, the resistance value of the resistor will increase irreversibly, and even the voltage breakdown will burn the film layer, eventually causing the resistor to open. The reasons for the drift of the electrical parameters of the resistor are more complicated, and the common reasons are the electrical load aging and temperature aging of the resistor. When an electrical load is applied to the resistor, electrolysis damages the thin film resistor and accelerates its aging process. In the same way, when high temperature stress is applied to the resistor, the resistance body of the resistor will accelerate oxidation, and the resistance parameter will also drift. Generally, the accelerated aging caused by the applied load is greater than the accelerated aging caused by increasing the ambient temperature. Because under the electrical load, the local temperature rise caused by the internal structural defects and inhomogeneity of the resistor will exceed the average heating temperature rise of the resistor. The main failure modes and failure mechanisms of common resistors are shown in Table 4.38.

4.7.2.2 Main Failure Modes of Capacitors

Due to the wide variety of capacitors, the materials, structures, manufacturing processes, performance and use environments of various capacitors are different, so the failure modes and failure mechanisms of capacitors are diverse. For capacitors, the common failure modes are short circuit, open circuit, electrical parameter degradation (including capacitance change, loss tangent increase and insulation resistance decrease), liquid leakage and lead corrosion fracture.

1. **Short Circuit**

The main failure mechanism of short circuit: ① There are defects and defects in the dielectric, impurities and conductive particles; ② Aging of the dielectric; ③ Electrochemical breakdown of the dielectric; ④ Ion migration; ⑤ Mechanical damage of the dielectric during the manufacturing process; Edge arcing between electrodes under wet and low pressure; ⑦ instantaneous short circuit of the dielectric under mechanical stress.

2. **Open Circuit**

The main failure mechanism of the open circuit: ① Due to the oxidation of the lead-out wire and the contact point of the electrode, resulting in low-level failure; ② Corrosion and fracture of the anode lead-out electrode (electrolytic capacitor); ③ Dry adjustment and freezing of the working electrolyte; ④ The working electrolyte and the Instantaneous open circuit between dielectrics.

3. **Electrical Parameter Degradation**

The main failure mechanisms of electrical parameter degradation: ① The influence of moisture; ②I on migration; ③ Residual stress relaxation (winding capacitor); ④ Surface contamination; ⑤ Internal defects.

The main failure modes and failure mechanisms of common capacitors are shown in Table 4.39.

4.7.2.3 Main Failure Modes of Inductors

Inductors have a wide range of applications, and can be used as the main device for tuning, oscillation, coupling, matching, filtering, delay and compensation in electronic circuits. The failure modes of inductors include open circuit, electrical parameter drift, etc. The main failure modes and failure mechanisms of common inductors are shown in Table 4.40.

4.7.2.4 Main Failure Modes of Electrical Connectors

Electrical connectors use mechanical pressure to make conductors contact each other and have the ability to conduct current. They are widely used in various digital medical equipment. The common failure modes and failure mechanisms are analyzed as follows.

1. **Open Circuit**

Table 4.39 Common main failure modes and failure mechanisms of capacitors

Capacitor category	Failure mode	Failure mechanism
Ceramic capacitor	Open circuit	Thermal stress; mechanical stress
	Short circuit	Dielectric material defects; production process defects; silver electrode migration
	Parameter drift	There are cracks, pores and other defects inside the medium
Aluminum electrolytic capacitors	Leakage	Poor sealing; aging and cracking of rubber; volatilization of electrolyte under high temperature and high pressure
	Burst	The AC component in the working voltage is too large; the dielectric defect of the oxide film; the presence of harmful ions such as chloride ions or sulfate radicals; the internal pressure is too high
	Open circuit	Electrochemical corrosion of electrode lead-out wire; poor contact between lead-out foil and electrode; partial oxidation of electrode lead-out foil and solder piece
	Breakdown	Anodic oxide film rupture; local damage to the oxide film; aging or drying of the electrolyte; process defects
	Leakage current increases	The compactness of the oxide film becomes poor; the oxide film is damaged; the chloride ion is seriously polluted; the working electrolyte formula is not good; the purity of raw materials is not high
	Decrease in capacitance and increase in loss	The loss of electrolyte is more; the viscosity of the electrolyte is higher at low temperature
Liquid tantalum electrolytic capacitor	Leakage	Poor seal; rough surface of anode tantalum wire; improper welding of negative nickel lead
	Momentary open circuit	Insufficient amount of electrolyte
	Changes in electrical parameters	Electrolyte consumption; moisture in the electrolyte diffuses outward through the sealing rubber under storage conditions; electrochemical dissociation of moisture occurs under working conditions
Solid tantalum electrolytic capacitor	Short circuit	Oxide film defects; relative displacement between the tantalum block and the anode lead-out wire; the tantalum lead-out wire of the anode shakes

There are many factors that cause open circuit, such as unreasonable material selection or poor heat treatment process quality, hard and brittle jack material causing jack reed breakage, jack material being too soft causing jack slack; poor bonding process quality causing jack There is excess glue sticking between the contact pins; the quality of the assembly process is poor, and the secondary locking assembly is not assembled in place. During the production process of the connector assembly, the

Table 4.40 Common main failure modes and failure mechanisms of inductors

Inductor category	Failure mode	Failure mechanism
Chip Multilayer Inductors	Open circuit	The printed pattern of the internal electrode is incomplete or partially missing; the connection point is incompletely printed or the connection with the internal electrode is unreliable; improper use or test operation
	Porcelain fracture	Thermal stress; mechanical stress
	Welding	Poor quality of terminal electrodes; tin-lead plating; incomplete or partially weak nickel interlayer; poor solder wettability or poor flux quality; terminal electrodes are oxidized or corroded
Wire Wound Inductor	Open circuit	Winding disconnection; overcurrent; electrochemical corrosion
	Electrical parameter drift	Bad wire insulation

wire core is broken or mechanically damaged, causing the wire core to be damaged. Mismatch, improper use of crimping pliers cause virtual pressure, etc. All of these will cause the failure of the contact part of the contact as the core part of the connector assembly.

2. **Poor Contact**

There are many factors that cause poor contact of the connector, unreasonable structural design of the contact piece, wrong material selection, out-of-tolerance machining dimensions, rough surface, unreasonable heat treatment, bonding and surface treatment processes, harsh storage and use environment, and improper operation. It will cause poor contact at the contact part and terminal part of the contact. All links such as design, manufacturing, inspection, storage and use may cause poor contact of the connector. On the basis of understanding the failure mechanism, targeted corrective measures must be put forward to avoid and prevent the recurrence of similar failure cases.

There is a difference between a bad contact and an open circuit. The purpose of poor contact detection is to detect and reject some products with poor contact and high-impedance contacts that lead to increased loop resistance. Because when the general conductance meter is used for conduction detection, when the circuit resistance is lower than the judgment value of the on-off resistance, the digital diagnosis and treatment equipment will reflect it as a circuit. In fact, there may be poorly connected high-impedance contacts in the conduction loop. For communication cable assemblies, some loop working currents and working voltages are only tens of milliamps and tens of millivolts, so the loop resistance is required to be as low as possible, and generally should not exceed several milliohms to tens of milliohms. If there are high-impedance contacts in the loop caused by virtual soldering, virtual voltage, or core damage, the loop resistance will exceed the specified value, which will affect the normal transmission of the signal.

3. **Momentary Power Failure**

The size of the contact resistance of the connector assembly terminal (contact piece) is mainly related to the contact pressure. Static contact resistance corresponds to when the contact pressure remains constant or its variation is negligible. When the connector is used in a dynamic environment such as vibration, shock, and collision, its contact resistance will change with the magnitude, direction, and time of the contact pressure, which is called dynamic contact resistance. Because this change is affected by the external dynamic environment and occurs in a very short period of time; a pair of mated contacts may be squeezed to reduce the contact resistance, or may be pulled to increase the contact resistance, and even cause Momentary power outage. This momentary power failure lasts only a few microseconds and is enough to cause the system to crash.

Instantaneous break detection is a further dynamic assessment of the product on the basis of static conduction, in order to assess the contact reliability of the connector assembly (wire harness) in a dynamic environment. In addition to selecting a transient detector that meets the requirements of product technical standards for transient detection, it must also be equipped with a device that can provide test conditions such as vibration, impact, and collision that meet the frequency and acceleration specified in product technical standards to assess connectors. Whether there is any instantaneous power failure of the mated contacts in its components (wiring harness) under dynamic stress conditions. It is generally believed that the voltage drop at both ends of a mated pair of contacts exceeds 50% of the power supply or the contact resistance instantaneously increases beyond the specified value, which can be judged as an instantaneous power failure failure. Therefore, there are two conditions for judging whether a drop-off occurs: duration and voltage drop (or contact resistance increment), both of which are indispensable.

4. **Poor Insulation**

By applying a high voltage to a certain detection point and measuring the leakage current between the non-conducting point to determine whether the insulation resistance is qualified. Leakage current greater than the set value is unqualified, less than or equal to the set value is qualified.

Insulation resistance is mainly affected by factors such as insulator material, temperature, humidity, contamination, test voltage and duration of continuous application of test electricity. There are metal residues on the surface or inside of the insulator, surface dust, flux, or pollution and moisture, organic material precipitates and harmful gases., will cause short circuit, leakage, breakdown, low insulation and other poor insulation.

5. **Short Circuit (Breakdown)**

Short circuit refers to the failure fault that the circuit that should not be conducted in the connector assembly is conducted, and it is a fatal defect that endangers the safe use performance. Poor quality of insulating materials, harsh environmental conditions such as damp heat, salt spray, dust, wrong wiring during assembly, and poor crimping quality are all direct causes of short circuit failures.

Breakdown means that there are defects in the insulator, and after the test voltage is applied, breakdown discharge or damage will inevitably occur. Sequence discharge manifests as failure phenomena such as arcing (surface discharge), spark discharge (air discharge) or breakdown (breakdown discharge).

6. **Miswiring**

Miswiring refers to the miswiring fault caused by the operator's human error during the production and assembly of connector components. For example, the normal wiring is A1-B1, A2-B2, and now the wrong wiring is A1-B2, A2-B1. If B1 is short-circuited, it can be judged as a miswiring fault.

7. **Poor Fixation**

If the fixation is poor, the mild one will affect the contact reliability, causing instantaneous power failure. In the severe case, the structure of the electrical connector component will be unreliable due to materials, design, process and other reasons in the mated state, which will cause the gap between the plug and the socket of the connector. Abnormal separation or even disintegration occurs between the insulator and the contact, between the pin and the socket, which will cause serious consequences of interruption of power transmission and signal control of the control system.

Unreliable design structure, wrong material selection, improper selection of molding process, poor quality of heat treatment, mold, crimping, assembly and other processes, deformation and fracture of elastic parts, failure of secondary locking mechanism and improper crimping and assembly will all cause poor fixation.

8. **Poor Seal**

For electrical connectors with tightness requirements, the tightness must be tested 100% one by one in strict accordance with the requirements of the standard, and products with excessive leakage rates must be eliminated. Due to the poor interchangeability of the shell, poor injection molding quality of the insulator, and poor mating of the contacts, etc., the stress concentration at the interface between the insulator and the contact, and defects such as micro-cracks and air bubbles will cause poor sealing and failure.

For example, a digital diagnosis and treatment equipment used to seal the electrical connector shell and insulator between the use of 771 adhesive adhesive curing, sealing test found air leakage, failure analysis, confirmed that the adhesive is not fully cured, poor bonding, curing shrinkage resulting in large cavities.

4.7.2.5 Discrete Main Failure Modes

With the improvement of the semiconductor production process, the failure of discrete devices caused by the production process is decreasing. More and more discrete devices fail due to improper use. According to the statistics of the use of digital medical equipment, the main failure models of discrete devices are as follows:

(1) Open circuit, including lead wire breakage, chip burnout, chip bonding and chip cracking, etc.
(2) Drift of electrical parameters, including reduction of withstand voltage, excessive leakage current, increase of saturation voltage drop, drift of turn-on voltage, degradation of DC amplification factor, increase of on-resistance, channel leakage and surface leakage, etc.
(3) Short circuit, including complete short circuit or exhibiting resistance characteristics.

Since there are many types of discrete devices, due to their different functions and processes, the failure performance is quite different and has its own particularity. However, as a basic device formed by semiconductor technology, its failure mechanism has certain similarities. The failure mechanism of semiconductor discrete devices in digital medical equipment is summarized as follows:

(1) Thermal breakdown. Thermal breakdown or secondary breakdown failure is the main failure mechanism affecting semiconductor power devices, and most of the damage during use is related to the secondary breakdown phenomenon. Secondary breakdown is divided into forward bias secondary breakdown and reverse bias secondary breakdown. The former is related to the thermal performance of the device itself, such as the doping concentration of the device, the intrinsic concentration, etc., and the latter is related to the carrier avalanche multiplication in the space charge region (such as near the collector). The two are always accompanied by the current inside the device concentrated.
(2) Overcurrent burnt. For rectifier diodes or thyristors (especially diodes with bonding process), instantaneous overcurrent pulses appear during operation, and the main failures caused by overcurrent pulses are melting of the top metallization; mechanical damage, device cracks, which are caused by thermal expansion The role of thermal and mechanical stress; due to the negative temperature effect of the resistance caused by the temperature rise, the forward voltage drop of the diode decreases, and the positive feedback is formed, resulting in the formation of hot spots in the local area.
(3) Overvoltage breakdown. The reverse breakdown voltage of the discrete device is limited by the avalanche breakdown, and it can work in the avalanche breakdown state for a short time. For planar junction devices, the edge position limits the maximum reverse voltage (except for MOSFETs, where the cell structure determines that avalanche breakdown initially starts below the cell), therefore, avalanche breakdown first starts from the edge. For example, for a planar junction diode with a guard ring, the electric field strength between the P-type anode and the nearest voltage ring is the largest, and if a breakdown occurs here, it is related to the voltage.
(4) Dynamic avalanche. During the dynamic turn-off process, the current-controlled impact ionization phenomenon affected by the free carrier concentration in the device causes dynamic avalanche, which may occur in bipolar devices, diodes and IGBTs.

(5) Chip welding failure. The ideal welding interface should have no internal stress, no cracks and voids, low ohmic contact and low ground contact thermal resistance. In fact, due to the pollution of the bottom surface of the silicon wafer and the gold-plated layer of the base, natural aging and the influence of the gold-plated layer, there are unreliable factors in the soldering interface of the chip.

    Since the chip and the solder are different materials with different coefficients of thermal expansion, there is a problem of thermal mismatch at high temperatures. In addition, the existence of solder voids will increase the thermal resistance of the device, make heat dissipation worse, form hot spots in local areas, increase the junction temperature, and cause temperature-related failures such as electromigration.

(6) Inner wire bonding failure. The corrosion failure of the bonding point is caused by corrosion under the action of water vapor, chlorine, etc. Thermal or vibration cycles lead to aluminum bond wire fatigue failure. The volume of the IGBT packaged in the module increases. If the installation method is improper, it is easy to form stress concentration, which will lead to fatigue fracture of the internal leads of the module. For power devices, an aluminum-aluminum bonding system is used, and excessive bonding pressure will cause damage such as bonding craters.

4.7.2.6 Main Failure Modes of Integrated Circuits

The failure modes of semiconductor integrated circuits are various, and the parts where the failure occurs of the integrated circuits are classified. The main failure modes of the integrated circuits are shown in Table 4.41.

It can be seen from Table 4.42 that there are various failure modes of integrated circuits, among which the more common failure modes are electrical parameter degradation, gate interlayer breakdown and short circuit, metallized interconnection open circuit, chip burnout, circuit leakage, and circuit non-function, storage data loss, protection circuit burnout, secondary breakdown, and aluminum penetration are described in detail below.

(1) Gate interlayer breakdown and short circuit. With the scaling down of VLSI devices, the high electric field on the thin gate oxide layer is a major factor affecting device yield and reliability during device production. When the oxide layer is injected before there is electricity, there will be structural changes (trap, interface state, etc.), which will cause an increase in local current. When enough charges are injected into the oxide layer, thermal damage will occur, resulting in a low line in the oxide layer. The resistance path of the dielectric layer produces an unrecoverable leakage, that is, a breakdown short circuit of the gate dielectric layer. This breakdown can be obtained by applying a current to the dielectric layer or applying a high electric field.

(2) Degradation of electrical parameters. The degradation of electrical parameters refers to the decrease of the current gain of the bipolar device, the increase of the

Table 4.41 Main failure modes of integrated circuits

Failure part	Failure model
Chip body	Electrical parameter degradation, secondary breakdown, chip crack, leakage or short circuit, parameter drift; open circuit, short circuit, leakage, and burning of metal interconnection lines (interconnection system)
Film loading	Chip disengagement cracks, hot spots
Bonding wire	Adhesion and delamination of bond lead frame, solder joints fatigue damage
Encapsulation	Encapsulation material rupture, encapsulation material fatigue cracks, chip surface leakage, aluminum penetration (corrosion of the aluminum film on the chip), open circuit or short circuit, chip crack, pin brittle open circuit, stored data loss
External factors (mechanical vibration, shock, over-voltage stress, power supply pulsation)	Gate dielectric breakdown short circuit, chip burnout, stored data loss, protection circuit burnout

reverse leakage current of the PN junction, and the change of the breakdown voltage terminal. For MOS devices, the flat-band voltage, threshold voltage drift, transconductance drop, linear region drain current and saturation region drain current decrease or even breakdown; for charge-trap devices, the transfer efficiency decreases; for optoelectronic devices, This is a decrease in luminous efficiency, etc.

(3) The metallized interconnection line is open. The open circuit of the metallized interconnection refers to the open circuit of the aluminum wiring used for electrical connection on the chip. The reason for the open circuit is related to the processing technology and use conditions of the chip.

In multi-layer metal wiring, the use of etching to etch the through holes on the aluminum and dielectric layers will cause uneven thickness of the second layer of metal film at the edge of the metal and the steps of the oxide layer, resulting in broken bars and open circuits.

During use, the current density flowing in the metal strip is too high, which causes the migration of metal atoms, which leads to the breakage of the metallized interconnection line and produces an open circuit.

(4) The chip is burned. When an excessive input signal or power supply voltage is applied to the chip, a large area of the device will be burned or a serious overstress breakdown point will be generated on the chip, which is chip burn.

There is an NPNP parasitic thyristor structure in the CMOS circuit, which will be triggered under certain conditions, and a large current will flow between the power supply and the ground, and a positive feedback process will be formed in the NPNP parasitic thyristor structure at the same time. At this time, the parasitic thyristor structure In the conduction state, as long as the

Table 4.42 *F* distribution critical value table

Degrees of freedom ($n-m-1$)	$\alpha = 0.05$ Total number of independent variables (m)				$\alpha = 0.01$ Total number of independent variables (m)				Degrees of freedom ($n-m-1$)
	1	2	3	4	1	2	3	4	
1	0.997	0.999	0.999	0.999	1	1	1	1	1
2	0.95	0.975	0.983	0.987	0.99	0.995	0.997	0.998	2
3	0.878	0.93	0.95	0.961	0.959	0.976	0.983	0.987	3
4	0.811	0.881	0.912	0.93	0.917	0.949	0.962	0.97	4
5	0.754	0.836	0.874	0.898	0.874	0.917	0.937	0.949	5
6	0.707	0.795	0.839	0.867	0.834	0.886	0.911	0.927	6
7	0.666	0.758	0.807	0.838	0.798	0.855	0.885	0.904	7
8	0.632	0.726	0.777	0.811	0.765	0.827	0.86	0.882	8
9	0.602	0.697	0.75	0.786	0.735	0.8	0.836	0.861	9
10	0.576	0.671	0.726	0.763	0.708	0.776	0.814	0.84	10
11	0.553	0.648	0.703	0.741	0.684	0.753	0.793	0.821	11
12	0.532	0.627	0.683	0.722	0.661	0.732	0.773	0.802	12
13	0.514	0.608	0.664	0.703	0.641	0.712	0.755	0.785	13
14	0.497	0.59	0.646	0.686	0.623	0.694	0.737	0.768	14
15	0.482	0.574	0.63	0.67	0.606	0.677	0.721	0.752	15
16	0.468	0.559	0.615	0.655	0.59	0.622	0.706	0.738	16
17	0.456	0.545	0.601	0.641	0.575	0.647	0.691	0.724	17
18	0.444	0.532	0.587	0.628	0.561	0.633	0.678	0.71	18
19	0.433	0.52	0.575	0.615	0.549	0.62	0.665	0.698	19
20	0.423	0.509	0.563	0.604	0.537	0.608	0.652	0.685	20
21	0.413	0.498	0.552	0.592	0.526	0.596	0.641	0.674	21
22	0.404	0.488	0.542	0.582	0.515	0.585	0.63	0.663	22
23	0.396	0.479	0.532	0.572	0.505	0.574	0.619	0.652	23
24	0.388	0.47	0.523	0.562	0.496	0.565	0.609	0.642	24
25	0.381	0.462	0.514	0.553	0.487	0.555	0.6	0.633	25
26	0.374	0.454	0.506	0.545	0.478	0.546	0.59	0.626	26
27	0.367	0.446	0.498	0.536	0.47	0.538	0.582	0.615	27
28	0.361	0.439	0.49	0.529	0.463	0.53	0.573	0.606	28
29	0.355	0.432	0.482	0.521	0.456	0.522	0.565	0.598	29
30	0.349	0.426	0.476	0.514	0.449	0.514	0.558	0.591	30
35	0.325	0.397	0.445	0.482	0.418	0.481	0.523	0.556	35
40	0.304	0.373	0.419	0.455	0.393	0.454	0.494	0.526	40
45	0.228	0.353	0.397	0.432	0.372	0.43	0.47	0.501	45
50	0.273	0.336	0.379	0.412	0.354	0.41	0.449	0.479	50

(continued)

Table 4.42 (continued)

Degrees of freedom (n − m − 1)	α = 0.05				α = 0.01				Degrees of freedom (n − m − 1)
	Total number of independent variables (m)				Total number of independent variables (m)				
	1	2	3	4	1	2	3	4	
60	0.25	0.308	0.348	0.38	0.325	0.377	0.414	0.442	60
70	0.232	0.286	0.324	0.354	0.302	0.351	0.386	0.413	70
80	0.217	0.269	0.304	0.332	0.283	0.33	0.362	0.389	80
90	0.205	0.254	0.288	0.315	0.267	0.312	0.343	0.368	90
100	0.195	0.241	0.274	0.3	0.254	0.297	0.327	0.351	100
125	0.174	0.216	0.246	0.269	0.228	0.266	0.294	0.316	125
150	0.159	0.198	0.225	0.247	0.208	0.244	0.27	0.29	150
200	0.138	0.172	0.196	0.215	0.181	0.212	0.234	0.253	200
300	0.113	0.141	0.16	0.176	0.148	0.174	0.192	0.208	300
400	0.098	0.122	0.139	0.153	0.128	0.151	0.167	0.18	400
500	0.088	0.109	0.124	0.137	0.115	0.135	0.15	0.162	500
1000	0.062	0.077	0.088	0.097	0.081	0.096	0.106	0.115	1000

power supply voltage does not drop below the critical value, even if the trigger signal disappears, the formed conduction current will not disappear, causing the device to burn out. The parasitic thyristor effect of CMOS circuits is also called door lock effect.

(5) Circuit leakage. Circuit leakage refers to a much larger current in the device that should be insulated or a small current, and it is an order of magnitude increase. The magnitude of the current is related to the damaged part of the device.

In multi-layer metal wiring, there are pinholes in the oxide layer between the two layers of wiring and cracks in the dielectric film caused by the unevenness of the first layer of metal or excessive thickness of the dielectric film, which destroys the insulation performance of the dielectric and generates leakage.

(6) The circuit has no function. The non-function of the circuit means that the circuit port that should have signal output becomes no signal output. The factors affecting the non-function of the circuit include internal and external factors: the internal cause is that the bonding wire of the output signal port is blown so that the signal cannot be output; Bypass to ground; the external cause is mainly insufficient power supply so that the circuit cannot output signals.

(7) Stored data is lost. Loss of stored data refers to the phenomenon of circuit misoperation caused by external factors, which causes the loss of charge stored in dynamic memory, the flipping of storage cells in static RAM (random access memory), and the loss of dynamic logic circuit information, which has nothing to do with the physical defects of the device itself.

(8) The protection circuit is burned out. During the processing, production, assembly, storage and transportation of microelectronic devices, they may come into contact with static-carrying containers, test equipment and operators, and the static electricity will be discharged to the ground through the device leads, causing damage or failure of the device. This is called Electrostatic discharge damage (ESD). It has damage to all kinds of devices, but is particularly sensitive to MOS devices. The antistatic ability of the device is related to the device type, input protection structure, layout design, manufacturing process and usage.

    The ESD of the device is divided into three grades of 1, 2 and 3, and its antistatic voltage is below 2000 V, 2000–3999 V and above 4000 V respectively. Under the action of overelectric stress or excessive static voltage, the protection circuit will be shocked or burned, so that the device will lose its function and cause failure.

(9) Secondary breakdown. When the device is biased at a special operating point, the voltage suddenly drops, the current suddenly rises, and the physical phenomenon of negative resistance is called secondary breakdown. At this time, if there is no limit current or other protective measures, the device will be burned. The secondary breakdown is different from the avalanche breakdown. The avalanche breakdown is an electrical breakdown. Once the reverse bias voltage drops, the device (if the breakdown occurs under current limiting control) can return to normal, which is reversible and non-destructive of. The secondary breakdown is a destructive thermal breakdown. It is an irreversible process. Excessive current flows through the PN junction, and the temperature is very high, which burns the PN junction.

(10) Aluminum penetration. When silicon dissolves into the overlying aluminum film, aluminum passes through the connection window when the connection hole is annealed. This phenomenon is often referred to as aluminum film spikes or connection pits. The silicon melted into the aluminum film will precipitate after the temperature of the silicon wafer drops, or form small islands on the oxide layer, or epitaxial silicon as a connection hole, resulting in a decrease in the effective contact area, an increase in the contact resistance, or even blocking the entire connection.

4.7.3 Acceleration Model of Components Under Typical Stress

The acceleration mechanisms and acceleration effects of various external stresses on various failure modes are different. The component acceleration model is used to describe the relationship between the reliability characteristics of the failure mode (such as average life, characteristic life, failure rate, etc.) and the accelerated stress level. Commonly used acceleration models include thermal aging (high temperature) acceleration model, thermal fatigue (temperature cycle) acceleration model, temperature-humidity two comprehensive stress acceleration model, mechanical stress or electrical stress inverse power law acceleration model, random vibration fatigue model, shock vibration fatigue model, temperature-vibration acceleration model, generalized Eyring acceleration model, etc. In this chapter, by analyzing the influence of external stresses such as different environmental stresses and electrical stresses on electronic components, an accelerated model of components under typical stress is given, which is used to describe the reliability characteristics of failure modes (such as average life, characteristic life, failure rate, etc.) and the accelerated stress level, to provide reference for readers to carry out accelerated life tests.

4.7.3.1 High Temperature Aging Model

In the nineteenth century, Arrhenius studied the chemical process excited by temperature stress, and proposed the Arrhenius acceleration model based on a large amount of data. This model is suitable for products whose accelerated stress is a single temperature stress. The most important stress suffered by digital medical equipment during the storage period is temperature stress, so the Aronis model has been widely used in the accelerated storage life test of electronic products.

The stress life model describing the influence of temperature effects on the life of digital medical equipment generally uses the Arrhenis accelerated life model, which accelerates the chemical reaction inside the product (such as electronic components and insulating materials of digital medical equipment, etc.) And the Eyring model derived from the principles of quantum mechanics. American MIL-HDBK-217F *MIL ITARY HANDBOOK RELIABILITY PREDICTION OF ELECTRONIC EQUIPMENT* The Arrhenius model is used to describe the effect of thermal stress on the reliability of semiconductor discrete devices. Many literatures also use this model to discuss the failures that occur when product performance degradation accumulates to a certain extent. This failure is caused by some physical and chemical changes in the microstructure inside the product.

The Arrhenius acceleration model is expressed as follows:

$$\xi = Ae^{E_a/kT} \tag{4.66}$$

In the formula, ξ is a certain lifetime characteristic, such as median lifetime, average lifetime, etc.; is a *A constant*, and $A > 0$; E_a is the activation energy, related to the material, ev expressed E_a/k in electron volts 8.617×10^{-5}ev/°C; The unit is temperature, so it is also called activation temperature; E_a/k T it is an absolute temperature, and its value is approximately equal to the Celsius temperature value plus 273. The Arrhenis model suggests that the lifetime signature will decrease exponentially with increasing temperature.

4.7.3.2 Temperature Cycle Thermal Fatigue Model

The Coffin-Manson model is widely used in the welding of metal materials to model the fatigue failure (usually crack growth) of products caused by repeated temperature cycles. A typical Coffin-Manson model mainly considers the following three factors: the maximum temperature of the cycle $T_{\max}$, the amount of temperature change ΔT, and the cycle frequency f. The specific form of the model is:

$$N = A \cdot f^{-a} \cdot (\Delta T)^{-b} \cdot G(T_{\max}) \tag{4.67}$$

In the formula, N is the number of cycles at the time of failure; f is the cycle frequency; ΔT is the range of temperature variation in one cycle; A is the model coefficient; a cycle frequency index, $-1/3$ usually takes b a value; $G(T_{\max}) = \exp\left(E_{\mathrm{a}}/kT_{\max}\right)$ The Arrhenius relation at the highest temperature of a cycle, k is the Boltzmann constant, and E_{a} is the activation energy.

This is a semi-empirical model and only gives a trend. The Coffin-Manson model uses cycle frequency f to comprehensively reflect the influence of temperature duration and temperature change time on product performance under each cycle, and does not point out the difference between temperature duration and temperature change time. At the same time, the Coffin-Manson model does not reflect the difference between temperature cycling and temperature shock, which is also a shortcoming of the Coffin-Manson model in engineering applications.

4.7.3.3 Temperature and Humidity Aging Model

1. **Eyrin Model of Damp-Heat Aging**

The Eileen model of single stress is derived from the principles of quantum mechanics, which expresses the life characteristics of some products as a function of absolute temperature. When the absolute temperature changes within a small range, the single-stress Aylin model is similar to the Aronis model. In many applications, these two models can be used to fit the data, and the acceleration model to be selected is determined according to the fit. Therefore, the Eileen model is often used in accelerated storage life tests of electronic products.

Glasstene, Laidler, and Eyring proposed an acceleration model in 1941, which is known as the generalized Eyring model. This model is applicable to the case where the product is subjected to both temperature stress and another environmental stress, but it is necessary to assume that the temperature stress and the other environmental stress do not interfere with each other. The generalized Eyring model can be used when the components and materials are subjected to both temperature and other stresses during the storage period of the digital medical equipment, such as transportation and periodic testing.

The generalized Eyring model has the form:

$$t_L = CT^{\alpha} \cdot e^{\frac{E_a}{kT} + \sum_i \left(B_i + \frac{A_i}{T}\right) S_i} \tag{4.68}$$

In the formula,

t_L Product storage life;
E_a Activation energy;
T Temperature stress (in Kelvin);
S_i Stresses other than temperature stress;
k Boltzmann constant;
C, α Constant.

Whether it is the single-stress Eileen model or the generalized Eileen model, they are all activation energy-based models like the Arrhenius model. Similarly, they are mainly used to describe non-mechanical (non-material fatigue) in electronic products that depend on chemical Failure mechanisms for reactive, corrosion, species diffusion or migration processes.

But their main difference from the Arrhenius model is reflected in two aspects:

(1) The Arrhenis model is an empirical formula based on experimental results, while the Eyrin model is a theoretical result based on chemistry and quantum mechanics;
(2) The Arrhenis model only describes the relationship between failure and temperature, while the Eyring model believes that the relationship between failure and other types of stress can also be given in the model through similar mathematical forms.

2. **Peck Model**

In the actual storage life of electronic products, an important factor affecting the storage life of non-sealed devices, that is, plastic-encapsulated devices, is the ambient humidity. Moisture in the environment can penetrate through the plastic packaging material to cause chip corrosion and failure. However, none of the single-stress models can give a specific expression of the impact of environmental humidity on the storage life of the device.

In the 1970s, researchers began to construct a new lifetime model by introducing humidity based on the Arrhenius model. The Peck model is a temperature and humidity model under steady-state conditions. Peck summarized the results of many steady-state experiments, and at 85 °C/The result of 85%RH was compared and analyzed as a benchmark. In 1986, the life expression of plastic-encapsulated devices was given in the following form:

$$t_L = C \cdot H^{-n} e^{\frac{E_a}{kT}} \tag{4.69}$$

In the formula,

t_L Product storage life;
$\Phi(x)$ Activation energy;

T Temperature stress (unit: Kelvin);
H Relative humidity (unit: %RH).
k Boltzmann constant;
C Constant;
n A unitless constant greater than 0.

The Peck model is suitable for product failures caused by two kinds of stresses, temperature and humidity. It is recommended to be used when the failure of non-hermetic electronic or electromechanical devices is caused by two kinds of stress, temperature and humidity.

3. **Shirley Model**

The focus of this model is based on the Peck model, which considers the unsteady effects of frequent power on and off during the actual working process of the device on the process of moisture in the air entering and exiting the plastic-encapsulated device. The model form is as follows:

$$u, \sigma \tag{4.70}$$

For the meaning of each parameter, see *THB Reliability Models And Life Prediction For Intermittently-powered Non-hermetic Components.*

This model is suitable for non-hermetic devices that often need to be turned on and off during the period of regular inspection or combat readiness, and the failure of the device is caused by the joint action of temperature and humidity.

4.7.3.4 Inverse Power Law Aging Model

When electrical stress (such as voltage, current, electric power, etc.) is used as the accelerating stress, it is generally believed that the relationship between life characteristics and stress conforms to the inverse power law model:

$$\xi = AV^{-c} \tag{4.71}$$

Among them ξ is a performance characteristic; A is a constant; c is a normal constant related to the activation energy; V is the accelerated stress, usually voltage.

4.7.3.5 Random Vibration Fatigue Model

Under actual working conditions, electronic equipment will be subject to vibrations caused by external factors, and the circuit board inside the equipment will also vibrate with the vibration of the whole equipment. Due to the unstable stress generated by vibration, it will cause the reliability of solder joints of components on the board, the reliability of plated through holes and the fatigue of the circuit board itself.

Although the external factors themselves are very complex, in most cases the external factors have stable statistical characteristics and can be modeled as random vibrations. By studying the vibration characteristics of the circuit board itself, external excitations with stable statistical characteristics can be obtained. And generate the response statistical characteristics of different positions of the whole circuit board, and these statistical characteristics can reflect the vibration intensity of different positions of the whole circuit board, so as to determine the vibration fatigue life of components at different positions. The random vibration fatigue model is shown in formula (4.72):

$$1 \leq i \leq, 3 \leq n \leq 50 \tag{4.72}$$

In the formula, N_f is the fatigue life of the device; x and y are the position coordinates of the device on the circuit board; C is a constant determined according to the standard test, for random vibration, $C = 2 \times 10^6$; b is the fatigue strength The indices, $z1$ and $z2$ are determined by Eqs. (4.73) and (4.74).

$$z_1 = \frac{0.00022B}{ct\sqrt{L}} \tag{4.73}$$

$$z_2 = \frac{36.85\sqrt{\text{PSD}_{\text{max}}}}{f_n^{1.25}} \tag{4.74}$$

Among them, PSD_{max} is the maximum power density of random vibration; f_n is the minimum natural frequency of random vibration; B is the maximum value (in inches) of the distance from the 4 sides of the device to the 4 sides of the circuit board; L is the length of the device (in inches); t is the thickness of the circuit board (in inches); c is a coefficient, for two-column pin devices (such as DIP, SIP, SOJ, SOP, SOT), $c = 1.0$, for four-sided pin devices (such as QFP, PGA, BGA), $c = 1.26$, for leadless devices (such as chip resistors and capacitors), $c = 2.25$.

4.7.3.6 Shock Vibration Fatigue Model

This is an overstress model and the failure criterion is:

$$Z_{\text{allow}} < Z_{\text{max}} \tag{4.75}$$

In the formula:

$$z_{\text{allow}} = \frac{0.00132B}{ct\sqrt{L}} \tag{4.76}$$

$$Z_{\text{max}} = \frac{9.8GP_F}{f_n^{1.5}} \sin(\pi x)\sin(\pi y) \tag{4.77}$$

Among them, B is the maximum value of the distance from the 4 sides of the device to the 4 sides of the circuit board (in inches); L is the length of the device (in inches); t is the thickness of the circuit board (in inches); the value of parameter c The value of the parameter c in random vibration is the same; x and y *are* the position coordinates of the device on the circuit board; f_n is the minimum natural frequency; G is the impact acceleration; the determination of the value of the parameter P_F is as follows: Let T be the impact time, then for a half sine wave, there is:

$$P_F = \begin{cases} \frac{4f_nT}{1-(2f_nT)^2\cos(\pi f_nT)}, \ f_nT < 0.5 \\ \frac{2f_nT}{2f_nT-1}\sin\left(\frac{2\pi}{2f_nT+1}\right), \quad 0.5 < f_nT < 1.5 \\ \frac{2f_nT}{2f_nT-1}\sin\left(\frac{4\pi}{2f_nT+1}\right), \quad 1.5 < f_nT < 2.5 \\ 1, \ f_nT > 2.5 \end{cases} \tag{4.78}$$

For pulse waveforms, there is:

$$P_F = \sqrt{\frac{\sin(\pi f_nT)}{\pi f_nT} - \frac{2}{\pi f_nT}\sin(\pi f_nT)\cos(3\pi f_nT) + 1} \tag{4.79}$$

4.7.3.7 Temperature-Vibration Acceleration Model

In 1991, Donald B. Barker and other experts proposed an acceleration model for the influence of temperature and vibration stress on product life after studying the solder joints of printed circuit boards. The formula is described as follows:

$$N_f = \frac{1}{2}\left[\frac{F}{2\varepsilon} \cdot \frac{L_D \Delta\alpha \Delta T_e}{h}\right]^{\frac{1}{c}} \tag{4.80}$$

In the formula,

- N_f Product storage life (F > 1.0 if the chip carrier uses lead-free solder, otherwise F = 1.0);
- ε Fatigue ductility coefficient;
- h Solder joint height;
- ΔT_e Equivalent temperature range;
- L_D The maximum distance between solder joints of the device;
- $\Delta\alpha$ Absolute error in TCE between part and substrate.

This model is recommended for failures of electronic, electromechanical, and optoelectronic equipment, such as failure causes related to transportation or loading and unloading, fatigue or shedding of solder joints caused by vibration and temperature stress, and other failure mechanisms.

4.7.3.8 Generalized Eyring Acceleration Model

Some acceleration tests are T carried out under the joint action of absolute temperature and another stress, and the general form of the acceleration model is: V

$$\xi = \beta \cdot \exp[-(\gamma/T) - \delta V - \varepsilon(V/T)] \tag{4.81}$$

Here β, γ and δ are constant characteristic parameters of the product and the accelerated process. This model is often used to simulate the acceleration process of electronic products and dielectric materials, where V V represents the breakdown voltage or its logarithm.

4.7.4 Physical Model of Component Failure

4.7.4.1 Time-Dependent Gate Oxide Breakdown Model (TDDB)

Generally, the breakdown of the gate oxide layer of a MOS device refers to the instantaneous breakdown that occurs when a high voltage is applied so that the electric field strength reaches or exceeds the critical breakdown electric field that the dielectric material can withstand. In MOS devices and their integrated circuits, there is a thin layer of $SiO_{2\ \text{under the gate}}$, which is commonly referred to as gate oxide. The leakage of the gate oxide has a great relationship with the quality of the gate oxide. If the leakage increases to a certain extent, it will form a breakdown and cause the device to fail. Gate oxide breakdown is divided into instantaneous breakdown and time-dependent dielectric breakdown (Time Dependent Dielectric Breakdown, TDDB), the latter means that the applied electric field is lower than the intrinsic breakdown field strength of the gate oxide, and does not cause intrinsic breakdown wear, but breakdown still occurred after a certain period of time. This is due to the generation and accumulation of defects (traps) in the oxide layer during the application of electrical stress.

The breakdown of the gate oxide layer is related to the external electric field applied to the oxide layer, activation energy and temperature. It is generally believed that the breakdown of the oxide layer is the result of the joint action of thermal stress and electrical stress. The breakdown time is also related to the gate capacitance area, gate voltage etc. Below are two TDDB models,

Thermochemical degradation model (E model) [19]:

$$\text{TTF} = A \exp(\gamma E) \exp\left(\frac{E_{\text{a1}}}{kT}\right) \tag{4.82}$$

Breakdown model related to hole injection (1/*E* model) [20]:

$$\mathrm{TTF} = \tau \exp\left(\frac{G}{E}\right) \exp\left(\frac{E_{\mathrm{a2}}}{kT}\right) \tag{4.83}$$

In the above two formulas, A and τ are proportional constants; γ is the electric field acceleration parameter; G is a constant; E is the electric field intensity applied to the gate oxide layer; E_{a1} and E_{a2} are the thermal activation energy of the formula; k is the glass Ertzmann's constant; T is the absolute temperature.

In actual prediction, the two models are usually combined to form a unified model of E model and $1/E$ *model* [21], see formula (4.84):

$$\frac{1}{\mathrm{TTF}} = \frac{1}{t_E} + \frac{1}{t_{\frac{1}{E}}} \tag{4.84}$$

4.7.4.2 Solder Joint Thermal Fatigue Model

The main reason for thermal fatigue failure of solder joints is: due to the difference in coefficient of thermal expansion (Coefficient of Thermal Expansion, CTE) of the surrounding materials of solder joints, the thermal strain generated by various materials does not match during thermal expansion or contraction, and when the strain is not The coordination produces stress concentration, which leads to the initiation and propagation of cracks.

There are many kinds of thermal fatigue models for solder joints, such as stress-based fatigue models, strain-based fatigue models, energy-based fatigue models, etc. Among them, the most widely used is the strain-based Engelmaier model, which is represented by formula (4.85) Sure.

$$N_f = \frac{1}{2}\left(\frac{\Delta\gamma}{2\varepsilon_f}\right)^{\frac{1}{c}} \tag{4.85}$$

In the formula, N_f is the fatigue life; ε_f is the material constant, for the widely used eutectic solder, $\varepsilon_f = 0.325$; c is a parameter related to the temperature cycle profile, determined by the formula (4.86),

$$c = -0.442 - 0.0006T_{\mathrm{sj}} + 0.0147\ln\left(1 + \frac{360}{t_{\mathrm{H}}}\right) \tag{4.86}$$

the formula, T_{sj} is the average temperature of the temperature cycle (°C); t_{H} is the high temperature holding time in the temperature cycle (min); $\Delta\gamma$ is the total shear strain range, which consists of three parts, namely:

$$\Delta\gamma = \gamma_{\mathrm{e}} + \gamma_{\mathrm{p}} + \gamma_{\mathrm{c}} \tag{4.87}$$

the formula, γ_e is the elastic strain component; γ_p is the plastic strain component; γ_c is the creep strain component; there are many ways to determine $\Delta\gamma$, for the simplified first-order fatigue model, for leadless packages and leads Foot package, $\Delta\gamma$ *are determined* by formula (4.88) and formula (4.89):

$$\Delta\gamma = F\frac{L_D}{h}\Delta\alpha\Delta T \tag{4.88}$$

$$\Delta\gamma = 0.5F\frac{K_D}{(200\text{psi})Ah}(\Delta\alpha_c L\Delta T - \Delta\alpha_s L\Delta T)^2 \tag{4.89}$$

Equation (4.88) applies to leadless package (such as LCC) solder joints.

In the formula, h is the height of the solder joint; L_D is the characteristic dimension; $\Delta\alpha$ is the difference between the CTE of the device packaging material and the circuit board material; ΔT is the difference between the highest temperature and the lowest temperature in the thermal cycle profile; F is the correction Coefficients generally take values within the range of 0.5 to 1.5.

Formula (4.89) is applicable to the solder joints of leaded packages (such as SOP, QFP). In the formula, K_D is the stiffness of the lead material (in lb/in); A is the area of the solder joint (in $^{2)}$; h is the height of the solder joint (in in); it α_c is the CTE of the device packaging material; α_s CTE of printed circuit board material; L is half of the length of the diagonal line of the pin (unit is in); ΔT is the difference between the highest temperature and the lowest temperature in the thermal cycle profile; F is the correction factor, generally in the range of 0.5 to 1.5 value within the range.

4.7.4.3 Electromigration Model

When a strong current flows through a metal wire, metal ions will move under the interaction of the current and other factors and form pores or cracks in the wire. This phenomenon is called electromigration.

Electromigration is caused by the diffusion of metal ions. It has three diffusion forms: surface diffusion, lattice diffusion, and grain boundary diffusion. The diffusion patterns involved will be different for different metallic materials. For example, the diffusion in bumps is mainly lattice diffusion; the diffusion in Al interconnects is mainly grain boundary diffusion; and the diffusion in Cu interconnects is mainly surface diffusion. The external forces that cause diffusion mainly include: the comprehensive force generated by the momentum exchange between electrons and metal ions and the external electric field, the diffusion force generated by the non-equilibrium ion concentration, the mechanical stress generated by the longitudinal pressure gradient, and the thermal stress generated by the temperature gradient. The presence of these stresses can lead to discontinuity in the ion current density and thus electromigration.

In addition to the above-mentioned external stress, electromigration is also affected by geometric factors. At high current densities, mechanical stress gradients are created on metal interconnect lines. At the same time, within a certain range of less than the current density, the electromigration lifetime decreases with the increase of the length, and beyond this limit, the increase of the length has little effect on the electromigration lifetime. At this time, when the line width becomes comparable to or even smaller than the grain size, the grain boundary diffusion will be reduced and converted to lattice diffusion and surface diffusion. In addition, the presence of corners, steps, and contact holes will increase the local stress gradient and accelerate the occurrence of electromigration.

The third type of factor that affects electromigration is the metal material itself. Usually alloys can effectively inhibit electromigration. For example, doping a little copper can greatly improve the life of an aluminum strip. Adding a small amount of silicon can also improve reliability, because copper atoms along the grain interface Absorption reduces the number of sites available for diffusion.

The traditional electromigration lifetime model often uses the Black equation, see formula (4.90) . This equation establishes the relationship between the electromigration of circuit components and the current density flowing through the metal, as well as the geometric size, material properties and temperature distribution of the metal.

$$\mathrm{MTTF} = \frac{Wd}{Cj^n} \exp\left(\frac{E_\mathrm{a}}{kT}\right) \tag{4.90}$$

the formula, W and d are the shape parameters of the metal, and it is generally considered that the product of the two is the cross-sectional area of the metal wire; T is the absolute temperature; j is the current density; m and n are the failure intensity index, at low current density, $n = m = 1$; at high current density, $n = m = 3$; C is a parameter related to the structure, geometric size and temperature of the metal; E_a is the electromigration activation energy of the material; k is the Boltzmann constant ($k = 8.617 \times 10^{-5}$ eV/°C).

4.7.4.4 Plated Through Hole (PTH) Thermal Fatigue Model

Plated Through Hole (PTH) refers to a through hole in a multilayer circuit board, which is electroplated with conductive materials such as copper, nickel or solder, and is used to provide electrical connections for conductive metals of different board layers. It is an important structural component of the circuit board.

PTH failure is mainly caused by CTE mismatch between coating material and substrate material. This mismatch is mainly manifested in the outermost pad and the thickness direction of the PWB, because the CTE of the outermost pad of a multilayer board is usually 3 to 4 times that of the plating. Due to the CTE mismatch, when the PWB experiences complex temperature environment conditions throughout its life cycle, the thermal stress generated in the PTH will cause damage to the metal coating, and eventually lead to thermomechanical overstress failure or fatigue failure of the

PTH. Fatigue failure of PTH will lead to poor electrical and mechanical properties of PTH. For example, PTH failure will lead to increased resistance, or even completely open the circuit, which will eventually lead to circumferential fracture and loss of specified function of the circuit. See formula (4.91) for the PTH thermal fatigue failure mechanism model.

$$N_f^{-0.6} D_f^{0.75} + 0.9 \times \frac{S_u}{E_p}\left[\frac{\exp(D_f)}{0.36}\right]^{0.1785 \lg \frac{10^5}{N_f}} - \Delta\varepsilon = 0 \tag{4.91}$$

In the formula, N_f is the expected average fatigue life (the number of cycles before failure); D_f is the fatigue durability coefficient of the PTH coating material; S_u is the fracture strength of the PTH coating material; E_p is the elastic modulus of the PTH coating material; $\Delta\varepsilon$ is the total strain.

4.8 Failure Distribution Model and Statistical Analysis

4.8.1 Overview

The failure distribution model is a mathematical description of system (or component) failure (or failure) characteristics. There are many types of failure distribution models with different uses. From the modeling method, there are "white box" and "black box" methods. From the modeling object, it can be divided into failure (failure) time model and failure (failure) number model. At present, for products, the modeling method of failure (failure) time is generally used in statistical methods, and the product has only two states: fault state and normal state. When using the failure (failure) time modeling method, the empirical modeling method is usually used, that is, combining product failure data and engineering experience, selecting a distribution model that matches the failure data information, and performing parameter estimation and fitting optimization on the model. degree test.

This section systematically summarizes the commonly used failure rate distribution functions (exponential distribution, Weibull distribution, lognormal distribution) and the solution method of distribution parameters. The final data processing results use the least squares method and maximum likelihood estimation.

4.8.2 Exponential Distribution Model

4.8.2.1 Introduction to Distribution

Exponential distribution is one of the commonly used distribution functions of digital medical equipment. It is usually used to describe the situation where the instantaneous failure rate is constant, and it can be used for the distribution function of the performance retention period of the product. The exponential distribution is often used to describe the life distribution of electronic components, and the life distribution of a complex system composed of many independent components is also commonly used to describe the exponential distribution. As long as the number of failures of a component or system within $[t_1, t_2]$ obeys the Poisson distribution, the lifetime of the component or system obeys the exponential distribution. The exponential distribution plays an important role in the field of reliability.

Exponential distribution has the following advantages: ① Simple parameter estimation; ② Convenient mathematical processing; ③ Wide applicability. The probability density function of the exponential distribution is

$$f(t) = \lambda e^{-\lambda t}, t > 0 \tag{4.92}$$

Among them, λ is the failure rate, and the reliability function is

$$R(t) = e^{-\lambda t} \tag{4.93}$$

The cumulative failure probability distribution function is

$$F(t) = 1 - e^{-\lambda t} \tag{4.94}$$

The failure rate function is

$$\lambda(t) = \frac{f(t)}{R(t)} = \frac{\lambda e^{-\lambda t}}{e^{-\lambda t}} = \lambda \tag{4.95}$$

from formula (4.92) that the failure rate function of a random variable subject to exponential distribution is a constant, that is, it belongs to accidental failure. This point is unique to random variables that obey exponential distribution. If the failure rate of a random variable is known to be constant, its distribution must be exponential.

The mean life and variance of the exponential distribution are

$$E(T) = \int_0^{\infty} tf(t)dt = \int_0^{\infty} t\lambda e^{-\lambda t}dt = \frac{1}{\lambda} \tag{4.96}$$

$$V(T) = \frac{1}{\lambda^2} \tag{4.97}$$

The average failure rate function of the exponential distribution is

$$m(t) = \frac{1}{t}\int_0^t \lambda(x)dx = \frac{1}{t}\int_0^t \lambda dx = \lambda \tag{4.98}$$

The biggest feature of the exponential distribution is no memory. The so-called no memory refers to the product whose service life obeys the exponential distribution.

If it is still intact when stored until t_0, the probability that the product can continue to be stored until t is the same as the probability that the product can be stored from the beginning until t. The same probability at work t.

For the exponential distribution, in addition to the simple exponential distribution, the exponential distribution with position parameters is also one of the commonly used life distribution models, that is, the two-parameter exponential distribution, and its distribution function is as follows

$$f(t) = \lambda e^{-\lambda(t-T)}, t \geq T \tag{4.99}$$

where is T a positional parameter.

The mean life and variance of the two-parameter exponential distribution are

$$E(T) = \int_0^{\infty} t f(t) dt = \int_0^{\infty} t\lambda e^{-\lambda(t-T)} dt = \frac{1}{\lambda} + T \tag{4.100}$$

$$V(T) = \frac{1}{\lambda^2} \tag{4.101}$$

4.8.2.2 Parameter Solution

The parameter estimation of the exponential distribution includes point estimation and interval estimation, among which point estimation usually adopts three methods: moment estimation method, least square method and maximum likelihood estimation method; interval estimation usually adopts Pearson estimation method.

1. **Moment Estimation**

If the failure (fault) data conforms to the exponential distribution after preliminary determination, the distribution parameters can be estimated by the moment estimation method (referred to as the moment method).

The basic idea of the method of moments is to make the population moment equal to the sample moment to obtain the model parameter equation, and then obtain the estimation of the unknown parameters of the model. Assuming that the probability density function of the model is $f(t)$, then the j-th order moment is defined as

$$u_j(\theta) = \int_0^{\infty} t^j f(t) dt \tag{4.102}$$

$j = 1, 2, \cdots, \theta$ representing an unknown parameter. It can be seen from the definition that the first-order overall moment is a mathematical expectation, and the first-order overall moment has a linear relationship with the variance. Assuming that there is a complete effective data sample $t_1, t_2, \cdots, t_n$, then the j-th order moment of the sample is defined as

$$\gamma_k = \frac{1}{n}\sum_{i=1}^{n} t_i^k \tag{4.103}$$

From the relationship between population moments and sample moments

$$u_j(\theta) = \int_0^{\infty} t^j f(t)\mathrm{d}t = \gamma_k = \frac{1}{n}\sum_{i=1}^{n} t_i^k \tag{4.104}$$

For the exponential distribution, it can be seen from the previous analysis that the mean and variance of the exponential distribution are respectively

$$E(T) = \int_0^{\infty} tf(t)\mathrm{d}t = \int_0^{\infty} t\lambda \mathrm{e}^{-\lambda t}\mathrm{d}t = \frac{1}{\lambda} \tag{4.105}$$

$$V(T) = \frac{1}{\lambda^2} \tag{4.106}$$

Therefore, the moment estimation equation of the exponential distribution can be obtained

$$E(T) = \frac{1}{\lambda} = \frac{1}{n}\sum_{i=1}^{n} t_i \tag{4.107}$$

Is

$$\lambda = \frac{1}{\frac{1}{n}\sum_{i=1}^{n} t_i} \tag{4.108}$$

Or

$$V(T) = \frac{1}{\lambda^2} = \frac{1}{n}\sum_{i=1}^{n} t_i^2 \tag{4.109}$$

Is

$$\lambda = \frac{1}{\sqrt{\frac{1}{n}\sum_{i=1}^{n} t_i^2}} \tag{4.110}$$

1. **Least Square Method**

The least squares method is to estimate the unknown parameters of the model by applying the principle of the least squares method after the model is properly transformed.

The cumulative distribution function of the exponential distribution $F(t) = 1 - e^{-\lambda t}$, let $y = \ln \frac{1}{1-F(t)}$, $x = t$. Transforming the cumulative distribution function into

$$y = \lambda x \tag{4.111}$$

Therefore, $(x_1, y_1), (x_2, y_2), \cdots, (x_r, y_r)$ a straight line is formed with a slope of λ. It can be solved by the following formula.

$$\hat{\lambda} = \frac{l_{xy}}{l_{xx}} \tag{4.112}$$

$$l_{xx} = \sum_{i=1}^{n} (x_i - \overline{x})^2 = \sum_{i=1}^{n} x_i^2 - n\overline{x}^2 \tag{4.113}$$

$$l_{xy} = \sum_{i=1}^{n} (x_i - \overline{x})(y_i - \overline{y}) = \sum_{i=1}^{n} x_i y_i - n\overline{x}\overline{y} \tag{4.114}$$

2. **Maximum Likelihood Method (MLE)**

Take n samples to test, and set the censoring time (timed censoring without replacement) as t_0. Within $[0, t_0]$, r products fail, and the failure time is

$$t_1 \le t_2 \le \cdots \le t_0 \tag{4.115}$$

The probability that a product fails within $[t_i, t_i + dt_i]$ is $f(t_i)dt_i$, $i = 1,2, \ldots, r$. The probability that the lifetime of the remaining n-r products exceeds t_0 is $[e^{-\lambda t_0}]^{n-r}$, so the probability of the experimental observation result is

$$C_n^r(\lambda e^{-\lambda t_1} dt_1)(\lambda e^{-\lambda t_2} dt_2) \cdots (\lambda e^{-\lambda t_r} dt_r)[e^{-\lambda t_0}]^{n-r} \tag{4.116}$$

Neglecting the constant term, the likelihood function of the exponential distribution can be established.

$$L(\lambda) = \lambda^r \exp\{-\lambda[\sum_{i=1}^{r} t_i + (n-r)t_0]\} \tag{4.117}$$

Taking logarithms on both sides, the log likelihood equation is established as

$$\ln L(\lambda) = r \ln \lambda - \lambda[\sum_{i=1}^{r} t_i + (n-r)t_0]\} \tag{4.118}$$

Deriving the log-likelihood equation and making it equal to 0, the maximum likelihood estimate of the exponential distribution parameter is obtained as

$$\hat{\lambda} = \frac{r}{S(t_0)} \quad (4.119)$$

Among them, $S(t_0) = \sum_{i=1}^{r} t_i + (n - r)t_0$.
The estimated average lifespan is

$$\hat{\mu} = \frac{S(t_0)}{r} \quad (4.120)$$

3. **Interval Estimation (MLE)**

The expression for the confidence limit for the failure rate with a confidence level of 1-α is as follows:

A one-sided confidence interval with an upper limit of:

$$T^* = \begin{cases} nt', & \text{Replacement timed ending} \\ \sum_{i=1}^{r} t_{(i)} + (n - r)t', & \text{No replacement timed ending} \end{cases} \quad (4.121)$$

Two-sided confidence interval:

$$\hat{\lambda}\frac{\chi^2_{\alpha/2}(2r)}{2r} < \lambda < \hat{\lambda}\frac{\chi^2_{1-\alpha/2}(2r)}{2r} \quad (4.122)$$

or

$$\frac{\chi^2_{\alpha/2}(2r)}{2S(t_0)} < \lambda < \frac{\chi^2_{1-\alpha/2}(2r)}{2S(t_0)} \quad (4.123)$$

4.8.2.3 Distribution Test

For a sample size of n and a censored number of r without replacement timing or fixed number of censors, r failure data are measured, taking the timed censored data as an example, the data form is as follows

$$t_{(1)} \leq t_{(2)} \leq \cdots \leq t_{(r)} \leq t', r \leq n \quad (4.124)$$

In the case of no replacement, $t_{(i)}$ is the order statistic of the out-of-tolerance time, and t' is the test termination time. Assuming that the given significance level is α, the test methaods for exponential distribution include χ^2 test method and Gendenko test method.

1. χ^2 **Test Method**

Take the null hypothesis H_0: the failure time obeys the exponential distribution, then the statistic is

$$\chi^2 = 2\sum_{k=1}^{d} \ln \frac{T^*}{T_k} \quad (4.125)$$

In the formula:

$$d = \begin{cases} r-1, & \text{Definite ending} \\ r, & \text{Timed ending} \end{cases}$$

T^* is the total test time until the end of the test, T_k and is the total test time to the first k failure, that is

$$T^* = \begin{cases} nt', & \text{Replacement timed ending} \\ \sum_{i=1}^{r} t_{(i)} + (n-r)t', & \text{No replacement timed ending} \end{cases} \quad (4.126)$$

It can be proved that when it is established, H_0 χ^2 it obeys χ^2_{2d} the distribution, that is, χ^2 it obeys the distribution with degrees of freedom $2d$. χ^2 For a given significance level α, if the observed value of the statistic is $\chi^2 < \chi^2_{2d,\alpha/2}$ either $\chi^2 > \chi^2_{2d,1-\alpha/2}$ rejected H_0, otherwise, it is accepted H_0.

2. **Gendenko Test**

The non-replacement fixed-number censored data whose sample size is n *and* the censored data is r;

$$t_{(1)} \leq t_{(2)} \leq \cdots \leq t_{(r)} \quad (4.127)$$

Take the null hypothesis H_0: the failure time obeys the exponential distribution, then the statistic is

$$F = \frac{r_2 \sum_{i=1}^{r_1} y_i}{r_1 \sum_{i=r_1-1}^{r} y_i} \quad (4.128)$$

In the formula: $r_1 = [r/2], r_2 = r - r_1, y_i = (n - i + 1)(t_{(i)} - t_{(i-1)}), i = 1, 2, \cdots, r(t_{(0)} = 0)$.

When the null hypothesis is established, it can be proved that F obeys the $2r_1, 2r_2$ F *distribution* with degrees of freedom. At that time $F < F_{2r_1,2r_2;\alpha/2}$, it indicates that the interval between adjacent failures tends to become larger, and the failure rate may be decreasing; at that time, the failure rate may be increasing. $F > F_{2r_1,2r_2;1-\alpha/2}$ Therefore, at that time, the null hypothesis is rejected $F < F_{2r_1,2r_2;\alpha/2}$或$F > F_{2r_1,2r_2;1-\alpha/2}$ H_0; otherwise, the null hypothesis is accepted H_0.

4.8.3 *Weibull Distribution Model*

4.8.3.1 Distribution Introduction

Weibull distribution is a relatively complex distribution commonly used in reliability research. This distribution was initially used to study the fatigue life of metal materials, and later it was widely used in the life distribution model of complex electromechanical products. Since the Weibull distribution can be transformed into other distributions due to different values of the scale parameters, the distribution has strong adaptability and can be used to describe the performance retention period of the fiber optic gyroscope. The probability density of the three-parameter Weibull distribution is as follows:

$$f(t) = \begin{cases} \frac{\beta}{\alpha}\left(\frac{t-\gamma}{\alpha}\right)^{\beta-1} \exp\left[-\left(\frac{t-\gamma}{\alpha}\right)^{\beta}\right], & t \geq \gamma \\ 0, \ t < \gamma \end{cases} \tag{4.129}$$

In the formula:

α Scale parameter;
β Shape parameters;
γ Positional parameters.

In the three-parameter Weibull distribution, the scale parameter is a random variable related to the average life of the product. For two Weibull distributions, when other parameters are the same, the change of the scale parameter is expressed as a probability density function on the horizontal axis on the function curve to the compression. The position parameter indicates that there will be no failure or failure within a certain period of time. When other parameters are the same, the change of the position parameter is expressed as moving left and right along the horizontal coordinate axis on the function curve. When the position parameter is a negative value, it means that the product has expired during the storage period. The shape parameter is a parameter representing the shape of the Weibull distribution curve. When the shape parameter takes different values, the Weibull distribution presents different characteristics. When the shape parameter is less than 1, the failure rate of the system decreases, showing typical early failure characteristics; when the shape parameter is equal to 1, the Weibull distribution can be transformed into an exponential distribution, which can characterize the life distribution characteristics of the product in the accidental failure period; when When the shape parameter is greater than 1, the failure rate of the system increases, which can characterize the system loss-type failure life distribution characteristics. When the Weibull distribution shape parameter is greater than 3, the Weibull distribution function is basically close to the normal distribution function. It is because of the strong adaptability of the Weibull distribution function that it has been widely used in the engineering field.

Usually, products may fail during storage or early working, so the three-parameter Weibull distribution can be simplified to a two-parameter Weibull distribution. The probability density function of the two-parameter Weibull distribution function is as follows:

$$f(t) = \begin{cases} \frac{\beta}{\alpha}\left(\frac{t}{\alpha}\right)^{\beta-1} \exp\left[-\left(\frac{t}{\alpha}\right)^{\beta}\right], & t \geq 0 \\ 0, & t < 0 \end{cases} \tag{4.130}$$

The reliability function of the two-parameter Weibull distribution is:

$$R(t) = \exp\left[-\left(\frac{t}{\alpha}\right)^{\beta}\right] \tag{4.131}$$

The cumulative distribution function is

$$F(t) = 1 - \exp\left[-\left(\frac{t}{\alpha}\right)^{\beta}\right] \tag{4.132}$$

The mean life and variance of the two-parameter Weibull distribution are

$$E(T) = \int_0^{\infty} tf(t)\mathrm{d}t = \int_0^{\infty} t\frac{\beta}{\alpha}\left(\frac{t}{\alpha}\right)^{\beta-1} \exp\left[-\left(\frac{t}{\alpha}\right)^{\beta}\right]\mathrm{d}t = \alpha\Gamma(1 + 1/\beta) \tag{4.133}$$

$$V(T) = \alpha^2[\Gamma(1 + 2/\beta) - \Gamma^2(1 + 1/\beta)] \tag{4.134}$$

4.8.3.2 Parameter Solution

The parameter estimation of the Weibull distribution includes point estimation and interval estimation, and the point estimation can usually use moment estimation method, least square method, maximum likelihood estimation method, best linear unbiased estimation (BLUE), simple linear unbiased estimation (GLUE) and other 5 methods; interval estimation can usually also use the Pearson estimation method.

1. **Moment Estimation**

The mean life and variance of the two-parameter Weibull distribution are

$$E(T) = \int_0^{\infty} tf(t)\mathrm{d}t = \int_0^{\infty} t\frac{\beta}{\alpha}\left(\frac{t}{\alpha}\right)^{\beta-1} \exp\left[-\left(\frac{t}{\alpha}\right)^{\beta}\right]\mathrm{d}t = \alpha\Gamma(1 + 1/\beta) \tag{4.135}$$

$$V(T) = \alpha^2[\Gamma(1 + 2/\beta) - \Gamma^2(1 + 1/\beta)] \tag{4.136}$$

Therefore, the moment estimation equation of the Weibull distribution can be obtained

$$E(T) = \alpha\Gamma(1 + 1/\beta) = \frac{1}{n}\sum_{i=1}^{n} t_i \tag{4.137}$$

Or

$$V(T) = \alpha^2[\Gamma(1 + 2/\beta) - \Gamma^2(1 + 1/\beta)] = \frac{1}{n}\sum_{i=1}^{n} t_i^2 \tag{4.138}$$

Solving Eqs. (4.135) and (4.136) jointly, α, β the estimated values of the parameters can be obtained, usually $\alpha > 0, \beta > 0$.

2. **Least Square Method**

The least squares method is to apply the principle of the least squares method to estimate the unknown parameters of the model after an appropriate transformation of the model. Take the two-number Weibull distribution as an example.

$$\ln\ln\frac{1}{1 - F(t)} = -\beta\ln a + \beta\ln t \tag{4.139}$$

make

$$y = \ln\ln\frac{1}{1 - F(t)} \tag{4.140}$$

$$x = \ln t \tag{4.141}$$

$$A = -\beta\ln\alpha \tag{4.142}$$

$$B = \beta \tag{4.143}$$

According to the principle of least square method

$$\hat{B} = \frac{l_{xy}}{l_{xx}} \tag{4.144}$$

$$\hat{A} = \overline{y} - \hat{B}\overline{x}$$

$$l_{xx} = \sum_{i=1}^{n} (x_i - \overline{x})^2 = \sum_{i=1}^{n} x_i^2 - n\overline{x}^2 \quad (4.145)$$

$$l_{xy} = \sum_{i=1}^{n} (x_i - \overline{x})(y_i - \overline{y}) = \sum_{i=1}^{n} x_i y_i - n\overline{x}\overline{y} \quad (4.146)$$

$$\overline{x} = \frac{1}{n} \sum_{i=1}^{n} x_i \quad (4.147)$$

$$\hat{\beta} = \hat{B}, \hat{\alpha} = \exp(-\hat{A}/\hat{B}) \quad (4.148)$$

Among them: $y = \ln\ln\frac{1}{1-F(t)}$, $x = \ln t$.

For a linearized model, it is necessary to test the regression effect to check whether the data meets the linear requirement. There are two testing methods: analysis of variance and correlation coefficient testing.

(1) Analysis of variance method

The test formula of the variance analysis method is

$$F = \frac{S_{回}}{S_{余}/(n-2)} \quad (4.149)$$

Among them, $S_{回} = \sum_{i=1}^{n} (\hat{y}_i - \overline{y})^2$, $S_{余} = \sum_{i=1}^{n} (y_i - \hat{y}_i)^2$.

For a given confidence level α, consult F the critical value of the distribution table $F_\alpha(1, n-2)$, if it is $F > F_\alpha(1, n-2)$, then the correlation is considered significant, otherwise, the correlation is not significant. Partial F distribution critical values are shown in Table 4.42.

2. **Correlation coefficient test method**

The correlation coefficient test test statistic is

$$r = \frac{\sum_{i=1}^{n} (x_i - \overline{x})(y_i - \overline{y})}{\sqrt{\sum_{i=1}^{n} (x_i - \overline{x})^2 \sum_{i=1}^{n} (y_i - \overline{y})^2}} = \frac{l_{xy}}{\sqrt{l_{xx} l_{yy}}} \quad (4.150)$$

The larger the $|r|$ is, the more significant the linear relationship is. When $|r| > c$, then c is a critical value, the linear relationship can be considered significant. See Table 4.43 for the critical value of the correlation coefficient.

3 **Maximum Likelihood Estimation**

A total of failure (fault) data $n = n_f + n_s$ is obtained, n, n_s, n_f are respectively the number of right-truncated data and failure data, which are respectively recorded as G, F, then the likelihood function is:

Table 4.43 Correlation coefficient critical value ($\alpha = 0.05, 0.01, 0.1$)

n 1 n 2	1	2	3	4	5	6	7	8	9	10	20	30	Infinite
1	161	200	216	225	230	234	247	239	241	242	248	250	254
	4052	4999	5403	5625	5764	5859	5928	5981	6022	6056	6208	6258	6366
	38.96	49.5	53.59	55.8	57.2	58.2	58.9	59.4	59.9	60.2	61.7	62.3	63.33
2	18.51	19	19.16	19.3	19.3	19.3	19.4	19.4	19.4	19.4	19.4	19.5	19.5
	98.49	99	99.17	99.3	99.3	99.3	99.3	99.4	99.4	99.4	99.5	99.5	99.5
	8.53	9	9.16	9.24	9.29	9.33	9.35	9.37	9.38	9.39	9.44	9.46	9.49
3	10.13	9.55	9.28	9.12	9.01	8.94	8.83	8.84	8.81	8.78	8.66	8.62	8.53
	34.12	30.8	29.46	28.7	28.2	27.9	27.7	27.5	27.3	27.3	27	26.5	26.12
	5.54	5.46	5.39	5.34	5.31	5.28	5.27	5.25	5.24	5.23	5.18	5.17	5.13
4	7.71	6.94	6.59	6.39	6.26	6.16	6.09	6.04	6	5.96	5.8	5.74	5.63
	21.2	18	16.96	16	15.5	15.2	15	14.8	14.7	14.5	14	13.8	13.16
	4.54	4.32	4.19	4.11	4.05	4.01	3.98	3.95	3.94	3.92	3.84	3.82	4.76
5	6.61	5.79	5.41	5.19	5.05	4.95	4.88	4.82	4.78	4.74	4.56	4.5	4.36
	16.26	13.3	12.06	11.4	11	10.7	10.5	10.3	10.2	10.1	9.55	9.38	9.02
	4.06	3.78	3.62	3.52	3.45	3.4	3.37	3.34	3.32	3.3	3.21	3.17	3.1
6	5.99	5.14	4.76	4.53	4.39	4.28	4.21	4.15	4.1	4.06	3.87	3.81	3.67
	13.74	10.9	9.78	9.15	8.75	8.47	8.26	8.1	7.98	7.87	7.39	7.23	6.88
	3.78	3.46	3.29	3.18	3.11	3.05	3.01	2.98	2.96	2.94	2.84	2.8	2.72
7	5.59	4.74	4.35	4.12	3.97	3.87	3.79	3.73	3.68	3.63	3.44	3.38	3.23
	12.25	9.55	8.45	7.85	7.46	7.19	7	6.84	6.71	6.62	6.15	5.98	5.65
	3.59	3.26	3.07	2.96	2.88	2.83	2.78	2.75	2.72	2.7	2.59	2.56	2.47
8	5.32	4.46	4.07	3.84	3.69	6.58	3.5	3.44	3.39	3.34	3.15	3.08	2.93
	11.26	8.65	7.59	7.01	6.63	6.37	6.19	6.03	5.91	5.82	5.36	5.2	4.86
	3.46	3.11	2.92	2.81	2.73	2.67	2.62	2.59	2.56	2.54	2.42	2.38	2.29
9	5.12	4.26	3.86	3.63	3.48	3.37	3.29	3.23	3.18	3.13	2.96	2.86	2.71
	10.56	8.02	6.99	6.42	6.06	5.8	5.62	5.47	5.35	5.26	4.8	4.64	4.31
	3.36	3.01	2.81	2.69	2.61	2.55	2.51	2.47	2.44	2.42	2.3	2.25	2.16
10	4.96	4.1	3.71	3.48	3.33	3.22	3.14	3.07	3.02	2.97	2.77	2.7	2.54
	10.04	7.56	6.55	5.99	5.64	5.39	5.21	5.06	4.95	4.85	4.41	4.25	3.91
	3.29	2.92	2.73	2.61	2.52	2.46	2.41	2.38	2.35	2.32	2.2	2.16	2.06
11	4.84	3.98	3.59	3.36	3.2	3.09	3.01	2.95	2.9	2.86	2.65	2.57	2.4
	9.65	7.2	6.22	5.67	5.32	5.07	4.88	4.74	4.63	4.54	4.1	3.94	3.6
	3.23	2.86	2.66	2.54	2.45	2.39	2.34	2.3	2.27	2.25	2.12	2.08	1.97
12	4.75	3.88	3.49	3.26	3.11	3	2.92	2.85	2.8	2.76	2.54	2.46	2.3
	9.33	6.93	5.95	5.41	5.06	4.82	4.65	4.5	4.39	4.3	3.86	3.7	3.36
	3.18	2.81	2.61	2.48	2.39	2.33	2.28	2.24	2.21	2.19	2.06	2.01	1.9
13	4.67	3.8	3.41	3.18	3.02	2.92	2.84	2.77	2.72	2.67	2.46	2.38	2.2
	9.07	6.7	5.74	5.2	4.86	4.62	4.44	4.3	4.19	4.1	3.67	3.51	3.16

(continued)

Table 4.43 (continued)

$n1$ $n2$	1	2	3	4	5	6	7	8	9	10	20	30	Infinite
	3.14	2.76	2.56	2.43	2.35	2.28	2.23	2.2	2.16	2.14	2.01	1.96	1.85
14	4.6	3.74	3.34	3.11	2.96	2.85	2.77	2.7	2.65	2.6	2.39	2.31	2.13
	8.86	6.5 1	5.56	5.03	4.69	4.46	4.28	4.14	4.03	3.94	3.51	3.34	3
	3.1	2.73	2.52	2.39	2.31	2.24	2.19	2.15	2.12	2.1	1.96	1.91	1.8
15	4.54	3.68	3.29	3.06	2.9	2.79	2.7	2.64	2.59	2.55	2.33	2.25	2.07
	8.68	6.36	5.42	4.89	4.56	4.32	4.14	4	3.89	3.8	3.36	3.2	2.87
	3.07	2.7	2.49	2.36	2.27	2.21	2.16	2.12	2.09	2.06	1.92	1.87	1.76
16	4.49	3.63	3.24	3.01	2.85	2.74	2.66	2.57	2.54	2.49	2.28	2.2	2.01
	8.53	6.23	5.29	4.77	4.44	4.2	4.03	3.89	3.78	3.69	3.26	3.1	2.75
	3.05	2.67	2.46	2.33	2.24	2.18	2.13	2.09	2.06	2.03	1.89	1.84	1.72
17	4.45	3.59	3.2	2.96	2.81	2.7	2.62	2.55	2.5	2.45	2.23	2.15	1.96
	8.4	6.11	5.18	4.67	4.34	4.1	3.93	3.79	3.68	3.59	3.16	3	2.65
	3.03	2.64	2.44	2.31	2.22	2.15	2.1	2.06	2.03	2	1.86	1.81	1.69
18	4.41	3.55	3.16	2.93	2.77	2.66	2.58	2.51	2.46	2.41	2.19	2.11	1.92
	8.28	6.01	5.09	4.58	4.25	4.01	3.85	3.71	3.6	3.51	3.07	2.91	2.57
	3.01	2.62	2.42	2.29	2.2	2.13	2.08	2.04	2	1.98	1.84	1.78	1.66
19	4.38	3.52	3.13	2.9	2.74	2.63	2.55	2.48	2.43	2.38	2.15	2.07	1.88
	8.18	5.93	5.01	4.5	4.17	3.94	3.77	3.63	3.52	3.43	3	2.84	2.49
	2.99	2.61	2.4	2.27	2.18	2.11	2.06	2.02	1.98	1.96	1.81	1.76	1.63
20	4.35	3.49	3.1	2.87	2.71	2.6	2.52	2.45	2.4	2.35	2.12	2.04	1.84
	8.1	5.84	4.94	4.43	4.1	3.87	3.71	3.56	3.45	3.37	2.94	2.77	2.42
	2.97	2.59	2.38	2.25	2.16	2.09	2.04	2	1.96	1.94	1.79	1.74	1.61
30	4.17	3.32	2.92	2.69	2.53	2.42	2.34	2.27	2.21	2.16	1.93	1.84	1.62
	7.59	5.39	4.51	4.02	3.7	3.47	3.3	3.17	3.06	2.98	2.55	2.38	2.01
	2.88	2.49	2.28	2.14	2.05	1.98	1.93	1.88	1.85	1.82	1.67	1.61	1.46
40	4.08	3.23	2.81	2.61	2.45	2.34	2.25	2.18	2.12	2.07	1.84	1.74	1.51
	7.31	5.18	4.31	3.83	3.51	3.29	3.12	2.99	2.88	2.8	2.37	2.2	1.8
	2.84	2.44	2.23	2.09	2	1.93	1.87	1.83	1.79	1.76	1.61	1.54	1.38
Endless	3.84	2.99	2.6	2.37	2.21	2.09	2.01	1.94	1.88	1.83	1.57	1.46	1
	6.64	4.6	3.78	3.32	3.02	2.8	3.64	2.51	2.41	2.32	1.87	1.69	1
	2.71	2.3	2.08	1.94	1.85	1.77	1.72	1.67	1.63	1.6	1.42	1.34	1

$$L(\theta) = \prod_{i \in F} f(t_i; \theta) \prod_{i \in G} R(t_i; \theta) \tag{4.151}$$

where θ is a parameter variable. The likelihood function for the two-parameter Weibull distribution is:

$$\ln[L(\beta,\alpha)] = n_f \ln(\beta) - n_f\beta\ln(\alpha) + (\beta-1)\sum_{i\in F}\ln(t_i) - \sum_{i\in F+G}\left(\frac{t_i}{\alpha}\right)^{\beta} \tag{4.152}$$

the two sides respectively to β, α obtain:

$$\frac{\partial \ln[L(\beta,\alpha)]}{\partial\beta} = \frac{n_f}{\beta} - n_f\ln(\alpha) + \sum_{i\in F}\ln(t_i) - \sum_{i\in F+G}\left(\frac{t_i}{\alpha}\right)^{\beta}\ln\left(\frac{t_i}{\alpha}\right) \tag{4.153}$$

$$\frac{\partial \ln[L(\beta,\eta)]}{\partial\eta} = \frac{-n_f\beta}{\eta} + \sum_{i\in F+G}\left(\frac{t_i}{\eta}\right)^{\beta}\cdot\frac{\beta}{\eta} \tag{4.154}$$

Setting the partial differential equal to zero, we get:

$$\alpha = \left(\frac{\sum_{i\in F+G} t_i^{\beta}}{n_f}\right)^{\frac{1}{\beta}} \tag{4.155}$$

$$\frac{n_f}{\beta} - n_f\ln(\alpha) + \sum_{i\in F}\ln(t_i) - \frac{1}{\alpha^{\beta}}\sum_{i\in F+G} t_i^{\beta}\ln\left(\frac{t_i}{\alpha}\right) = 0 \tag{4.156}$$

The maximum likelihood estimates of the parameters are obtained by solving.

4 **Best Linear Unbiased Estimation (BLUE)**

The cumulative distribution function of the two-parameter Weibull distribution is

$$F(t) = 1 - \exp\left[-\left(\frac{t}{\alpha}\right)^{\beta}\right] \tag{4.157}$$

Usually, it is difficult to directly calculate β, α the estimated value, so the cumulative distribution function can be changed, and the logarithmic transformation of the investigated life can be carried out, so that $\sigma = 1/\beta$, $\mu = \ln\alpha$.

then there is

$$F(x) = 1 - \exp(-e^{\frac{x-u}{\sigma}}) \tag{4.158}$$

This distribution becomes an extreme value distribution, so that

$$y = \frac{x-u}{\sigma} \tag{4.159}$$

then there is

$$F(y) = 1 - \exp(-e^{y}) \tag{4.160}$$

When $\mu = 0, \sigma = 1$ it is the standard extreme value distribution.

If there are n test samples put into the life test, $t_1 \leq t_2 \leq \cdots \leq t_r$ it is the first r order statistics. Due to the monotonicity of the logarithmic function, if it is set $X_k = \ln t_k$, it $X_1 \leq X_2 \leq \cdots \leq X_r$ can be regarded as a $F_x(x)$ first r order statistics with a capacity of n from it. If it is assumed that $y_k = (x - \mu_k)/\sigma$, then $Y_1 \leq Y_2 \leq \cdots \leq Y_r$ can be regarded as the r-th order statistics from the standard extreme value distribution $F_y(y)$ whose capacity is n. Since $F_y(y)$ does not contain any unknown parameters, the mathematical expectation, variance and covariance of $Y_1 \leq Y_2 \leq \cdots \leq Y_r$ can be obtained through the distribution of order statistics.

$$E(y_k) = a_k \tag{4.161}$$

$$\mathrm{Var}(y_k) = v_{kk} \tag{4.162}$$

$$\mathrm{Cov}(y_k, y_l) = v_{kl} \tag{4.163}$$

then there is

$$\left\{\begin{array}{l} E(x_k) = \mu + \sigma a_k \\ \mathrm{Var}(x_k) = \sigma^2 v_{kk} \\ \mathrm{Cov}(x_l, x_l) = \sigma^2 v_{kl} \end{array}\right\} \tag{4.164}$$

For convenience, set

$$X = \begin{pmatrix} x_1 \\ x_2 \\ \vdots \\ x_r \end{pmatrix}, M = \begin{pmatrix} 1 & a_1 \\ 1 & a_2 \\ \vdots & \vdots \\ 1 & a_r \end{pmatrix}, \theta = \begin{pmatrix} \mu \\ \sigma \end{pmatrix}, V = \begin{pmatrix} v_{11} & v_{12} & \cdots & v_{1r} \\ v_{21} & v_{22} & \cdots & v_{2r} \\ \vdots & \vdots & \vdots & \vdots \\ v_{r1} & v_{r2} & \cdots & v_{rr} \end{pmatrix} \tag{4.165}$$

Combined with the Gauss-Markov theorem, it can be calculated that

$$\hat{\theta} = \begin{pmatrix} \hat{\mu} \\ \hat{\sigma} \end{pmatrix} = (M'V^{-1}M)^{-1}(M'V^{-1}X) \tag{4.166}$$

and have

$$M'V^{-1}M = \begin{pmatrix} \sum_k \sum_j v_{kl} & \sum_k \sum_k a_k v_{kl} \\ \sum_k \sum_j a_l v_{kl} & \sum_k \sum_l a_k a_{kl} v_{kl} \end{pmatrix} \tag{4.167}$$

$$(M'V^{-1}M)^{-1} = \begin{pmatrix} A_{r,n} & B_{r,n} \\ B_{r,n} & l_{r,n} \end{pmatrix} \tag{4.168}$$

$$A_{r,n} = \{(\sum_k \sum_l v_{kl})(\sum_k \sum_l a_k a_l v_{kl}) - (\sum_k \sum_l a_k v_{kl})^2\}^{-1} \sum_k \sum_l a_k a_l v_{kl} \tag{4.169}$$

$$B_{r,n} = \{(\sum_k \sum_l v_{kl})(\sum_k \sum_l a_k a_l v_{kl}) - (\sum_k \sum_l a_l v_{kl})^2\}^{-1} \sum_k \sum_l a_k v_{kl} \tag{4.170}$$

$$l_{r,n} = \{(\sum_k \sum_l v_{kl})(\sum_k \sum_l a_k a_l v_{kl}) - (\sum_k \sum_l a_k v_{kl})^2\}^{-1} \sum_k \sum_l v_{kl} \tag{4.171}$$

The final σ_i estimate and variance are:

$$\hat{\sigma} = \sum_{k=1}^{r} C(n, r, l)x_k = \sum_{k=1}^{r} C(n, r, l) \ln t_k \tag{4.172}$$

$$\hat{\mu} = \sum_{k=1}^{r} D(n, r, k) \ln t_k \tag{4.173}$$

$$D(n, r, k) = \sum_{l=1}^{r} A_{r,n} v_{kl} + \sum_{l=1}^{r} B_{r,n} \alpha_l v_{kl} \tag{4.174}$$

$$C(n, r, k) = \sum_{l=1}^{r} B_{r,n} v_{kl} + \sum_{l=1}^{r} l_{r,n} \alpha_l v_{kl} \tag{4.175}$$

final β, α estimate is

$$\hat{\alpha} = \exp(\hat{\mu}), \hat{\beta} = 1/\hat{\sigma} \tag{4.176}$$

5. **Simple Linear Unbiased Estimation (GLUE)**

When $n > 25$, due to the calculation deviation, the BLUE coefficient in the extreme value distribution has not been calculated, but μ, σ $n > 25$ is often encountered in engineering practice. To solve this problem, simple linear unbiased estimation is introduced.

Assuming that the life *T of the product* obeys the Weibull distribution with parameter α, β, then $X = \ln t$ it obeys the extreme value distribution with parameter μ, σ, $Y = (X - \mu)/\sigma$ where $\sigma = 1/\beta$. $\mu = \ln \alpha$ Obey the standard extreme value distribution with parameters (0, 1).

Because $\sigma > 0$ it is a scale parameter in the extreme value distribution, the distance between any two order statistics $|X_i - X_j|$ contains σ information. If an order statistic is selected X_S, then other order statistics X_i and their distance

$$|X_i - X_s|, i = 1, 2, \cdots, r \tag{4.177}$$

contained in all σ of them can be combined to obtain σ a better estimate. Take the average of these distances

$$\hat{\sigma} = \frac{1}{nk}\sum_{i=1}^{r}|X_i - X_s| = \frac{1}{nk}[(2s - r)X_s - \sum_{i=1}^{s} X_i + \sum_{i=s+1}^{r} X_i] \tag{4.178}$$

As the estimation of σ, $\hat{\sigma}$ is the linear estimation of σ. In order to make $\hat{\sigma}$ an unbiased estimation, then

$$E\left(\frac{1}{nk}\sum_{i=1}^{r}|X_i - X_s|\right) = \sigma \tag{4.179}$$

Or

$$E\left(\frac{1}{nk}\sum_{i=1}^{r}\left|\frac{X_i - \mu}{\sigma} - \frac{X_s - \mu}{\sigma}\right|\right) = \sigma \tag{4.180}$$

$$k = \frac{1}{n}E\left\{(2s - r)Y_s - \sum_{i=1}^{r} Y_i + \sum_{i=r+1}^{r} Y_i\right\} \tag{4.181}$$

In this way, it is determined k to only rely on n, r, s, so remember $k = k_{s,r,n}$. For a given n, r, s, can be $E(Y_i)$ calculated according to $k = k_{s,r,n}$. Any one of them can be taken, and usually can be selected according to the following formula $i = 1, 2, \cdots, ri = 1, 2, \cdots, r$

$$s = \begin{cases} r, & r \leq 0.9n \\ n, & r > 0.9n, n \leq 15 \\ n - 1, & r > 0.9n, 16 \leq n \leq 24 \\ [0.892n] + 1, & r > 0.9n, n \geq 25 \end{cases} \tag{4.182}$$

The resulting σ simple linear unbiased estimate

$$\begin{aligned} \hat{\sigma} &= \frac{1}{nk}\sum_{i=1}^{r}|X_i - X_s| = \frac{1}{nk}\left[(2s - r)X_s - \sum_{i=1}^{s} X_i + \sum_{i=s+1}^{r} X_i\right] \\ &= \frac{2.3026}{nk_{r,n}}\left[(2s - r)\lg t_s - \sum_{i=1}^{s} \lg t_i + \sum_{i=s+1}^{r} X_i\right] \end{aligned} \tag{4.183}$$

μ A simple linear unbiased estimate of

$$\hat{\mu} = X_s - E(Y_s)\hat{\sigma} \tag{4.184}$$

The estimated value obtained is β, $\alpha\beta$, α

$$\hat{\alpha} = \exp \tilde{\mu},\ \hat{\beta} = 1/\hat{\sigma} \tag{4.185}$$

6. **Interval Estimation**

(1) β Interval estimation of shape parameters

Given a confidence level of $(1 - a)$, β the confidence interval for the parameter is: $[\omega_1 \hat{\beta}, \omega_2 \hat{\beta}]$

$$\omega_1 = \left(\frac{k_1}{rc}\right)^{\left(\frac{1}{1+q}\right)^2} \tag{4.186}$$

$$\omega_2 = \left(\frac{2}{rc}\right)^{\left(\frac{1}{1+q}\right)^2} \tag{4.187}$$

In the formula:

$$c = 2.14628 - 1.361119 * q \tag{4.188}$$

$$k_1 = \chi^2_{\frac{a}{2}}[c \cdot (r - 1)] \tag{4.189}$$

$$k_2 = \chi^2_{1-\frac{a}{2}}[c \cdot (r - 1)] \tag{4.190}$$

$$q = \frac{r}{n} \tag{4.191}$$

In the formula:

r number of complete failures;
n The total number of data (including censored data).

$\chi^2_a(\upsilon)$ is χ^2 the quantile value of a the distribution with degrees of freedom. υ When the degree of freedom is large, $\chi^2_a(\upsilon)$ it is inconvenient to find, it can be approximated by the following formula:

$$\chi^2_a(\upsilon) \approx \upsilon\left[1 - \frac{2}{9\upsilon} + Z_a\sqrt{\frac{2}{9\upsilon}}\right]^2 \tag{4.192}$$

(2) Interval estimation of scale parameters

At a confidence level of $(1 - a)$, a the confidence interval for the scale parameter is: $[A_1 \hat{\alpha}, A_2 \hat{\alpha}]$.

For different censored samples, the method of calculating the sum is A_1 also A_2 different. When timing truncation is used, that is $r < n$, then:

$$A_1 = \exp\left(-\frac{d_1}{\wp}\right) \tag{4.193}$$

$$A_2 = \exp\left(-\frac{d_2}{\wp}\right) \tag{4.194}$$

In the formula:

$$d_1 = \frac{A_3 + x\sqrt{x^2(A_6^2 - A_4A_5) + rA_4}}{r - A_5x^2} \tag{4.195}$$

$$d_2 = \frac{A_3 - x\sqrt{x^2(A_6^2 - A_4A_5) + rA_4}}{r - A_5x^2} \tag{4.196}$$

in:

$$A_3 = -A_6x^2 \tag{4.197}$$

$x = N_{1-\frac{q}{2}}$ is the quantile of the normal distribution.

$$A_4 = 0.49q - 0.134 + 0.622q^{-1} \tag{4.198}$$

$$A_5 = 0.2445(1.78 - q)(2.25 + q) \tag{4.199}$$

$$A_6 = 0.029 - 1.083\ln(1.325q) \tag{4.200}$$

4.8.3.3 Distribution Test

The Weibull distribution can usually be tested by using the Van Montfort test, χ^2 test and other test methods.

The common method used to test the goodness of fit of the Weibull distribution is the Van Montfort test. Assuming that there is n a sample put into the test, r a total of failure times are obtained, respectively $t_1 < t_2 < \cdots < t_r$, the test time $t_i, i = 1, 2, \cdots, r$ obeys the Weibull distribution, which can be set

$$x_i = \ln t_i; \Lambda_i = \frac{x_i - \mu}{\sigma}, i = 1, 2, \cdots, r; \mu = \ln\alpha, \sigma = 1/\beta \tag{4.201}$$

Then the corresponding statistics can be constructed as:

$$F = \frac{\sum_{i=[r/2]+1}^{r} \Upsilon_i/(r-[r/2]-1)}{\sum_{i=1}^{[m/2]} \Upsilon_i/[r/2]}, i = 1, 2, \cdots, r-1 \tag{4.202}$$

in:

$$\Upsilon_i = \frac{x_{i+1} - x_i}{E(\Lambda_{i+1}) - E(\Lambda_i)}, i = 1, 2, \cdots, r-1 \tag{4.203}$$

$E(\Lambda_{i+1})$ Can be obtained from the Table Then the statistic asymptotically obeys the distribution with degrees of freedom F of F "Table for Reliability Test" $2(r - [r/2]-1)$,$2[m/2]$. When experimenting with sample size $n > 100$, $E(\Lambda_{i+1})-E(\Lambda_i)$ the BLOM approximation method can be used.

$$E(\Lambda_{i+1}) - E(\Lambda_i) \approx \ln\left\{\ln\left[\frac{4(n-i-1)+3}{4n+1}\right]/\ln\left[\frac{4(n-i)+3}{4n+1}\right]\right\} \tag{4.204}$$

For a given confidence level $1-\alpha$, the corresponding rejection region is

$$F \le F_{1-\alpha/2}((r-[r/2]-1), 2[r/2]) = \frac{1}{F_{\alpha/2}((r-[r/2]-1), 2[r/2]} \tag{4.205}$$

Or

$$F \ge F_{\alpha/2}((r-[r/2]-1), 2[r/2]) \tag{4.206}$$

4.8.4 Lognormal Distribution Model

4.8.4.1 Introduction to Distribution

The lognormal distribution is a form in which the natural logarithm of the random variable is normally distributed, and it is also one of the commonly used life distribution models of the system, especially widely used in the field of maintainability analysis. The probability density function of the lognormal distribution is

$$f(t) = \frac{1}{\sigma t\sqrt{2\pi}} \exp\left[-\frac{1}{2}\left(\frac{\ln(t)-\mu}{\sigma}\right)^2\right], t \ge 0 \tag{4.207}$$

The cumulative distribution function of the lognormal distribution is

$$F(t)=\int_0^t \frac{1}{\sigma t\sqrt{2\pi}}\exp\left[-\frac{1}{2}\left(\frac{\ln(t)-\mu}{\sigma}\right)^2\right]dt \tag{4.208}$$

The reliability function is

$$R(t)=1-F(t)=1-\int_0^t \frac{1}{\sigma t\sqrt{2\pi}}\exp\left[-\frac{1}{2}\left(\frac{\ln(t)-\mu}{\sigma}\right)^2\right]dt \tag{4.209}$$

The failure rate function is

$$\lambda(t)=\frac{\phi\left(\frac{\ln(t)-\mu}{\sigma}\right)}{t\sigma R(t)} \tag{4.210}$$

The mean life and variance of the lognormal distribution are

$$E(T)=\int_0^\infty tf(t)dt=e^{\mu+\sigma^2/2} \tag{4.211}$$

$$V(T)=e^{2\mu+\sigma^2}(e^{\sigma^2}-1) \tag{4.212}$$

4.8.4.2 Parameter Solving

The parameter estimation of the Weibull distribution includes point estimation and interval estimation, and the point estimation can usually use four methods such as moment estimation method, least square method, best linear unbiased estimation (BLUE), and simple linear unbiased estimation (GLUE).

1. **Moment Estimation**

The mean and variance of the lognormal distribution are

$$E(T)=\int_0^\infty tf(t)dt=e^{\mu+\sigma^2/2} \tag{4.213}$$

$$V(T)=e^{2\mu+\sigma^2}(e^{\sigma^2}-1) \tag{4.214}$$

Therefore, the moment estimation equation of the lognormal distribution can be obtained

$$E(T)=e^{\mu+\sigma^2/2}=\frac{1}{n}\sum_{i=1}^{n}t_i \tag{4.215}$$

$$V(T) = \mathrm{e}^{2\mu+\sigma^2}(\mathrm{e}^{\sigma^2} - 1) = \frac{1}{n}\sum_{i=1}^{n} t_i^2 \tag{4.216}$$

Jointly solve the available $\hat{\mu}$, $\hat{\sigma}$ moment estimates.

2. **Least Square Method**

The cumulative distribution function of the lognormal distribution is

$$F(t) = \int_0^t \frac{1}{\sigma t\sqrt{2\pi}} \exp\left[-\frac{1}{2}\left(\frac{\ln(t) - \mu}{\sigma}\right)^2\right] \mathrm{d}t \tag{4.217}$$

After transformation, the above formula can be transformed into a standard overall distribution

$$F(t) = \int_{-\infty}^{\frac{\ln t - \mu}{\sigma}} \frac{1}{\sqrt{2\pi}} \mathrm{e}^{-\frac{x^2}{2}} \mathrm{d}x = \Phi\left(\frac{\ln t - \mu}{\sigma}\right) \tag{4.218}$$

Since the standard normal distribution function $\Phi(x)$ is strictly monotonously rising, it has an inverse function, and the inverse function is

$$\Phi^{-1}[F(t)] = \frac{\ln t - \mu}{\sigma} \tag{4.219}$$

Assuming

$$\Phi^{-1}[F(t)] = Y, X = \ln t \tag{4.220}$$

then there is

$$Y = \frac{1}{\sigma}X - \frac{\mu}{\sigma} \tag{4.221}$$

This is an equation of a line that can be solved by the method of least squares.

$$l_{xx} = \sum_{i=1}^{n} (x_i - \overline{x})^2 = \sum_{i=1}^{n} x_i^2 - n\overline{x}^2 \tag{4.222}$$

$$l_{xy} = \sum_{i=1}^{n} (x_i - \overline{x})(y_i - \overline{y}) = \sum_{i=1}^{n} x_i y_i - n\overline{xy} \tag{4.223}$$

$$\overline{x} = \frac{1}{n}\sum_{i=1}^{n} x_i \tag{4.224}$$

The final solution is:

$$\hat{\sigma} = \frac{l_{xx}}{l_{xy}} \quad (4.225)$$

$$\hat{\mu} = \overline{x} - \hat{\sigma}\overline{y} \quad (4.226)$$

3. **Best Linear Unbiased Estimation (BLUE)**

T of the product obeys the logarithmic normal distribution $LN(u, \sigma^2)$, then

$$X = \ln t \sim N(\mu, \sigma^2) \quad (4.227)$$

$$Y = \frac{\ln t - \mu}{\sigma} \sim N(0, 1) \quad (4.228)$$

n samples are randomly selected from this batch of products for life test, the censored number is r. If there are n test samples put into life test, $t_1 \leq t_2 \leq \cdots \leq t_r$ it is the first r order statistics. Due to the monotonicity of the logarithmic function, if set $X_k = \ln t_k$, then $X_1 \leq X_2 \leq \cdots \leq X_r$ It can be seen as the $N(u, \sigma^2)$ first r order statistics with a capacity of n from it. If set $Y_k = (X - \mu_k)/\sigma$, $Y_1 \leq Y_2 \leq \cdots \leq Y_r$ can be regarded as the first r order statistics from the standard normal $N(0, 1)$ distribution with capacity n. Since it does not contain any unknown parameters, $N(0, 1)$ the mathematical expectation, variance and covariance can be obtained through the distribution of order statistics $Y_1 \leq Y_2 \leq \cdots \leq Y_r$

$$E(y_k) = a_k \quad (4.229)$$

$$\mathrm{Var}(y_k) = u_{kk} \quad (4.230)$$

$$\mathrm{Cov}(y_k, y_l) = u_{kl} \quad (4.231)$$

Using the Gauss-Markov theorem and matrix operations, u, σ the best linear unbiased estimate available.

$$\hat{\sigma} = \sum_{k=1}^{r} C'(n, r, k) X_k \quad (4.232)$$

$$\hat{\sigma} = \sum_{k=1}^{r} D'(n, r, k) X_k \quad (4.233)$$

The corresponding coefficients can be obtained by looking up the Table

4. **Simple Linear Unbiased Estimation (GLUE)**

In the simple linear unbiased estimator of two parameters u, σ in the lognormal distribution, when $r \leq 0.9n$, the simple linear unbiased estimator of u, σ is:

$$\hat{\sigma} = \frac{1}{nk_{r,n}}\left[r \ln t_r - \sum_{i=1}^{r} \ln t_i\right] \tag{4.234}$$

$$\hat{\mu} = \ln t_r - E(Y_r)\hat{\sigma} \tag{4.235}$$

Interval estimates:

Referring to the standard normal distribution, the interval estimates of u, σ for the log-normal distribution can be obtained as the expressions for the confidence limits of u with confidence level $1 - \alpha$, respectively, as follows.

A one-sided confidence interval with an upper limit of:

$$\mu < \overline{X} + t_\alpha \sqrt{\frac{S^2}{n(n-1)}} \tag{4.236}$$

A one-sided confidence interval with a lower bound of:

$$\mu > \overline{X} - t_\alpha \sqrt{\frac{S^2}{n(n-1)}} \tag{4.237}$$

Two-sided confidence interval:

$$\overline{X} - t_{\alpha/2}\sqrt{\frac{S^2}{n(n-1)}} < \mu < \overline{X} + t_{\alpha/2}\sqrt{\frac{S^2}{n(n-1)}} \tag{4.238}$$

Confidence limits with a confidence level of 1—are expressed as σ follows: $\alpha\alpha$.

Two-sided confidence interval:

$$S^2/\chi^2_{\alpha/2}(n) < \sigma^2 < S^2/\chi^2_{1-\alpha/2}(n) \tag{4.239}$$

A one-sided confidence interval with an upper limit of:

$$\sigma^2 < S^2/\chi^2_{1-\alpha}(n) \tag{4.240}$$

A one-sided confidence interval with a lower bound of:

$$\sigma^2 > S^2/\chi^2_\alpha(n) \tag{4.241}$$

4.8.4.3 Distribution Test

For a n complete sample with a sample size of or a n censored r sample with a censored data of, test whether the data $t_{(1)} \leq t_{(2)} \leq \cdots \leq t_{(r)} \leq t', r \leq n$ come from a lognormally distributed population. It can be divided into two categories: when it is a complete sample, there are multiple test methods, such as Shapiro-Wilk's W test method and D'Agostino's D test method; for the censored data, there is currently no The corresponding numerical method is generally tested by the method of probability drawing. In addition, for normal distribution or lognormal distribution, there are more intuitive skewness test and kurtosis test methods.

1. **W Test**

Take the null hypothesis H_0: the failure time obeys the lognormal distribution, then the statistic $t_{(i)}, i = 1, 2, \cdots, n$ W is

$$W = \left\{ \sum_{i=1}^{d} a_i [\ln t_{(n+1-i)} - \ln t_{(i)}] \right\}^2 / \sum_{i=1}^{n} (\ln t_i - \ln \bar{t})_2 \tag{4.242}$$

The scope of use of the W test is $3 \leq n \leq 50$, where $d = [n/2]$ is $\ln \bar{t}$ the sample mean: $\ln \bar{t} = n^{-1} \sum_{i=1}^{n} \ln t_{(i)}$ the coefficient a_i can be obtained by looking up the table, and its range is $1 \leq i \leq, 3 \leq n \leq 50$.

It has been proved that, $\bar{a} = n^{-1} \sum_{i-1}^{n} a_i = 0, a_i = -a_{n+1-i}$ and $\sum_{i-1}^{n} a_i^2 = 1$. Therefore there

$$W = \left\{ \sum_{i=1}^{n} (\ln t_i - \ln \bar{t})(a_i - \bar{a}) \right\}^2 / \left\{ \sum_{i=1}^{n} (\ln t_i - \ln \bar{t})^2 (a_i - \bar{a})^2 \right\} \tag{4.243}$$

That is, when W is n the number $(\ln t_{(i)}, a_i), i = 1, 2, \cdots, n$ the square of the correlation coefficient between them, therefore $0 \leq W \leq 1$. When the null hypothesis H_0 is established, $(\ln t_{(i)}, a_i)$ there is a good linear relationship, and the value of W is close to 1. Therefore, at that time, the null hypothesis can be rejected $W \leq W_\alpha H_0$, and vice versa. W_α Can be obtained from the Table

2. **D Test**

$n > 50$ At that time, the coefficient calculation of the W test was very cumbersome, so D'Agostino proposed the D test method, the test statistic is

$$D = T/(n^{3/2} Q) \tag{4.244}$$

In the formula:

$$T = \sum_{i=1}^{n} \left(i - \frac{n+1}{2} \right) \ln t_{(i)} \tag{4.245}$$

$$D = \sqrt{\sum_{i=1}^{n} (\ln t_i - \ln \bar{t})^2} \tag{4.246}$$

The scope of the inspection is $50 \leq n < 1000$.
D are

$$E(D) = 0.28209479 \tag{4.247}$$

$$\sqrt{Var(D)} = 0.02998598/\sqrt{n} \tag{4.248}$$

Its standardized variable is denoted as

$$Y = [D - E(D)]/\sqrt{\text{Var}(D)} \tag{4.249}$$

When $Y \leq Y_{\alpha/2}$ or $Y \geq Y_{1-\alpha/2}$, the null hypothesis is rejected, and the failure data does not obey the lognormal distribution; otherwise, it is accepted.

3. **Skewness Test**

The sample is $t_{(i)}, i = 1, 2, \cdots, n$, then the skewness of the sample is

$$b_s = \frac{\sqrt{n}\left[\sum_{i=1}^{n} (\ln t_i - \ln \bar{t})^3\right]}{\left[\sum_{i=1}^{n} (\ln t_i - \ln \bar{t})^2\right]^{3/2}} \tag{4.250}$$

Suppose $Y = \ln t$, if it Y obeys a normal distribution, then its skewness

$$\beta_s = E(Y - EY)^3/[E(Y - EY)^2]^{3/2} = 0 \tag{4.251}$$

If you suspect that the parent population does not belong to the normal distribution, you can do the following test

$$H_0\ \beta_s = 0\ \beta_s > 0 \tag{4.252}$$

Or

$$H_0\ \beta_s = 0\ H_1\ \beta_s < 0 \tag{4.253}$$

Compared to the above two cases.
like

$$b_s > Z_{1-\alpha} \text{ or } b_s > -Z_{1-\alpha} \tag{4.254}$$

reject the null hypothesis H_0; otherwise, accept the null hypothesis H_0. $Z_{1-\alpha}$ You can refer to the corresponding statistical tables.

4. **Kurtosis Test**

Suppose the sample observation sample is $t_{(i)}, i = 1, 2, \cdots, n$, and the sample after logarithmic transformation is $\ln t_{(i)}, i = 1, 2, \cdots, n$, then the sample kurtosis is

$$b_k > n\sum_{i=1}^{n}(\ln t_i - \ln \bar{t})^4 \Big/ \left[\sum_{i=1}^{n}(\ln t_i - \ln \bar{t})^2\right]^2 \tag{4.255}$$

Suppose $Y = \ln t$, if it Y obeys a normal distribution, its kurtosis

$$\beta_k = E(Y - EY)^4/[E(Y - EY)^2]^2 = 3 \tag{4.256}$$

If you suspect the kurtosis of $\beta_k > 3$ the parent population or $\beta_k < 3$, and therefore suspect that the model is not a normal distribution, you can do the following kurtosis test

$$H_0\ \beta_k = 3\ H_1\ \beta_k > 3 \tag{4.257}$$

Or

$$H_0\ \beta_k = 3\ H_1\ \beta_k < 3 \tag{4.258}$$

Corresponding to the above two cases, if

$$b_k > Z'_{1-\alpha} \text{ or } b_k < Z'_{\alpha}$$

the null hypothesis is rejected H_0; otherwise, the null hypothesis is accepted H_0. $Z'_{1-\alpha}$, Z'_{α} you can refer to the corresponding statistical tables.

4.8.5 *Distribution Model Selection and Testing*

Considering that there are usually multiple typical distributions such as exponential distribution, Weibull distribution, and lognormal distribution, which distribution is the best, the best model can be selected through the goodness of fit test for various distribution models.

4.8.5.1 Selection of Distribution Model

The distribution model generally selects an appropriate failure distribution model based on the experience of the modeler and the preliminary analysis results of the failure (or failure) data. From the above chapters, we can see that the commonly used models include exponential distribution, Weibull distribution, lognormal distribution, etc., where exponential distribution and Weibull distribution are widely used in mechanical system modeling. The empirical selection of the distribution model can firstly analyze the frequency histogram of the failure (or failure) data based on the obtained failure (or failure) data to obtain the general trend of the probability density function; the cumulative distribution can also be drawn according to the grouping method of the frequency histogram function trend graph, combined with the frequency histogram and cumulative distribution function trend graph, preliminarily determine the appropriate model; Boolean probability graphs, lognormal distribution probability graphs, etc. determine whether failure (or failure) times follow the distribution.

The relationship between $f(t) = F'(t)$ the cumulative distribution function $F(t)$ of failure (or failure) time and its density function $f(t)$ *is.*

If the probability density function $f(t)$ of failure (or failure) time is peak-shaped, such as normal distribution and lognormal distribution, then

$$f'(t) = 0$$

That is

$$F''(t) = 0$$

It can be seen that if the probability density function $f(t)$ of the failure (or failure) time is peak-shaped, the distribution function $F(t)$ will have an inflection point.

If the probability density function $f(t)$ of the failure (or failure) time shows a monotonous downward trend, then

$$f'(t) < 0$$

That is

$$F''(t) < 0$$

It can be seen from this that if the probability density function $f(t)$ of failure (or failure) time presents a monotonous downward trend, its distribution function $F(t)$ will be convex on the positive semi-axis.

In the same way, if the probability density function $f(t)$ of failure (or fault) time shows a monotonous upward trend, its distribution function $F(t)$ will be concave on the positive semi-axis.

From the estimable theoretical distribution function $F(t)$, the shape of $f(t)$ can be preliminarily judged.

4.8.5.2 Distribution Model Compliance Test

After the failure distribution model is initially selected, the parameters of the distribution model should be solved and the distribution inspection should be carried out to ensure that the actual product failure distribution is consistent with the built model. Common failure distribution models for digital medical equipment: exponential distribution model, Weibull distribution Model, lognormal distribution model, etc., are given in the above chapters for detailed distribution introduction, parameter solution and distribution test methods. In addition to the distribution test methods in the above chapters, the distribution model test can be implemented by using the probability drawing method, graph method, Pearson test (χ^2 test) method, and Kplmogorov-Smirnov test method (also known as K-S test method or D test method). The general method for the goodness of fit of each distribution model is introduced in detail below:

(1) The probability drawing method is a simple graphical inspection method for testing the goodness of fit of the model. The basic idea of this method is to make a special inspection drawing for commonly used distribution models such as lognormal distribution and Weibull distribution. After deforming the commonly used distribution model, transform the obtained failure data to draw points on the drawing, and judge whether the failure data conforms to a certain distribution function through the curve trend of the drawn points.

Take the two- parameter Weibull distribution as an example. The CDF variant of the two-parameter Weibull distribution gives

$$\ln \frac{1}{1-F(t)} = -\beta \ln a + \beta \ln t \tag{4.259}$$

Make

$$y = \ln \frac{1}{1-F(t)} \tag{4.260}$$

$$x = \ln t \tag{4.261}$$

$$\begin{Bmatrix} A = -\beta \ln \alpha \\ B = \beta \end{Bmatrix} \tag{4.262}$$

Then the above formula can be transformed into:

$$y = A + Bx \tag{4.263}$$

If it is the abscissa and x y the ordinate, then the obtained data point is a straight line $(x_1, y_1), (x_2, y_2), \cdots, (x_n, y_n)$ whose slope is B and y the axis intercept is A, as shown in Fig. 4.20. With the help of this feature, a suitable distribution model can be preliminarily determined.

(2) Graphical method. The basic idea of the graphic method is to take the estimated reliability as the abscissa and the fitting value of the reliability as the ordinate. If the fitting effect is good, these points should be a standard straight line. By judging the trend of the data points, it can be used as a preliminary test of the goodness of fit.
(3) Goodness-of-fit analytical method. The above two methods may have different test results due to the different influences of subjective factors in different individuals' drawing. Therefore, the above two methods are not recommended.

The Pearson test (χ^2 test) method is suitable for the test of the discrete distribution model, and the Kplmogorov-Smirnov test method is suitable for the test of the continuous distribution model. The life distribution model generally adopts the continuous distribution model, so the Pearson test method is often used. In the following, we focus on explaining these two testing methods.

(1) Pearson test (χ^2 test) method

Let the distribution function of the parent be $F(x)$, and use the sample of the parent to test the hypothesis

$$H_0 : F(x) = F_0(x) \tag{4.264}$$

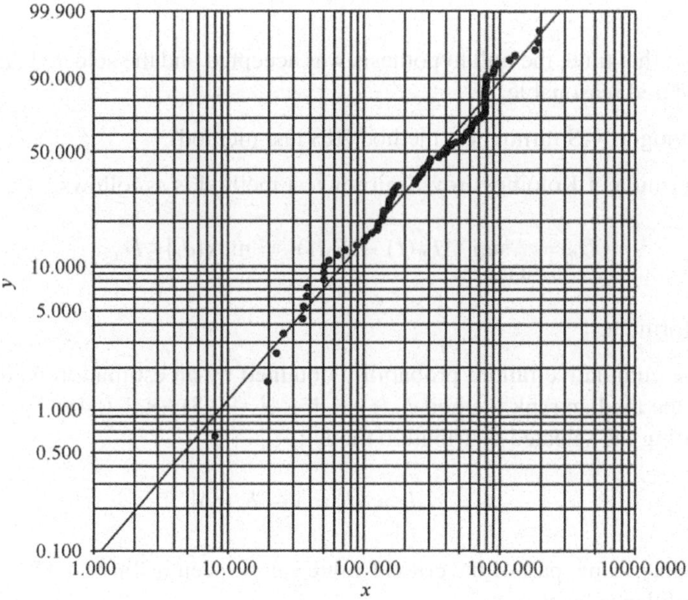

Fig. 4.20 Example of a Weibull probability graph

In order to find the test statistic, X the value range of the matrix is divided k into intervals, namely $(a_0, a_1), (a_1, a_2), \cdots, (a_{k-1}, a_k)$, λ_i is $F_0(x)$ the continuation point of the distribution function, a_0 can be taken $-\infty$, can be taken $+\infty$. recorded as

$$p_i = F_0(a_i) - F_0(a_{i-1}), i = 1, 2, \cdots, k \tag{4.265}$$

It p_i represents the probability that the parent population X falls into the i- th interval. If the size of the sample is n, it is np_i the theoretical frequency that the random variable X falls into. (a_{k-1}, a_k) If the actual frequency of n_i n observed values is (a_{k-1}, a_k), then when it is established, H_0 $(n_i - np_i)^2$ it is a small value, and the statistics can be constructed

$$\chi^2 = \sum_{i=1}^{k} \frac{(n_i - np_i)^2}{np_i} \tag{4.266}$$

Its extreme value distribution is a distribution with degrees of $k - 1$ freedom $\chi^2(k-1)$. For a given significance level α, given by

$$P_0(\chi^2 > c) = \alpha \tag{4.267}$$

Get the critical value

$$c = \chi^2_\alpha(k-1) \tag{4.268}$$

$\chi^2 \leq c$ At that time, the null hypothesis was accepted and the selected distribution was considered reasonable.

(2) Kolomogorov-Smirnov test method (KS test method).

The test formula of Kolomogorov-Smirnov test method is as follows:

$$D_n = \sup_{0 \leq t < +\infty} |F_n(t) - F_0(t)| = \max\{d_i\} \leq D_{n,\alpha} \tag{4.269}$$

In the formula:

$F_n(t)$ The cumulative failure probability obtained by an estimation method, such as the median rank method $F_n(t) = 1 - (i - 0.3)/(n + 0.4)$;
$F_0(t)$ Fitting the selected distribution model;

$$d_i = |F_0(t_i) - F_n(t_i)| \tag{4.270}$$

$D_{n,\alpha}$ Critical value, part of the critical value can be seen in Table 4.44;
α Confidence level;
n The number of faults.

Table 4.44 Partial critical value of KS test

Number of faults (n)	The critical value corresponding to the confidence level (α)				
	$\alpha = 0.200$	$\alpha = 0.150$	$\alpha = 0.100$	$\alpha = 0.05$	$\alpha = 0.01$
1	0.900	0.925	0.950	0.975	0.995
2	0.684	0.726	0.766	0.842	0.929
3	0.565	0.597	0.642	0.708	0.828
4	0.494	0.525	0.564	0.624	0.733
5	0.446	0.474	0.510	0.565	0.669
6	0.410	0.436	0.470	0.521	0.618
7	0.381	0.405	0.438	0.486	0.577
8	0.358	0.381	0.411	0.457	0.543
9	0.339	0.360	0.338	0.432	0.514
10	0.322	0.342	0.368	0.410	0.490
11	0.307	0.326	0.352	0.391	0.468
12	0.295	0.313	0.338	0.375	0.450
13	0.284	0.302	0.325	0.361	0.433
14	0.274	0.292	0.314	0.349	0.418
15	0.266	0.283	0.304	0.338	0.404
16	0.258	0.274	0.295	0.328	0.392
17	0.250	0.266	0.286	0.318	0.381
18	0.244	0.259	0.278	0.309	0.371
19	0.237	0.252	0.272	0.301	0.363
20	0.231	0.246	0.264	0.294	0.356
25	0.210	0.220	0.240	0.270	0.320
30	0.190	0.200	0.220	0.240	0.290
35	0.180	0.190	0.210	0.230	0.270
Greater than 35	$1.07/\sqrt{n}$	$1.14/\sqrt{n}$	$1.22/\sqrt{n}$	$1.36/\sqrt{n}$	$1.63/\sqrt{n}$

Distribution Model Identification and Optimization

When performing reliability modeling on failure data, it is often encountered that multiple models can fit the same batch of data, and can pass the goodness of fit test of a single model. Selecting the best distribution model among the distribution models of the goodness test is the key to ensure reliability modeling and evaluation accuracy. So far, there is no uniform optimization method in engineering applications, and the optimization criteria are generally set according to the actual needs of the product. Multiple model optimization criteria can be divided into single-criteria model optimization method and multi-criteria model optimization method according to different judgment criteria.

1. **Single Criterion Model Optimization Method**

The basic idea of the single-criteria model optimization method is to select the optimal model by setting a single judgment criterion to screen the models that pass the goodness-of-fit test. Commonly used screening criteria include: minimum error range, error coefficient of variation, minimum error variance, minimum maximum deviation, minimum average error of cumulative distribution function, minimum average error of probability density function, etc.

(1) The error range is the smallest

At t_i time, assuming that the observed value of the basic function of product reliability is $\phi'(t_i)$ the value obtained after fitting $\phi(t_i)$, there are K models selected, and for the obtained failure data $t_1 < t_2 < \cdots < t_r$, the minimum error range can be defined as

$$E_{\min} = \min_{1\le j\le k}\{\max_{1\le i\le r}\left|\phi'(t_i) - \phi(t_i)\right| - \min_{1\le i\le r}\left|\phi'(t_i) - \phi(t_i)\right|\} \tag{4.271}$$

When selecting the basic function, reliability function, cumulative distribution function, probability density function and failure rate function can be used as discrimination objects. Among the selected distribution models, the distribution function with the smallest error range is selected.

(2) The error coefficient of variation is the smallest

At t_i time, assuming the observed value of the basic function of product reliability $\phi'(t_i)$, the value obtained after fitting $\phi(t_i)$, for the obtained failure data $t_1 < t_2 < \cdots < t_r$, the minimum error range can be defined as:

$$Cv_{\min} = \min_{1\le j\le k}\left[\frac{\sqrt{\frac{1}{r-1}\sum_{i=1}^{r}(t_i - \bar{t})^2}}{\frac{1}{r}\sum_{i=1}^{r} t_i}\right] \times 100\% \tag{4.272}$$

When testing the lognormal distribution, just t replace in the formula with $\ln t$. Among the selected distribution models, the distribution function with the smallest error coefficient of variation is selected.

(3) The error variance is the smallest

At t_i time, the observed value of the basic function of product reliability is $\phi'(t_i)$ assumed to be the obtained value after fitting $\phi(t_i)$. For the obtained failure data $t_1 < t_2 < \cdots < t_r$, the minimum error variance can be defined as

$$\sigma^2_{\min} = \min_{1\le j\le k}\left\{\sum_{i=1}^{r}[\phi'(t_i) - \phi(t_i)]^2\right\} \tag{4.273}$$

Among the selected distribution functions, the distribution function with the smallest error variance is selected as the best fitting model.

(4) The maximum deviation is the smallest

At t_i time, the observed value of the basic function of product reliability is $\phi'(t_i)$ assumed to be the value obtained after fitting $\phi(t_i)$. For the obtained failure data $t_1 < t_2 < \cdots < t_r$, the maximum deviation can be defined as

$$\begin{aligned} D_{\min} &= \min_{1 \le j \le K} \{ \sup_{0 \le t < +\infty} |\phi'(t_i) - \phi(t_i)| \} \\ &= \min_{1 \le j \le K} \{ \max_{1 \le i \le r} [|\phi'(t_i) - \phi(t_i)|, |\phi'(t_{i+1}) - \phi(t_i)|] \} \end{aligned} \tag{4.274}$$

Among the selected distribution models, the distribution model with the largest deviation and the smallest is selected as the optimal fitting distribution model.

(5) The average error of the function is the smallest

At t_i time, the observed value of the basic function of product reliability is $\phi'(t_i)$ assumed to be the obtained value after fitting $\phi(t_i)$. For the obtained failure data $t_1 < t_2 < \cdots < t_r$, the minimum average error of the function can be defined as

$$\delta_F = \min_{1 \le j \le k} \left[\frac{1}{b-a} \int_a^b |\phi'(x) - \phi(x)| \mathrm{d}x \right] = \min_{1 \le j \le k} \left[\frac{1}{r} \sum_{i=1}^{r} |\phi'(t_i) - \phi(t_i)| \right] \tag{4.275}$$

When selecting the basic function, the reliability function, cumulative distribution function and failure rate function can be used as the object of discrimination. Among the selected distribution models, the distribution function with the smallest average error is selected.

(6) The average error of the probability density function is the smallest

At t_i time, assuming that the observed value of the product reliability basic function is $\phi'(t_i)$ the value obtained after fitting $\phi(t_i)$, for the obtained failure data $t_1 < t_2 < \cdots < t_r$, the minimum average error of the probability density function can be defined as

$$\delta_f = \min_{1 \le j \le k} \left[\sqrt{\frac{1}{b-a} \int_a^b |f(x) - g(x)|^2 \mathrm{d}x} \right] = \min_{1 \le j \le k} \left[\frac{1}{r} \sqrt{\sum_{i=1}^{r} |f(t_i) - g(t_i)|^2} \right] \tag{4.276}$$

where: $f(x)$ is the estimated probability density function, $g(x)$ and is the probability density function obtained by fitting.

For the lognormal distribution, just t replace in the formula with $\ln t$. Finally, the distribution with the smallest average error of the probability density function is selected as the optimal distribution function.

2. **Multi-Criteria Model Optimization Method**

The basic idea of the multi-criteria model optimization method is to synthesize the judgment criteria in the above-mentioned single-criteria optimization model.

There are two synthesis methods: cumulative method and comprehensive evaluation method.

(1) Accumulation method

The basic idea of the accumulation method is to accumulate two or more judgment values in a single criterion, and select the one with the smallest sum as the optimal distribution model. For example, the sum of the judging values of the above six criteria is selected as the judging criterion, see formula (4.277):

$$\rho_{\min} = \min_{1 \le j \le k} [E_{\min} + Cv_{\min} + \sigma^2_{\min} + D_{\min} + \delta_F + \delta_f] \tag{4.277}$$

(2) Comprehensive evaluation method

The comprehensive evaluation method is an evaluation method that considers multiple judgment criteria and the weight of each judgment criterion is different. The basic idea of this method is to give the weight of each single criterion through expert judgment, and then obtain the total value of the judgment criterion, and take the smallest one as the optimal model. See formula (4.278):

$$\rho_{\min} = \min_{1 \le j \le k} [w_1 E_{\min} + w_2 Cv_{\min} + w_3 \sigma^2_{\min} + w_4 D_{\min} + w_5 \delta_F + w_6 \delta_f] \tag{4.278}$$

4.9 Summary

This chapter elaborates on the relevant technologies required for the design and analysis of failure models of medical equipment. For digital medical equipment, fault tree modeling and analysis technology can be selected to analyze the root causes of unexpected events and improve the safety and effectiveness of medical equipment.; For newly developed core components, reliability modeling and prediction, failure mode impact criticality analysis techniques can be used to predict the failure rate level, analyze the main failure reasons, and take necessary preventive and improvement measures to improve its reliability. In addition, for two types of typical materials of mechanical parts and components, this chapter gives the main failure modes, and gives the calculation methods of the failure life of several types of mechanical parts and the accelerated test model method of several types of components. At the same time, A typical life distribution model is also given, which can provide reference for readers to study component failure and component life.

Chapter 5
Reliability Simulation Calculation and Analysis Method of Digital Diagnosis and Treatment Equipment

5.1 Overview

Reliability simulation calculation and analysis method refers to that in the design stage, with the help of professional simulation analysis software tools, the thermal stress, vibration stress and durable life models of products are established, and the thermal environment, vibration response and durable life of products are simulated to find out whether there are weak links in heat resistance and vibration resistance and whether the durable life can meet the requirements.

By means of reliability simulation calculation and analysis, the traditional test method of relying on physical prototype to obtain improvement opportunities through test exposure problems is broken, and the digital prototype of product design is used to analyze exposure problems through simulation calculation, so as to obtain improvement opportunities and effectively quantify the improved effect. Reliability simulation calculation and analysis not only greatly advance the opportunity of product improvement, but also significantly reduce the difficulty and cost of improvement, greatly shorten the improvement cycle and make it more convenient to verify the improvement effect.

Considering that all kinds of reliability simulation calculation and analysis need modeling and have a large workload, in order to reduce the workload and obtain the maximum working effect, this book suggests selecting the most necessary simulation items according to the product characteristics, such as thermal simulation calculation and analysis for power-consuming components with obvious heating, vibration stress simulation calculation and analysis for structural load-bearing parts bearing vibration stress, and durability life simulation calculation and analysis for more obvious wear-consuming components.

X. Li et al., *Reliability Engineering Technology of Digital Diagnosis and Treatment Equipment*, https://doi.org/10.1007/978-981-99-5522-0_5

5.2 Thermal Simulation Calculation and Analysis of Power Consumption Components

5.2.1 Purpose

Through the thermal simulation of the power consumption prototype, the temperature distribution inside the prototype is obtained, the weak links are found out, and the improvement suggestions are put forward to guide the thermal design improvement of power consumption components.

5.2.2 Simulation Calculation Process

The thermal simulation calculation and analysis process is shown in Fig. 5.1.

5.2.3 Working Steps

5.2.3.1 Information Collection

Before thermal simulation, some necessary information and data of the prototype should be collected, focusing on the information collection of the electronic control board and power devices of the prototype, including components, component information (model, size, power consumption, etc.), structural parts information, etc.

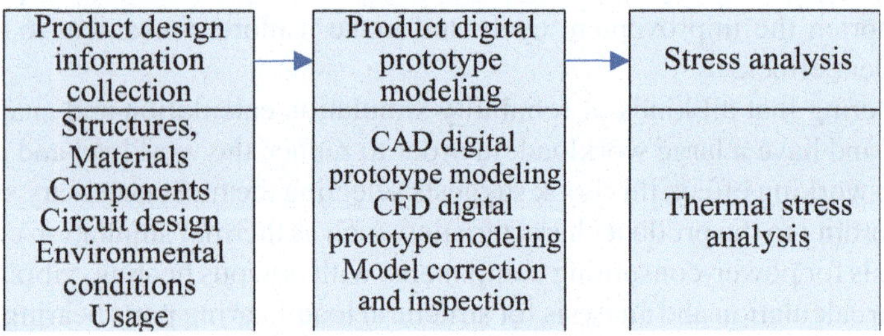

Fig. 5.1 Thermal simulation calculation and analysis process

5.2.3.2 Digital Prototype Modeling

According to the design documents of power consumption components, the CFD digital prototype model is established after proper simplification.

5.2.3.3 Grid Division

The grid is divided by structured grid and local encrypted grid, and the prototype is divided to ensure the grid quality can meet the requirements.

5.2.3.4 Parameter Setting

Set the ambient temperature and gravity direction of the power consumption component.

5.2.3.5 Preliminary Analysis of Thermal Stress

Under the condition that the ambient temperature has been set, the temperature result data of power consumption components are obtained by simulation, and the positions with higher temperature are found out to mark the position and temperature value, which provides data for the subsequent thermal design effect analysis.

5.2.4 Thermal Analysis and Improvement of Products

Compare the simulated temperature of components at higher temperature with the maximum operating temperature specified in the component specification to determine whether there is enough margin. Judge whether the current thermal design scheme conforms to relevant regulations according to the device withstand temperature and derating design criteria given in the component specification.

Take thermal design improvement measures to make its thermal environment meet relevant requirements in view of exceeding the specified maximum temperature or insufficient margin. Improvement usually includes three aspects:

(1) Adjust the layout of product components, and move components that cannot withstand high temperature to a better position in thermal environment;
(2) Strengthen the heat dissipation measures of the heat source near the position of the component, improve the local thermal environment, and reduce the temperature to the range that the component can bear;
(3) Replace the components of this model with those with stronger high temperature resistance to meet the working requirements at this temperature.

5.2.5 Examples

Taking a power consumption component as an example, the thermal simulation calculation and analysis are carried out by Flotherm software.

By collecting the simulation information of power consumption components, the reliability simulation model of power consumption components is established, and some geometric information which has little correlation with heat dissipation characteristics is omitted by further simplification. The reliability simulation model of power consumption components is shown in Fig. 5.2.

The circuit board of power consumption components is modeled according to actual geometric and material parameters, and the reliability simulation model of the circuit board is shown in Fig. 5.3.

Further modeling of each component in Flotherm, the modeling of components can choose thermal resistance model or detailed model, and the reliability simulation model of components is shown in Fig. 5.4.

On this basis, the reliability simulation model of power consumption components grid is divided. Taking Flotherm software as an example, the grid division is shown in Fig. 5.5. The grid distribution in the chassis is dense, which ensures that the complex heat dissipation process in the chassis can be fully analyzed. The computing space

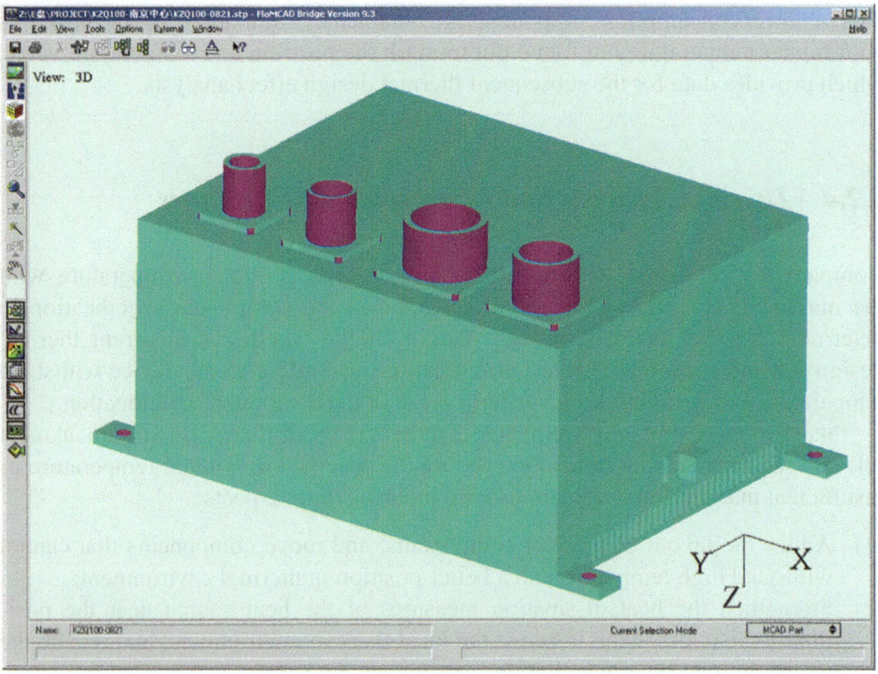

Fig. 5.2 Reliability simulation model of power components

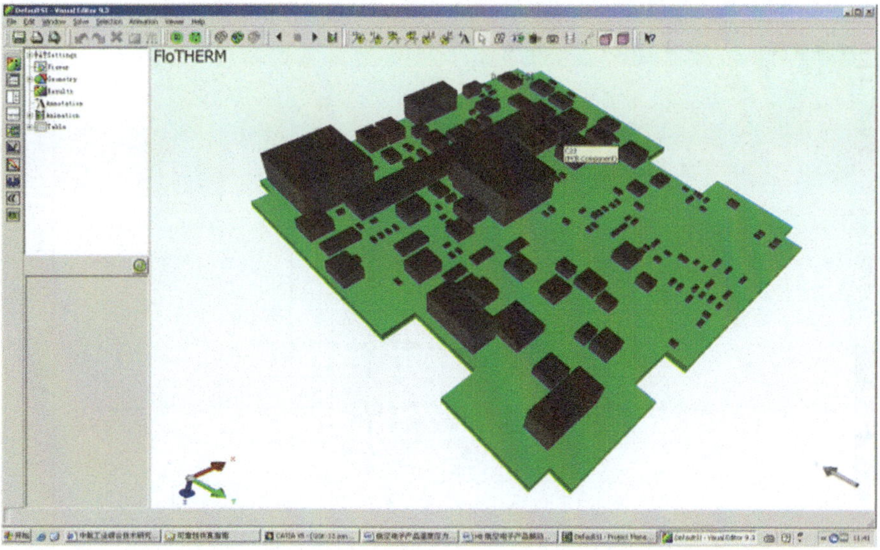

Fig. 5.3 Reliability simulation model of circuit board

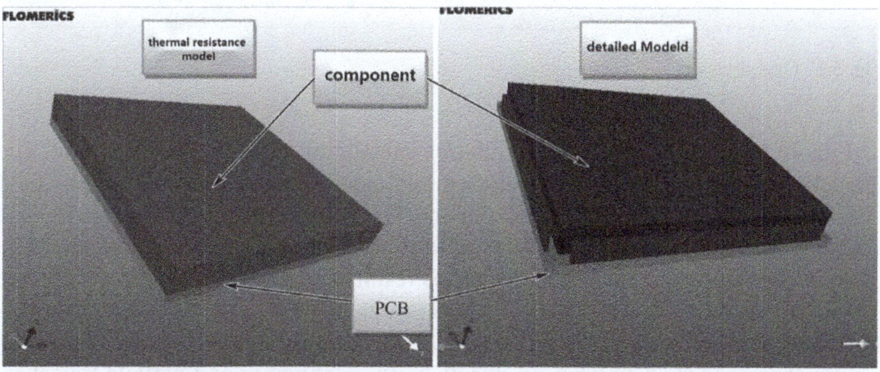

Fig. 5.4 Reliability simulation model of components

around the chassis is not the focus, and the grid distribution is loose. The length–width ratio of the grid is controlled at about 20, and the number of grids is controlled at about 1.5 million.

Select the corresponding solution domain, as shown in Fig. 5.6.

According to the solution domain, the temperature and flow field are solved and calculated. The convergence curve of the solution process is shown in Fig. 5.7.

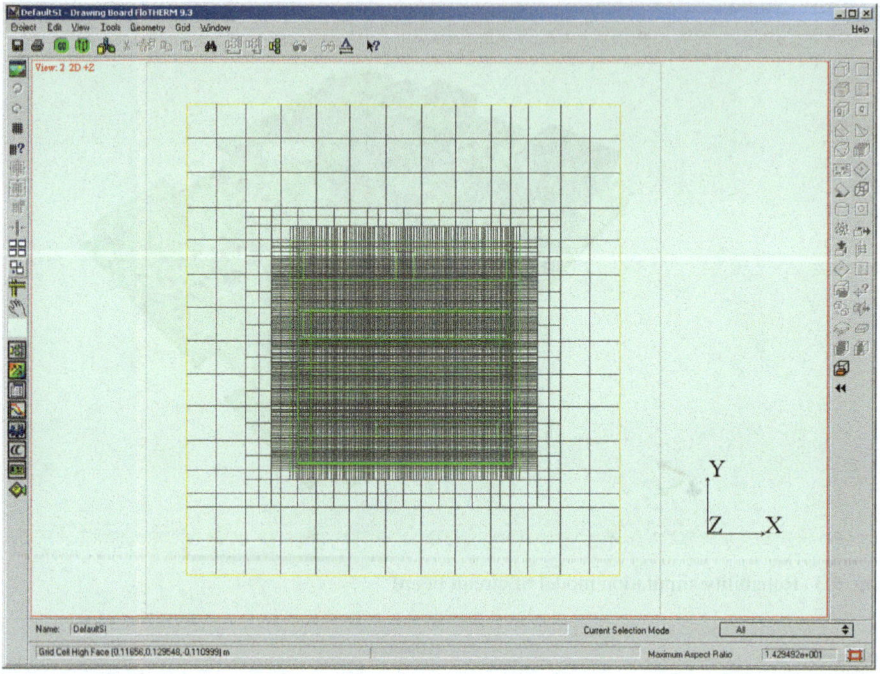

Fig. 5.5 Grid division

Finally, the results of thermal simulation calculation and analysis are output. The temperature field analysis results include the temperature values and temperature field distribution of power consumption components, circuit boards and components. The analysis results can be expressed in the form of data tables and nephograms. The thermal simulation calculation and analysis results are shown in Fig. 5.8.

It can also output the flow field analysis results, including the flow velocity, pressure value and flow field distribution inside or outside the product. The analysis results can be expressed by data table, vector diagram, nephogram and particle trajectory diagram. The flow field analysis results are shown in Fig. 5.9.

By analyzing the results of thermal simulation calculation, it can be seen that the middle structure of the main body bracket of the power consumption component hinders the air flow, and the air flow can be enhanced by increasing the number of through holes and modifying the aperture size; On the other hand, the structure and size of the heat sink in the power consumption component need to be re-optimized to increase the gas flow rate and improve the heat exchange capacity.

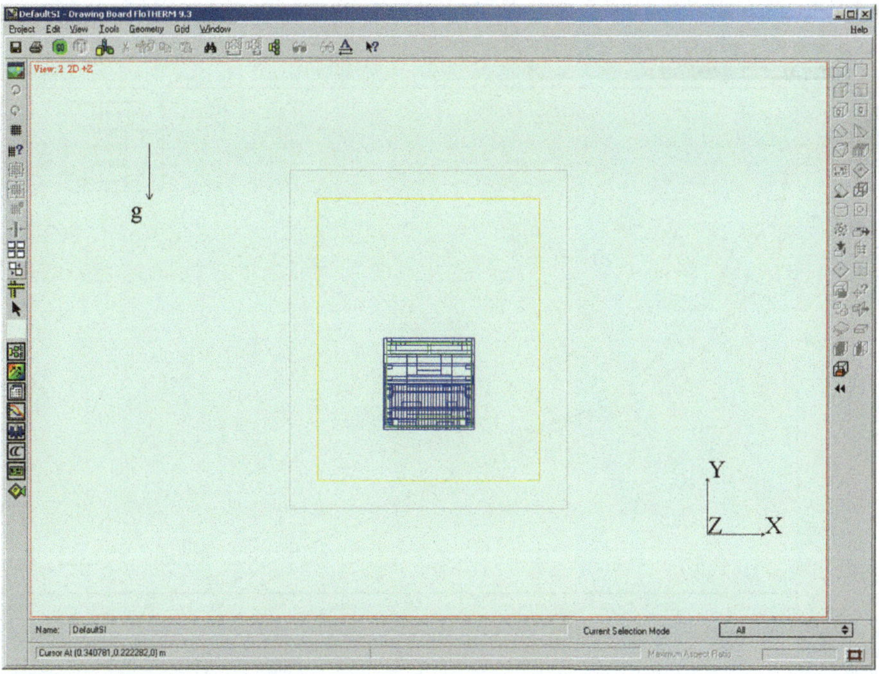

Fig. 5.6 Selecting the solution domain

5.3 Simulation Calculation and Analysis of Vibration of Vibration-Bearing Parts

5.3.1 Purpose

Through the vibration simulation of the vibration bearing parts, the vibration stress distribution of the prototype under the specified conditions is obtained, which provides reference for stress damage analysis and weak link determination of the prototype. In view of the weak links, the improvement suggestions are put forward to guide the anti-vibration design improvement of vibration-bearing components.

Generally speaking, the fixed digital diagnosis and treatment equipment is mainly subjected to vibration during transportation, but basically does not bear vibration stress during use. Of course, if there is a vibration source in the equipment, it will produce certain vibration stress, which will have an impact on the components near the vibration source. For mobile (vehicle-mounted and airborne) digital diagnosis and treatment equipment, the vibration stress in use can not be ignored.

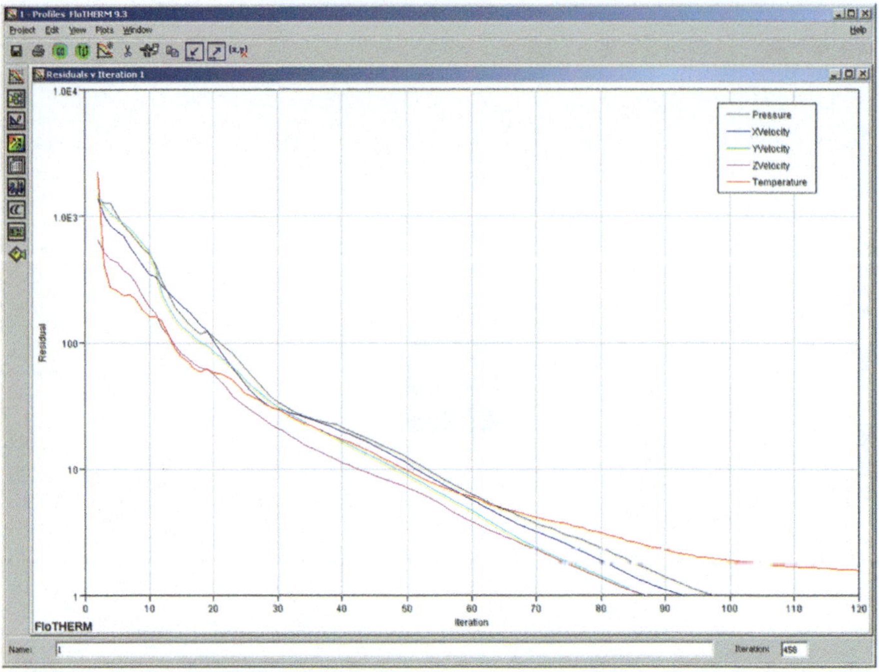

Fig. 5.7 Convergence curve of solution process

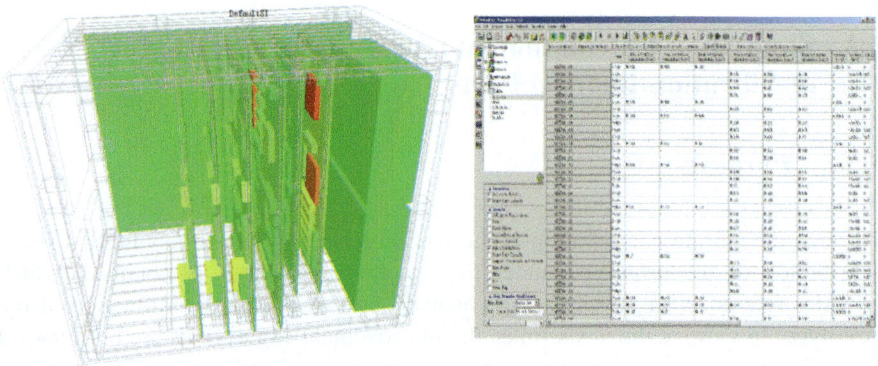

Fig. 5.8 Thermal simulation calculation and analysis results

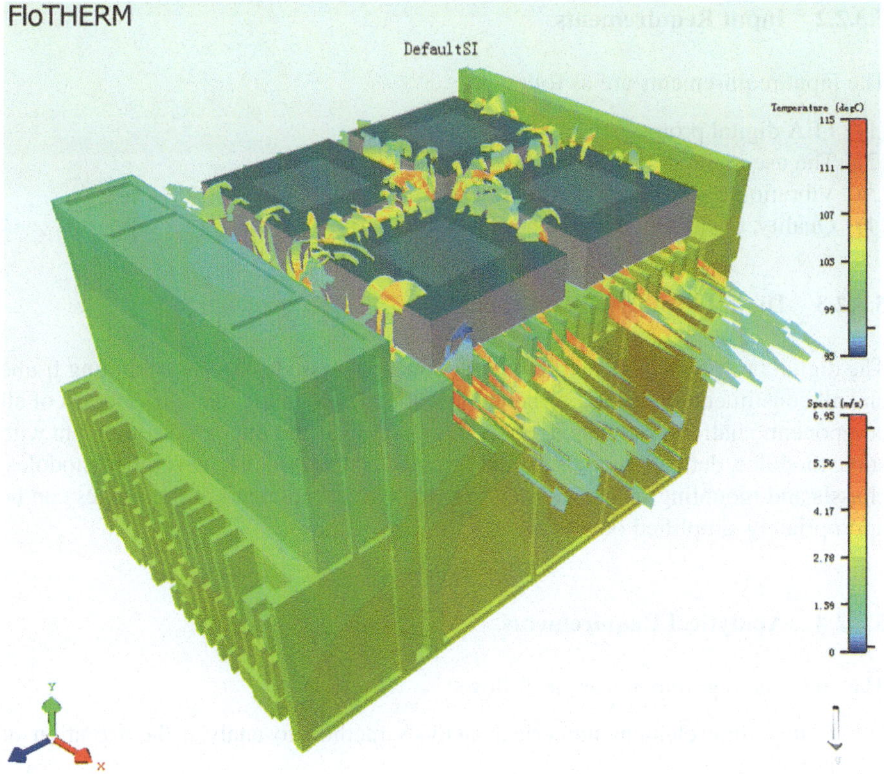

Fig. 5.9 Flow field analysis results

5.3.2 *General Requirements*

5.3.2.1 Software and Hardware Requirements

The following software conditions should be met:

(1) Common CAD software, such as CATIA V5, PRO-E, UG, etc.;
(2) FEA software, such as NASTRAN, ANSYS, ABAQUS;
(3) Electronic component database and material database suitable for reliability simulation test.

The following hardware conditions should be met:

(1) Workstations or computing servers running common CAD and FEA software;
(2) Terminal computer.

5.3.2.2 Input Requirements

The input requirements are as follows:

(1) FEA digital prototype;
(2) The use method of product life cycle;
(3) Vibration environmental conditions of products;
(4) Quality, environment and material information.

5.3.2.3 Digital Prototype Requirements

The digital prototype of reliability simulation shall include chassis, mounting frame and all constituent modules. For newly developed equipment, detailed models of all components shall be established. For newly developed and improved equipment with some modules, detailed models should be established for newly developed modules, chassis and mounting racks, and other outsourced components and modules can be appropriately simplified or equivalent.

5.3.2.4 Analytical Requirements

The analysis requirements are as follows:

(1) Using finite element numerical analysis method to analyze the vibration of products;
(2) Modal analysis and random response analysis of the product (including all components of the product) shall be included at least;
(3) It is necessary to analyze the vibration response distribution of products under the maximum vibration condition.

5.3.2.5 Output Requirements

(1) Modal information such as modal frequency and modal shape of products;
(2) Distribution of random vibration response (including root mean square acceleration value and root mean square displacement value) in the product under specified conditions.

5.3.3 Analytical Methods

The vibration stress analysis process is as follows:

(1) Information collection: collect data information related to vibration stress analysis;

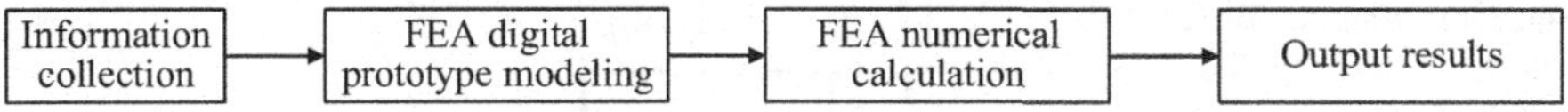

Fig. 5.10 Vibration stress analysis process

(2) FEA digital prototype modeling: Establishing FEA digital prototype of product vibration characteristics;
(3) FEA numerical calculation: Modal analysis and random vibration response analysis of FEA digital prototype;
(4) Output results: the simulation results are clearly displayed.

The vibration stress analysis process is shown in Fig. 5.10.

5.3.3.1 Information Collection

The following information should be added to the data collected by CAD digital prototype.

1) Quality Information

    (1) Total product quality;
    (2) Quality of each electronic module;
    (3) Quality of each component.

2) Material Properties

    (1) Elastic modulus of material;
    (2) Poisson's ratio;
    (3) Material density;
    (4) Material damping coefficient.

3) Environmental Conditions

    (1) The vibration value of the product;
    (2) The vibration environment spectrum of the product;
    (3) Excitation position and direction of vibration load.

5.3.3.2 FEA Digital Prototype Modeling

1. Modeling Requirements of FEA Digital Prototype

(1) Naming rules for digital prototypes

The FEA digital prototype naming format requirements are shown in Fig. 5.11.

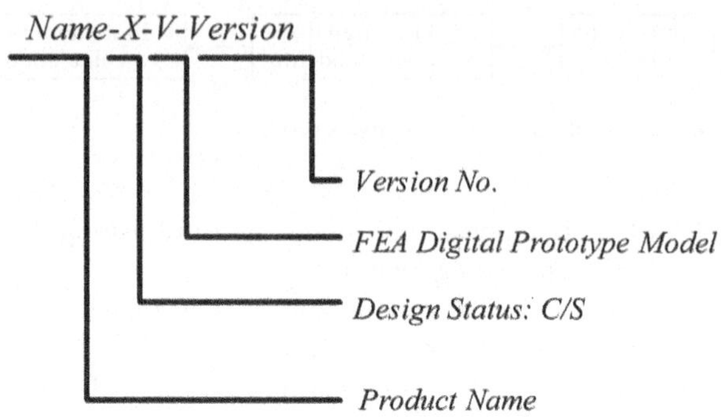

Fig. 5.11 Naming format requirements for FEA digital prototype

(2) Geometric Model Requirements

There are two methods to create geometric model for vibration stress analysis: one is to create geometric model by using geometric modeling function of FEA software; The second is to import CAD digital prototype model by using FEA software data interface.

(1) Modeling requirements of structural parts

- All structural parts models should be three-dimensional solid models;
- The model size should be consistent with the original actual size, without considering the dimensional deviation;
- There must be no defects in the model, and it must be continuous and complete;
- Remove the decorative features of small size;
- Remove non-connecting holes with smaller size;
- Remove smaller rounding and chamfering;
- The features of connecting screws and threads are omitted, but the connection relationship cannot be removed;
- The assembly relationship of parts must be accurate, and there must be no interference of parts and inadequate assembly;
- The simplified model weight should be close to the actual product weight.

(2) Board modeling requirements

- Printed circuit boards are generally treated as mean boards;
- Printed circuit boards with cold plates, which should retain physical characteristics;
- For printed circuit boards with reinforcing ribs, the reinforcing ribs should retain solid characteristics;
- The connection features of printed circuit boards should be retained.
- Component modeling requirements

(3) Component modeling requirements

- All component models shall be three-dimensional solid models;
- The pins of integrated circuit components can be omitted;
- The pins of double-lead components can be omitted;
- Leads or pins of connectors can be omitted;
- Remove smaller components;
- The mass of omitted components should be distributed on the electronic module.

3) Grid Division Requirements

(1) Semi-automatic grid division method should be adopted;
(2) The grid in the model area should be homogenized as much as possible;
(3) The nodes between grids should ensure good continuity;
(4) The symmetrical structure should ensure the symmetry of the grid;
(5) Under the condition of satisfying the accuracy, the grid form with fewer nodes should be selected;
(6) The density of grid should be divided according to the structural characteristics to reduce the amount of calculation;
(7) The load and constraint positions should coincide with the node positions to ensure the accuracy of boundary conditions.

4) Grid Quality Inspection

(1) Length–width ratio inspection: the ratio of long side to short side of quadrilateral grid should be less than 5;
(2) Warpage inspection: the smaller the diagonal distance of quadrilateral grid, the better;
(3) Distortion angle inspection: The distortion angle of triangular mesh should be less than 60°The twist angle of the quadrilateral grid should be less than 45°;
(4) Internal angle inspection: The angle of triangular mesh should be between 30 and 150°The inner angle of the quadrilateral grid should be between 45° and 135°;
(5) Jacques ratio check: quadrilateral unit should keep regular polygon as far as possible, and Jacques ratio should be greater than 0.7;
(6) Coincidence node inspection: ensure that the common nodes between cell grids are not coincidence points, but the same point;
(7) Free edge inspection: there can be no discontinuous points and edges in grid nodes and elements;
(8) T-edge inspection: there can be no interlaced cells between grids.

5) Parameter Setting

(1) Material attribute setting

- Setting the structural parts without equivalent treatment according to the actual material attributes;
- The equivalent structural parts are set according to the equivalent material attributes.

(2) Unit attribute setting

- The bar, beam, spring and damping are set according to the attributes of one-dimensional element;
- Set shell elements for two-dimensional elements of triangle and quadrilateral;
- The three-dimensional unit is set as a volume unit.

(3) Constraint Setting

- Set the constraint position;
- Set the degree of freedom.

6) Setting of environmental conditions

Set the excitation position, excitation direction and vibration environment spectrum of the product.

2. **Model Modification**

(1) Correcting Parameters

The parameters of FEA digital prototype which have great influence on the results of vibration stress analysis are modified. The main modified parameters are as follows:

(1) Material parameters, including density, elastic modulus and Poisson's ratio;
(2) Result parameters, including equivalent thickness;
(3) Damping parameters.

(2) Correction Method

According to the vibration test results, the FEA digital prototype is modified, and the model parameters of the FEA digital prototype are adjusted to meet the requirements of model modification. The FEA digital prototype correction process is shown in Fig. 5.12.

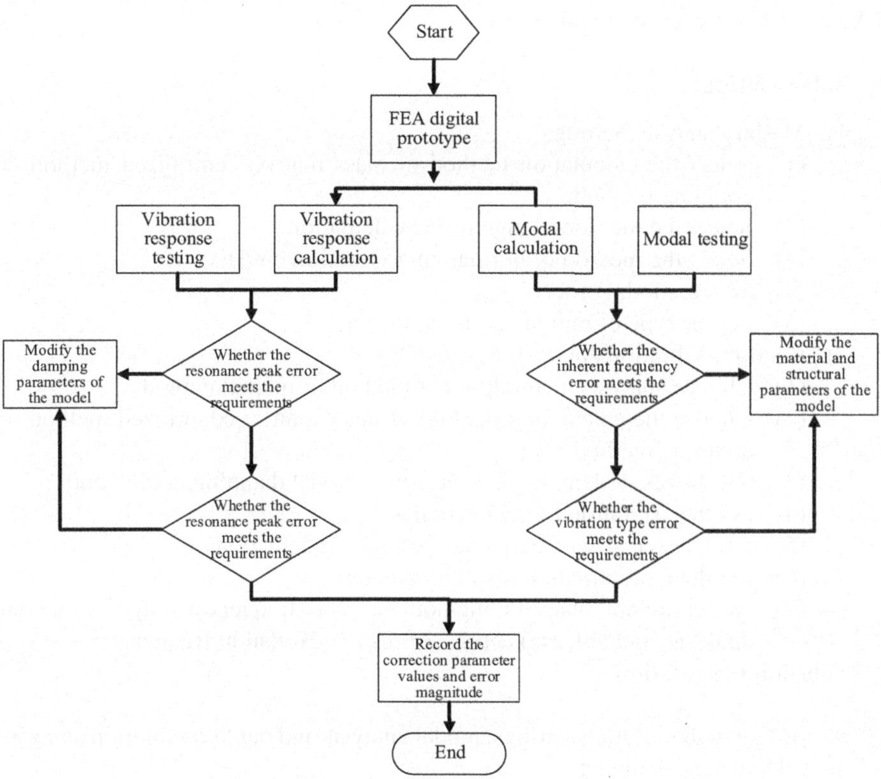

Fig. 5.12 FEA digital prototype correction process

(3) Amendment Requirements

The amendment requirements are as follows:

(1) It is generally required that the relative error between the first three natural frequencies and the test values should not exceed 10%;
(2) Modal correlation coefficient (MAC) is generally required to be greater than 0.75;
(3) It is generally required that the relative error of the first formant-peak of the response curve is less than or equal to 20%;
(4) It is generally required that the relative error of the first resonance frequency of the response curve is less than or equal to 15%.

5.3.3.3 FEA Numerical Calculation

1. **Solve Settings**
   1) Modal Analysis Settings
      (1) Select the calculation method of mass matrix: centralized method or coupling method;
      (2) Select the method of eigenvalue calculation;
      (3) Select the method of normalizing vibration mode;
      (4) Set the modal order;
      (5) Set the type of output result parameter.
   2) Random Vibration Analysis Setting
      (1) Choose analysis method: direct method or modal method;
      (2) Choose the calculation method of mass matrix: centralized method or coupling method;
      (3) Set the result damping coefficient or modal damping coefficient;
      (4) Set the excitation frequency range;
      (5) Set the step size of frequency response calculation;
      (6) Set the type of output result parameter;
      (7) Adopt modal analysis method, set the frequency range of modal analysis, and at least keep 2– 3 times of excitation frequency.
2. **Solution Calculation**

   According to the solution settings, modal analysis and random vibration analysis are solved and calculated.
3. **Computing Breakdown Handling**

   In case of error prompt, interruption information or no result in the solution process, the calculation process record file should be checked, the corresponding problems should be analyzed, and the model, load and boundary conditions should be checked for modification and recalculation.
4. **Output Result**

1) Modal Analysis Results

   The modal analysis results include natural frequencies and modes, and the specific requirements are as follows:

   (1) The mode order shall include at least the first mode of the chassis;
   (2) The modal phase should include the first three modes of each module;
   (3) The natural frequency results can be presented in the form of data list;
   (4) The results of mode shape should be presented in the form of cloud picture or grid deformation diagram.

2) Random Vibration Analysis Results

Random vibration analysis results refer to the random vibration response results of products, and the specific requirements are as follows:

(1) The output results should include the root mean square values of acceleration response and displacement response;
(2) The output results should be presented by cloud map or grid deformation map;
(3) The results of each point in the sub product model can be expressed in the form of a curve to represent the self power spectral density.

5.3.4 Examples

Taking a certain type of vibration-bearing component as an example, simulation calculation and analysis are carried out.

First, establish the digital prototype model of the vibration-bearing components, as shown in Fig. 5.13.

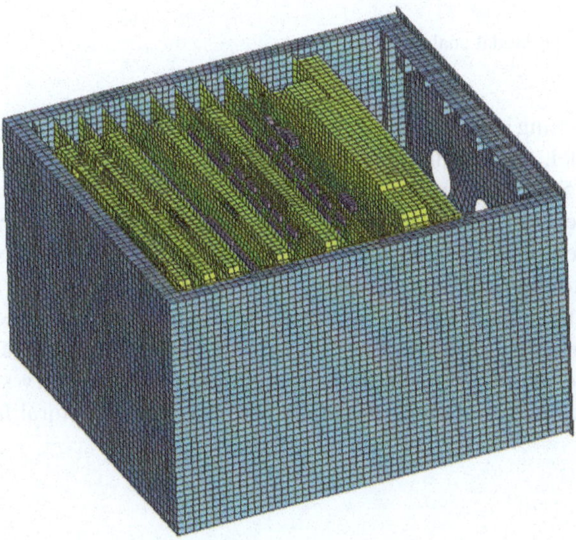

Fig. 5.13 Digital prototype model of vibration-bearing parts

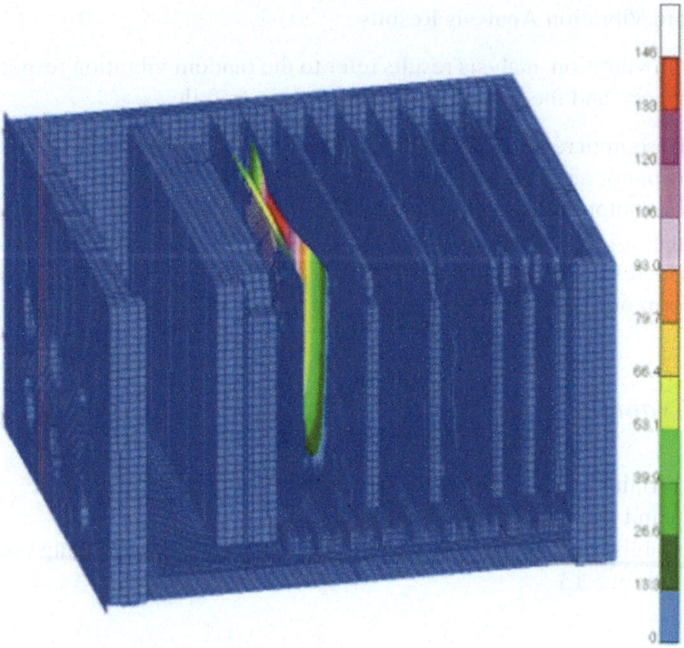

Fig. 5.14 First-order modal analysis results

Parameter setting, model modification and model simulation analysis are carried out on the model, and the first three modal analysis results are output, as shown in Figs. 5.14, 5.15 and 5.16 respectively.

At the same time, the random vibration analysis results of vibration bearing components are obtained, as shown in Figs. 5.17, 5.18 and 5.19 respectively.

According to the results of vibration simulation calculation and analysis of the vibration-bearing parts, the stress, strain and acceleration responses of the vibration-bearing parts are very small under the action of vibration load. Because the stress produced in the structure of vibration-bearing components is very small under the action of vibration load, the vibration load will not cause structural fatigue.

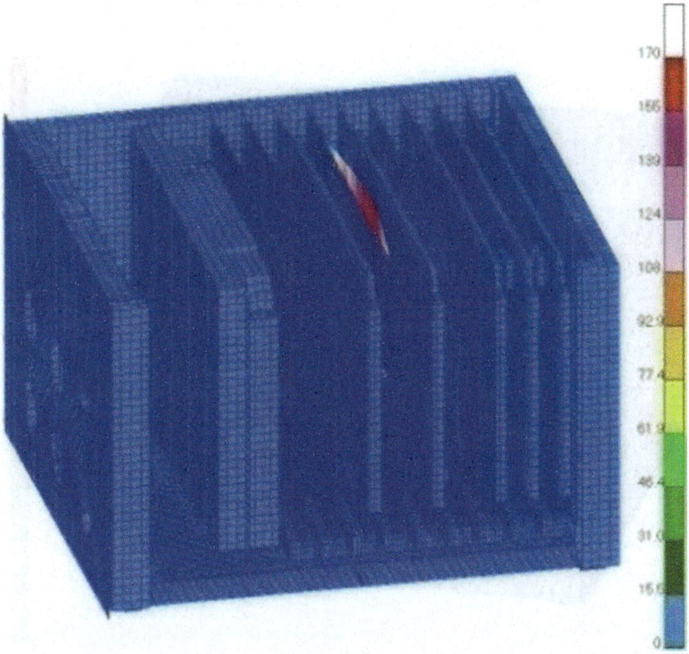

Fig. 5.15 Second-order modal analysis results

5.4 Simulation Calculation and Analysis of Durability Life of Worn Parts

5.4.1 Purpose

Through the analysis of the durable life of the wear-out parts in the product, the durable life of each wear-out part under the specified conditions is obtained, and whether the durable life of the wear-out parts meets the overall requirements of the product is judged, which provides reference for determining the weak links of the product durable life, and takes necessary improvement measures to meet the overall life requirements of the product.

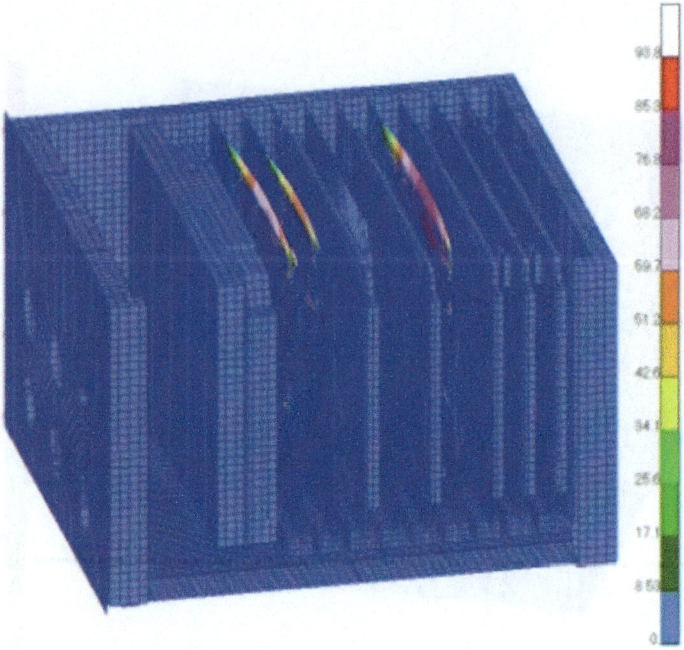

Fig. 5.16 Third-order modal analysis results

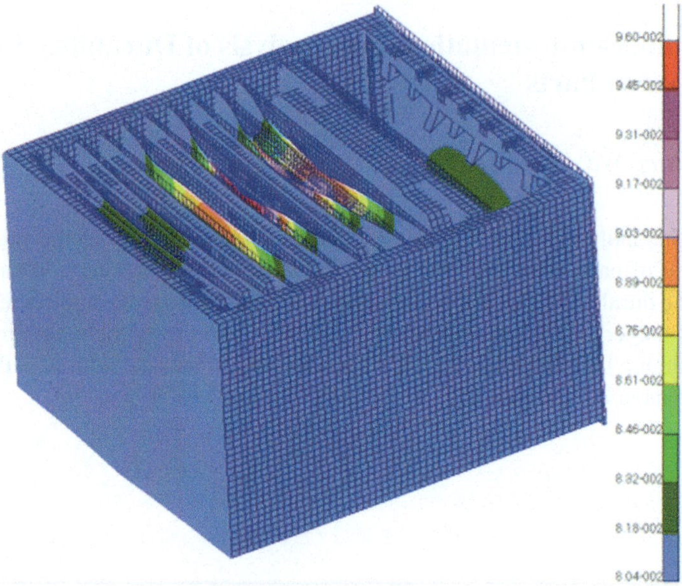

Fig. 5.17 Displacement root mean square nephogram

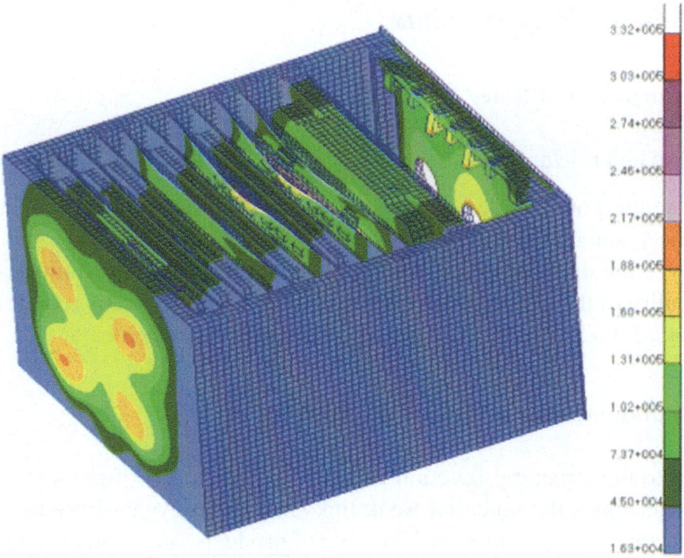

Fig. 5.18 Nephogram of root mean square acceleration

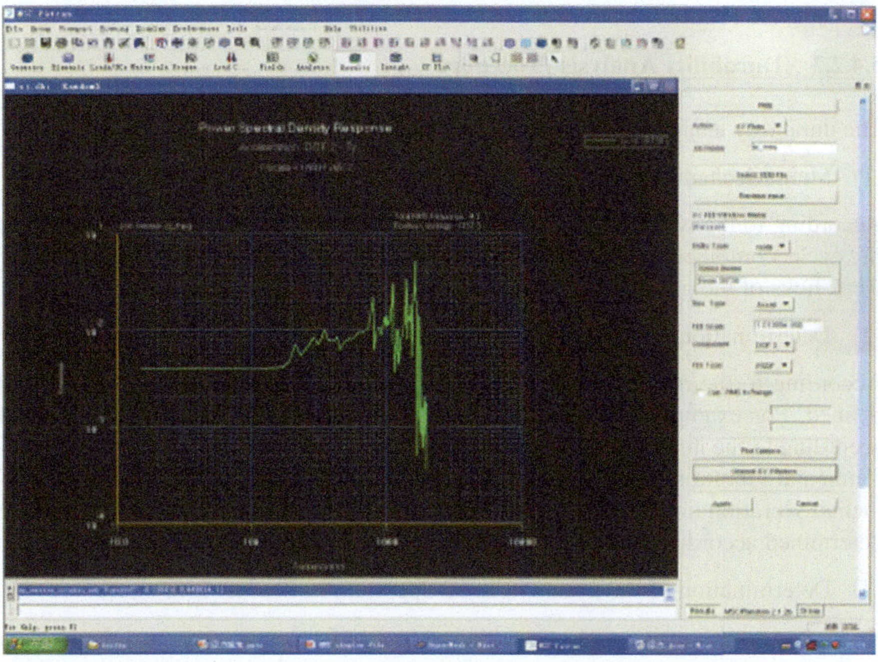

Fig. 5.19 Self-power spectral density function curve of response point

5.4.2 General Requirements

5.4.2.1 Purpose and Role

The purpose and role are as follows:

(1) Expose the potential design defects of products, determine the weak links of products, and clarify the main wear-out mechanism of products;
(2) Analyze the durability design level of the product and determine whether the durability of the product meets the specified durability index requirements;
(3) It lays a foundation for the design of durability test scheme.

5.4.2.2 Fundamentals of Durability Analysis

According to the structure, function and service conditions of products, durability analysis determines the potential weak links in the life cycle of products, clarifies the wear mechanism affecting the life cycle of products, and evaluates the life cycle of products quantitatively or qualitatively by using corresponding life quantitative analysis technology or similar product analogy method.

5.4.2.3 Durability Analysis Procedure

The durability analysis procedure is as follows:

(1) Main Mechanism Analysis of Durability

According to the working conditions and working environment during the product life cycle, combined with the composition, structure and principle of the product, the weak links of the product and its corresponding main mechanism are determined.

(2) Determination of Product Life Index

According to the main mechanism, the corresponding life index of the product is defined. For example, for fatigue and wear, the life index should be determined according to the number of working cycles of products; For fatigue caused by environmental vibration, the life index should be determined according to the environmental vibration time in the product life period; For aging, the life index should be determined according to the working time in the product life period.

(3) Determination of Environment/Load Spectrum in Product Life Cycle

According to the main mechanism, the corresponding environment/load spectrum is determined in combination with the environmental conditions and working conditions during the product life cycle.

(4) Selection of Durability Analysis Method

According to the determined main mechanism, the corresponding life quantitative analysis technology or qualitative evaluation method are selected. Common analysis methods include fatigue life analysis, wear life analysis, aging life analysis and comparative analysis of similar products.

(5) Durability Analysis and Evaluation

Using the determined durability analysis method, analyze whether the product reaches the expected durability index. If it is not achieved, the design scheme should be improved, and then the durability analysis should be carried out again.

5.4.2.4 Durability Analysis Report

The results of durability analysis shall be reported and used as information for product design review and later durability test scheme design. The durability analysis report should reflect the main contents and results of the analysis. Generally, it should include the following contents:

(1) Product function and working principle;
(2) Main mechanism analysis of durability;
(3) Durability analysis;
(4) Summary of durability analysis results;
(5) Analysis conclusions and corresponding suggestions;
(6) Analytical methods.

5.4.2.5 Main Mechanism Analysis of Durability

The purpose of main mechanism analysis is to analyze and determine the main mechanism affecting product durability. Its main tool is Failure Mode Mechanisms and Effects Analysis (FMMEA). FMMEA is a reliability analysis method to study the possible failure modes and failure mechanism of each component of a product and determine the influence of each failure mode on other components of the product and the required functions of the product. The purpose of FMMEA is to determine various potential failure modes and failure mechanisms of products, and to determine the main failure mechanism and its corresponding sensitive stresses (working stress and environmental stress) and characteristic parameters by comprehensive influence sequencing. Based on the comprehensive analysis of FMMEA, quantitative analysis of durability should be carried out for the weak links and their main mechanisms corresponding to the severe failure modes and the failure modes that have occurred before.

The main mechanism analysis flow of FMMEA is shown in Fig. 5.20, and the FMMEA comprehensive influence determination matrix and severity level are given, and the FMMEA table is formed by summary analysis.

(1) Determine the Functional Structure and Working Principle of the Product

FMMEA analysis should be carried out on the basis of clear product structure, working principle and working characteristics. For products with many parts, the structure level should be divided into initial agreed level, agreed level and lowest agreed level, and the product structure level diagram should be drawn to determine the lowest agreed level of mechanism analysis. The above-mentioned division of convention hierarchy is directly reflected in the FMMEA table, and the component names in the table should correspond to the convention hierarchy one by one.

(2) Identify Potential Failure Modes

Failure mode is defined as a certain expression of parts (or components), subsystems or the whole system can not achieve a certain function. The purpose of failure mode analysis is to find out all possible failure modes of products, and its main contents include:

1. Determine all possible failure modes according to the characteristics of the analyzed products, and then analyze each failure mode;
2. The results of FMEA can be used to analyze the potential failure modes of products.

(3) Determine the Impact of potential Failures

According to the structure, corresponding functions and potential failure modes of the product, the influence of each possible failure mode on the function, performance and structural parameters of the product is found out, which provides the basis for determining the failure cause and mechanism.

(4) Determine Potential Failure Causes and Sensitive Stresses

According to the life cycle load and action mode, the causes of each failure mode are analyzed, and the sensitive stress types and action modes are determined, which provides the basis for the stress types of subsequent durability tests.

(5) Determine the Potential Failure Mechanism

Fault mechanism is the physical, electrical, chemical, mechanical or other process that causes fault. On the basis of comprehensive consideration of failure modes and failure causes, according to load types and action modes, it is determined whether the corresponding mechanism of each failure mode is overstress type or wear type.

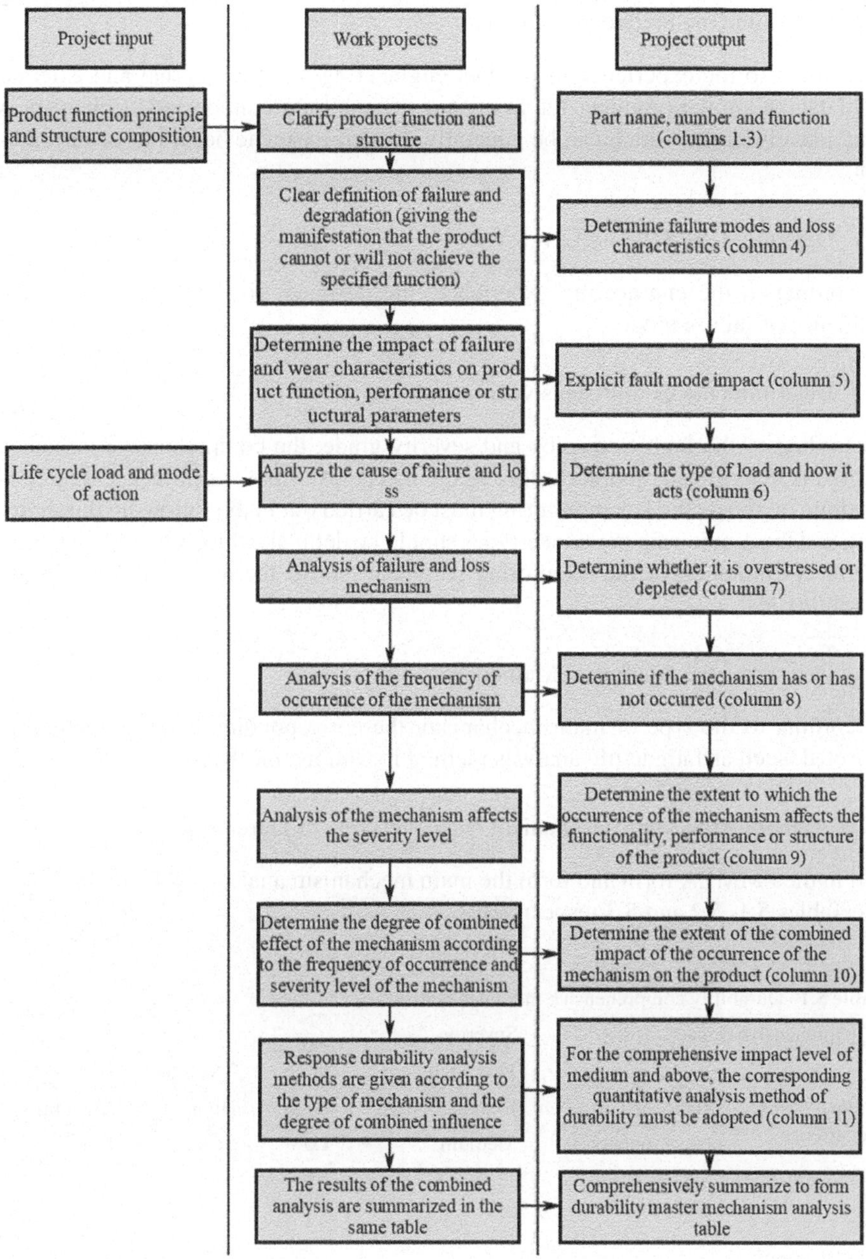

Fig. 5.20 FMMEA main mechanism analysis flow

(6) Determine the Frequency of Failure

According to the experience of product engineering and the internal and external field data of similar products, the frequency of each failure mode and mechanism is qualitatively given, which can be generally divided into whether it has occurred or not.

(7) Determine the Severity Level

According to the engineering experience, the designer gives the severity of the influence of failure mode.

(8) Determine the Comprehensive impact level

According to the fault frequency and severity grade, the comprehensive influence degree is determined, and according to the mechanism that the influence degree is medium or above, the key monitoring must be carried out in the follow-up durability test, and the monitoring parameter types should be defined, which provides the basis for the formulation of the monitoring parameter set of the tested products in the durability test.

(9) Determine the Analytical Method

According to the type of main mechanism, the corresponding analysis method is selected, such as fatigue life analysis method for fatigue mechanism.

(10) Generate the Main Mechanism Analysis Table of Durability

Fill in the FMMEA form and form the main mechanism analysis table of durability, see Tables 5.1, 5.2 and 5.3 respectively.

Table 5.1 Durability comprehensive influence matrix

Comprehensive impact		Severity			
		Very high	High	Medium	Low
Frequency of occurrence	Happened	Extremely high	High	High	Medium
	Never happened	Medium	Low	Low	Low

Table 5.2 Severity rating

Severity	Describe
Very high	Cause the loss of key or main functions of equipment, or cause harm to space environment, working environment and staff
High	Loss of some main functions or some key functions of equipment
Moderate or obvious	Indicators that cause partial function loss of equipment but do not affect main functions
Low or very small	Causing equipment performance degradation or unplanned maintenance and repair

5.4.2.6 Strength Analysis

Strength analysis refers to the ability of a structure or member to bear load at room temperature, which is usually referred to as strength analysis. It is one of the basic requirements of mechanical design, and the durability analysis of its wear characteristics can only be carried out after the strength requirements are met. The static strength analysis here includes:

(1) Check whether the bearing capacity of the structure meets the requirements of strength design;
(2) Check whether the ability of resisting deformation of the structure meets the requirements of strength design;
(3) Calculate and analyze the distribution law of stress and deformation of the structure under static load.

A large number of experimental results about material failure and examples of strength failure of engineering members show that although the failure phenomenon is complex, the failure caused by insufficient strength is mainly yield and fracture. Accordingly, there are currently four major strength theories to explain these two types of failure phenomena, as shown in Table 5.4.

Generally speaking, under normal temperature and static load conditions, brittle materials often occur brittle fracture, so the first and second strength theories are usually adopted; Plastic materials often yield plastically, so the third and fourth strength theories should be adopted; No matter plastic material or brittle material, when the three-dimensional tensile stress is close to equal, it is destroyed in the form of fracture, so the maximum tensile stress theory should be adopted; No matter plastic material or brittle material, when the three-dimensional compressive stress is nearly equal, plastic deformation will be caused, so the third or fourth strength theory should be adopted.

Strength analysis should determine the dangerous points of components in turn, calculate the equivalent stress, compare the strength conditions in the table, and finally judge whether the strength of components meets the design requirements. For complex structures and complex stress situations, finite element static analysis is usually used.

Table 5.3 FMMEA principal mechanism analysis table

Number	Part name	Function	Failure mode and loss characteristics	Effect of failures	Sensitive stress	Failure/loss mechanism	Frequency of occurrence	Harshness	Comprehensive impact	Analytical method
–	–	–	–	–	–	–	–	–	–	–
–	–	–	–	–	–	–	–	–	–	–
–	–	–	–	–	–	–	–	–	–	–
–	–	–	–	–	–	–	–	–	–	–

Table 5.4 Summary of four strength theories

Classification and name of strength theory		Strength condition	Failure form
The first strength theory	Maximum tensile stress theory	$\sigma_{r1} = \sigma_1 \leq \sigma_b / n = [\sigma]$	Fracture
The second strength theory	Maximum tensile strain theory	$\sigma_{r1} = \sigma_1 - \mu(\sigma_2 + \sigma_3) \leq \sigma_b / n = [\sigma]$	
The third strength theory	Maximum shear stress theory	$\sigma_{r3} = \sigma_1 - \sigma_3 \leq \sigma_s / n = [\sigma]$	Yield
The fourth strength theory	Specific energy theory of shape change	$\sigma_{r4} = \sqrt{(\sigma_1 - \sigma_2)^2 + (\sigma_2 - \sigma_3)^2 + (\sigma_3 - \sigma_1)^2} \leq \sigma_s / n = [\sigma]$	

5.4.2.7 Fatigue Life Analysis

Fatigue is one of the important wear-out failure modes of mechanical, electromechanical and hydraulic products. For mechanical products, adopting reasonable fatigue design is an important link and necessary guarantee to improve design level and product quality. For products with fatigue failure modes, besides the necessary strength, for products with fatigue failure modes, in addition to considering necessary strength, the most important thing is to consider fatigue strength, which means that the structure must undergo fatigue analysis and be designed from a fatigue perspective. The commonly used fatigue analysis methods are as follows *S*–*N* nominal stress method based on curve and *ε*-*N* local stress–strain method based on curve: the former is suitable for high cycle fatigue; The latter is suitable for low cycle fatigue. For mechanical products, most of them belong to high cycle fatigue. The calculation process of nominal stress is introduced in detail below.

The nominal stress method was first formed based on *S*–*N* fatigue design method of curve. It is based on the *S*–*N* curve of materials or parts, comparing the nominal stress and stress concentration factor of the fatigue dangerous parts of the specimen or structure, combined with the theory of fatigue cumulative damage, to verify the fatigue strength or calculate the fatigue life. It mainly describes the relationship between constant amplitude stress range and failure cycle of standard smooth specimen. The analysis process includes the following four processes. The calculation flow of nominal stress method is shown in Fig. 5.21.

(1) **Determine the Weak Fatigue Key Parts/parts of the Product**

Fatigue mainly occurs in components subjected to alternating loads, and the location of fatigue failure usually occurs at the sudden change in the cross-section of the component. The nominal stress at the failure point is not high, lower than the tensile strength and yield point of the material.

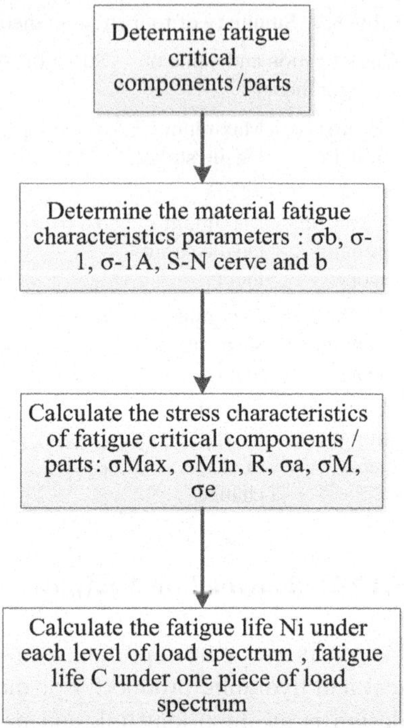

Fig. 5.21 Nominal stress calculation process

(2) **Determine the Fatigue Characteristics of Materials at Weak Parts** (*S–N Curve)*

The fatigue properties of the material, including material tensile strength σ_b, fatigue limit σ_{-1}, permissible fatigue limitσ_{-1A}, *S–N* curves, etc. can be obtained by consulting material properties manuals, material libraries that come with various software, such as ANSYS WORKBENCH, NCODEDesignLife, MSC.Fatigue, etc. If necessary, fatigue performance tests can also be performed on the material Fatigue. The *S–N* curves for the component materials are shown in Fig. 5.22.

Material *S–N* curves and fatigue limits σ_{-1} It can only represent the fatigue performance of standard smooth specimens, but the actual dimensions, shapes and surface conditions of parts are various, which are quite different from standard parts. Allowable fatigue limit σ_{-1A} After considering the factors affecting the fatigue limit, the fatigue limit of standard parts is modified by the influence coefficient. The fatigue limit reflects the actual fatigue performance of parts.

$$\sigma_{-1A} = k_a k_b k_e \sigma_{-1} \tag{5.1}$$

where:

k_a— Surface coefficient ($\leq$1);
k_b— Dimension coefficient ($\leq$1);
k_e— Reliability coefficient ($\leq$ 1).

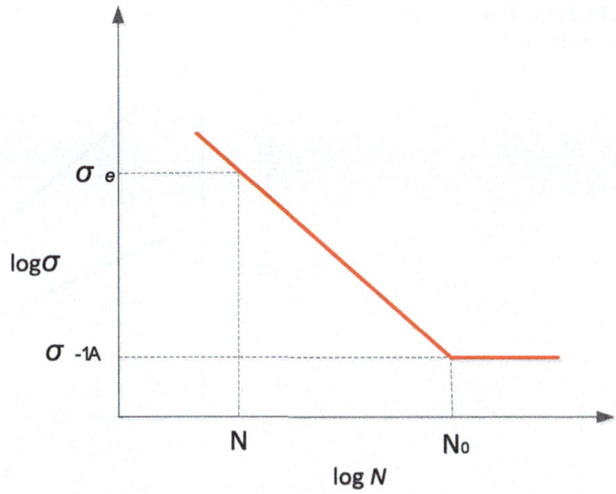

Fig. 5.22 Component material *S–N* curve

Surface coefficient and dimension coefficient can be found on pages 1157 and 1159 of *China Mechanical Design Grand Ceremony Volume 2*. For the reliability factor, see *Mechanical Engineering Design 8th Ed*, p. 288.

(3) Determine the Load Spectrum of Fatigue Analysis

According to the mission profile of the product, the stress cycle characteristics of the key components/parts of weak fatigue are obtained, including the maximum stress $\sigma_{\max}$, minimum stress σ_{Min} and calculate the corresponding stress ratio $R = \sigma_{\min}/\sigma_{\max,}$ stress amplitude $\sigma_a = (\sigma_{\max}\text{-}\sigma_{\min})/2$, average stress $\sigma_m = (\sigma_{\max} + \sigma_{\min})/2$. For uniaxial fatigue, $\sigma_{\max} = \sigma_1$, $\sigma_{\min} = \sigma_3$; For multiaxial fatigue, $\sigma_{\max} = \sigma_{\text{von mises max}}$, $\sigma_{\min} = \sigma_{\text{Von mises min}}$. Only two of the above five stress cycle parameters are independent, and the stress cycle level can be determined if only any two of them are known.

Most fatigue data are used in the laboratory under symmetrical loads ($\sigma_m = 0$), and most field service conditions contain non-zero average stress. A large number of studies have shown that under given stress amplitude, the average stress increases and the fatigue life decreases (Haigh curve is shown in Fig. 5.23). Through Haigh curve, the stress amplitude corresponding to non-zero average stress can be modified to the stress amplitude equivalent to zero average stress on the premise of keeping the life unchanged. The famous correction method is Goodman method:

$$\sigma_e = \frac{\sigma_b}{\sigma_b - \sigma_m}\sigma_a \tag{5.2}$$

(4) Calculation of Fatigue Cumulative Life

Assuming that the structure has no initial damage, once the structure has engineering detectable cracks, it is considered that the safe life is terminated. Safe life analysis

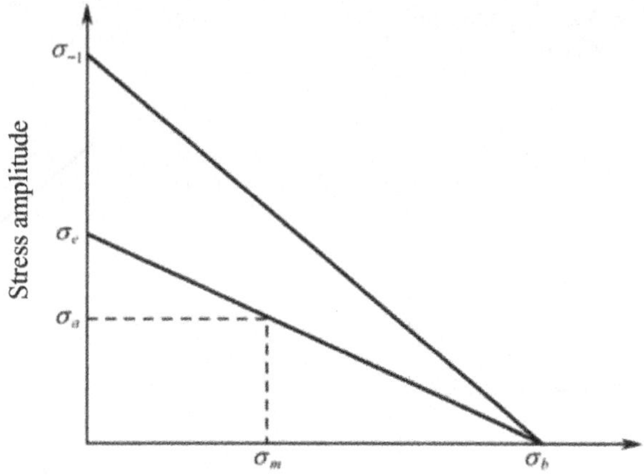

Fig. 5.23 Haigh curve (Goodman Curve)

estimates fatigue life according to the load spectrum in the life period and Miner linear cumulative damage theory. According to *S–N* Oblique line section of curve, it can be calculated that the corresponding fatigue life of equivalent stress amplitude (also called equivalent average stress) σe is:

$$N = N_0\left(\frac{\sigma_e}{\sigma_{-1A}}\right)^{\frac{1}{b}} \quad (5.3)$$

where:

N—Fatigue life under load (cycle times);

N_0—The fatigue life (cycle times) corresponding to the fatigue limit of the material is generally taken as 10^7;

b—The slope of the *S–N* curve. $b = \frac{\log\sigma - \log\sigma_{-1A}}{\log N - \log N_0}$ is the constant related to fatigue properties of materials.

In the known *S–N* Curve, the value of b can be calculated from two points on the diagonal line or obtained by consulting relevant manuals, such as page 17 of the Guide for Durability/Damage Tolerance Analysis and Design of Military Aircraft Structures. Note: In different data, The form of b may vary, and some definitions $|b|$ or $1/b$ is a material constant, where $b < 0$.

Calculate the fatigue damage caused by a load spectrum as follows:

$$\sum D_i = \sum \frac{n_i}{N_i} \quad (5.4)$$

where:

D_I—Damage under various load spectra;

N_I—Cycle times under load spectrum at all levels;

N_I—Fatigue life (number of cycles) under various load spectra.

According to Miner rule, when the damage sum is 1, the fatigue life of the product under a load spectrum C is calculated by

$$C = \frac{1}{\sum D_i} \tag{5.5}$$

According to the relative Miner rule, the critical damage sum is determined by using the damage and test values of similar parts under similar load spectrum D_f. The accuracy of life estimation can be greatly improved.

$$C = \frac{D_f}{\sum D_i} \tag{5.6}$$

If a load spectrum represents 2000Fh, the corresponding fatigue life of the product is $C \times 2000$ Fh.

The above fatigue analysis process can be implemented by commercial finite element software, such as MSC. Fatigue, ANSYS/FE-Fatigue or ANSYS nCode DesignLife.

5.4.2.8 Wear Life Analysis

Wear is one of the important failure modes that cause the failure of moving mechanism, and it belongs to wear failure. Wear mainly occurs on parts with relative motion, which is related to friction and lubrication, such as bearings, gears, hinges and guide rails, etc. Its consequences are to increase the clearance of parts, reduce the matching accuracy, increase noise, cause material consumption and damage, and finally lead to the degradation of equipment performance, even unable to complete the specified functions.

Abrasion and functional degradation of mechanical parts are usually a gradual process, except for severe abrasions that lead to sudden bite to death. Wear can be divided into three types: adhesive wear, abrasive wear and etching wear.

Wear life analysis methods usually adopt analogy analysis method, life calculation method based on wear model and empirical formula method.

1) **Similarity Analogy Analysis Method**

Use only when there is wear monitoring information of similar/similar products. The wear life of the product is determined by comparing the material, running speed, lubricating condition, surface contact stress and allowable limit wear amount of the friction pair.

2) **Life Calculation Method Based on Wear Model**

According to the wear model, the wear life of friction pair is obtained by dividing the allowable limit wear amount by the wear speed. At present, there are many

Table 5.5 Wear rate of different friction pair materials

k (10–15 m2/N)	Classification
0.0001–0.001	0
0.001–0.01	1
0.01–0.1	2
0.1–1	3
1–10	4
10–100	5
100–1000	6
1000–10000	7

known wear models, among which Archard model is the most widely used. This model indicates the relationship between wear and sliding distance, load and material properties, and is suitable for other wear types on sliding surfaces. The calculation formula is as follows:

$$V = kF_N s \tag{5.7}$$

where:

V—Wear volume after running-in period;

F_N—When the normal load can not be obtained directly, it can be calculated by Hertz contact theory;

s—Sliding distance;

k—Wear rate (m^2/N), depending on material combination, surface roughness, contact temperature, friction pair, etc.

Usually *k* Test can be used for determination. When the material's *K* Value less than $10^{-15}M^2/N$, it belongs to hard wear level. Table 5.5 shows *K* value classification reflects the different wear resistance of high/low anti-friction pair combination.

(2) **Empirical Formula Method**

This kind of method is mostly used for the calculation of standard parts, such as bearings. For life calculation of sliding bearings, plain bearings and rolling bearings, please refer to the fifth edition and second volume of Mechanical Design Manual, or the Grand Ceremony of Mechanical Design published by Jiangxi Science Press.

5.4.2.9 Aging Life Analysis

Aging is one of the important failure modes of rubber, plastic, adhesive and other polymer materials, which is characterized by the gradual deterioration of performance during storage and use, resulting in failure that cannot meet the use requirements, and belongs to wear-out failure. Similarity analogy method and empirical model method are usually used to analyze aging life.

(1) Similarity Analogy Method

It is only used when there is aging monitoring information of similar/similar products, and the aging life of products is determined by environmental stress, protective measures and materials of parts themselves.

(2) Empirical Model Method

According to the accelerated aging test data of materials, the aging curve of performance and time is established, and then the aging life of materials is predicted according to the corresponding life model. In the stage of life design and analysis, the aging problem is usually considered simply, and the aging situation is mainly detected in the later development test and appraisal test, and its durability is verified.

Rubber aging has an important relationship with storage environment and service state. The properties of rubber sealing ring such as hardness, tensile strength, elongation at break, compression set and stress relaxation gradually deteriorate. This is the aging process of rubber, and its main influencing factors are temperature, pretightening force, oil pressure impact and immersion. Among them, the compression set rate and compression stress relaxation rate have the most significant influence on the service life of rubber sealing ring.

Compression set rate y (%) is defined as follows (see GB 1683):

$$y = \frac{h_0 - h_2}{h_0 - h_1} \times 100\,\% \tag{5.8}$$

where:

h_0—Original height (mm) of sample;

h_1—Height of sample after compression (mm);

h_2—The recovery height (mm) of the sample after decompression.

Rubber aging process is a chemical reaction process. At present, empirical formulas are generally used to describe the relationship between compression set rate and aging time in engineering. This formula not only reflects the principle of reaction kinetics, but also accords with the actual situation:

$$1 - y = A_1 \mathrm{e}^{-kt^{\alpha}} \tag{5.9}$$

where:

A_1—Constant (considering $t = 0$, if the compression set is 0, then $A_1 = 1$);

k—Aging rate constant;

t—Aging time (d);

α—Aging reaction time index.

As a polymer material, the rate constant of internal chemical reaction process of rubber k And temperature T The relationship of obeys Arrhenius equation:

$$k = A_2 \mathrm{e}^{-\frac{E}{RT}} \tag{5.10}$$

where:

A_2—Frequency factor, constant;

E—Apparent activation energy (J/mol);

R—Gas constant, 8.314 J/(mol·k);

T—Aging reaction temperature (K).

The life of rubber sealing ring can be deduced from the above two types:

$$t = \left(\frac{\ln \frac{A_1}{1-y}}{A_2 e^{-\frac{E}{RT}}} \right)^{\frac{1}{\alpha}} \tag{5.11}$$

Assuming that when $y > 0.7$, the rubber sealing ring leaks, and then $y = 0.7$ is the failure threshold of rubber sealing ring. Thus, the life of rubber sealing ring can be obtained by substituting the y value and the related value. Unknown coefficients in models A_1, A_2, E And α can be calculated from aging test data.

5.4.2.10 Corrosion Life Analysis

Corrosion is a kind of important failure mode that causes the failure of metal products, which belongs to wear failure. Corrosion will lead to the decrease of structural strength and fatigue life, and shorten the service life of products. For equipment which is mainly in storage state or not used frequently, storage corrosion plays a leading role, and the corrosion life of equipment mainly depends on storage corrosion; For the equipment with high frequency of use, the environmental impact should not be ignored, and the corrosion life of the equipment should be determined by comprehensively considering the storage corrosion impact and the environmental impact. Commonly used analysis methods include similarity analogy method, accelerated test analysis method and so on.

(1) **Similarity Analogy Method**

It is only used when there is corrosion monitoring information of similar/similar products, and the corrosion life of products is determined by comparing corrosion environment, protective measures and products' own materials.

(2) **Accelerated Test Analysis Method**

Through accelerated corrosion test, the corrosion life of products is calculated by using equivalent acceleration relation. Electricity can be used for equivalent conversion Q as variables of corrosion amount, there are:

$$Q = \frac{1}{F} \int_0^t I_c \mathrm{d}\tau \tag{5.12}$$

where:

F—Faraday constant, 96514C/mol;

I_C—Current in different environments;

t—Action time.

For different corrosion environments, the corrosion current is I_c', then:

$$Q' = \frac{1}{F}\int_0^{t'} I_c' \mathrm{d}\tau \tag{5.13}$$

A large number of experimental measurement results show that, I_c And I_c' If the change in the corrosion process is small and can be regarded as constant, the laboratory and corrosion environment should be equal, and there must be:

$$I_c t = I_c' t' \tag{5.14}$$

$$t' = k_I t \tag{5.15}$$

where:

k_I—Is the conversion coefficient, $k_I = I_c / I_c'$.

Refer to Tables 5.6, 5.7 and 5.8 for the conversion coefficient between commonly used laboratory corrosion environmental parameters and standard air and water media.

Table 5.6 Conversion coefficient of humid air and standard humid air

Materials	RH%	T/°C				
		20	25	30	35	40
Aluminum alloy	70	0.16380	0.24400	0.32500	0.62526	0.92552
	80	0.16707	0.29053	0.42600	0.73177	1.03753
	90	0.11045	0.20700	0.29995	0.64997	1
Steel	70	0.09836	0.01454	0.17077	0.24143	0.55212
	80	0.08934	0.10057	0.31608	0.42364	0.73048
	90	0.05837	0.22919	0.40647	0.70959	1

Table 5.7 Conversion relationship between NaCl solution with different concentrations and water medium

NaCl solubility (%)	Aluminum alloy	Steel
0.35	0.643	0.558
0.5	0.612	0.485
1.72	0.335	0.417
3.5	0.121	0.320
7	0.0969	0.310

Table 5.8 Conversion coefficients of different acid concentrations with water medium

Materials	Acid concentration	HNO3	HCl	H2SO4
Aluminum alloy	0.1	0.267	0.454	0.635
	1	0.318	0.235	0.348
	2	0.353	0.110	0.302
Steel	0.1	0.571		
	1	0.467	0.368	0.467
	2	0.233	0.292	

Fig. 5.24 Simplified schematic diagram of corrosion pit

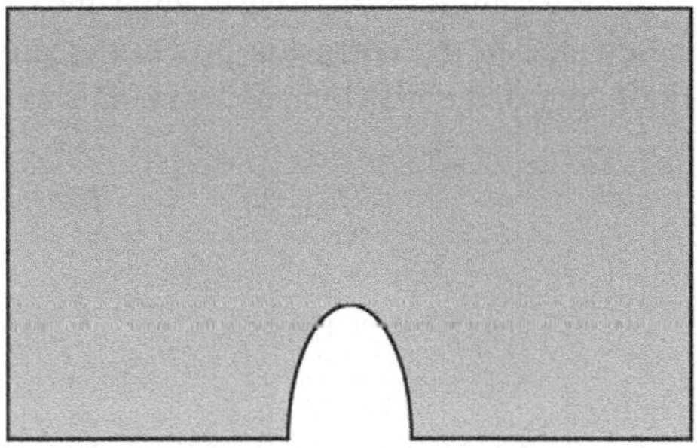

The simplified diagram of corrosion pits is shown in Fig. 5.24, and the expression of corrosion pits rate is:

$$dV/dt = MI_p/nF\rho \tag{5.16}$$

where:
V—Corrosion pore volume;
M—Atomic weight of material;
n—Valence of materials;
ρ—Density of material.

5.4.3 *Examples*

The endurance life simulation calculation and analysis of a certain type of transmission shaft are carried out.

The finite element model and grid section of the transmission shaft are shown in Figs. 5.25 and 5.26 respectively.

The transmission shaft is simulated and analyzed, and the strain nephogram and stress nephogram are shown in Figs. 5.27 and 5.28 respectively.

The fatigue life nephogram of transmission shaft is shown in Fig. 5.29.

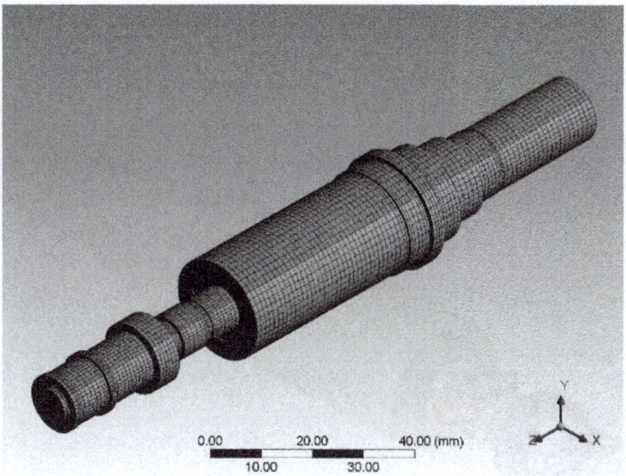

Fig. 5.25 Finite element model of transmission shaft

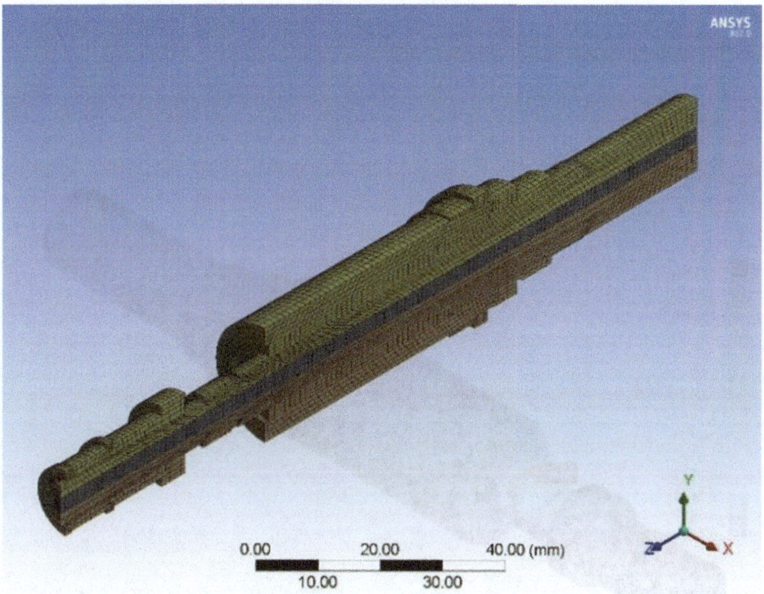

Fig. 5.26 Grid section of transmission shaft

According to the calculation and analysis results of the durability life of the transmission shaft, it can be concluded that, the lowest life of the transmission shaft also occurs at the supporting position of the inner bearing, and the life is 2.7×10^{10} turn. Because the speed value corresponding to the minimum life of the transmission shaft is 9×10^9 Therefore, the fatigue life of the transmission shaft meets the requirements.

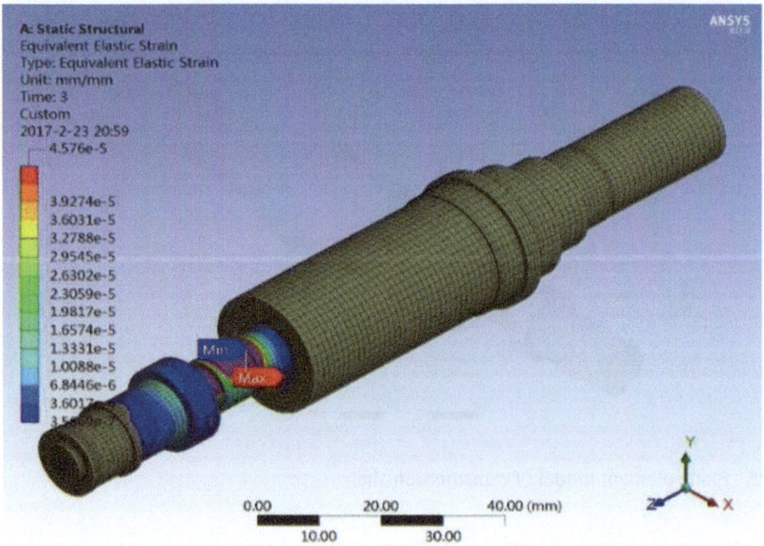

Fig. 5.27 Strain nephogram of transmission shaft

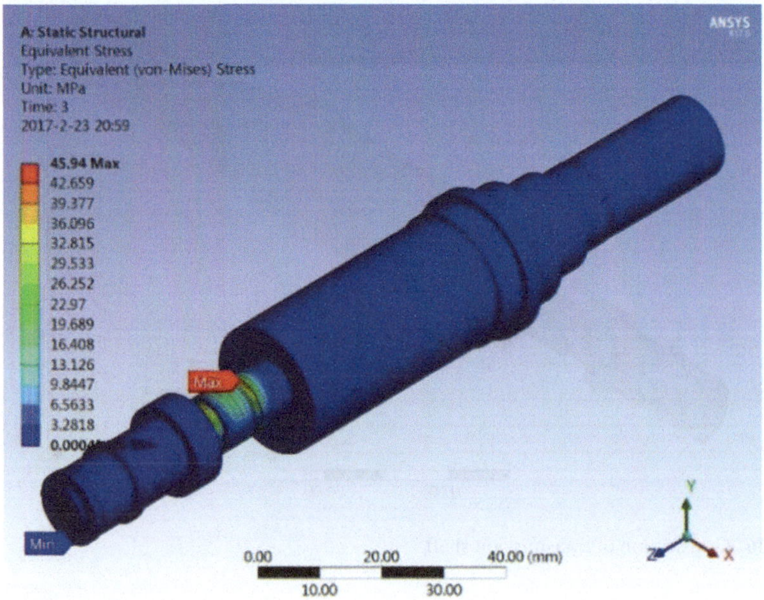

Fig. 5.28 Stress nephogram of transmission shaft

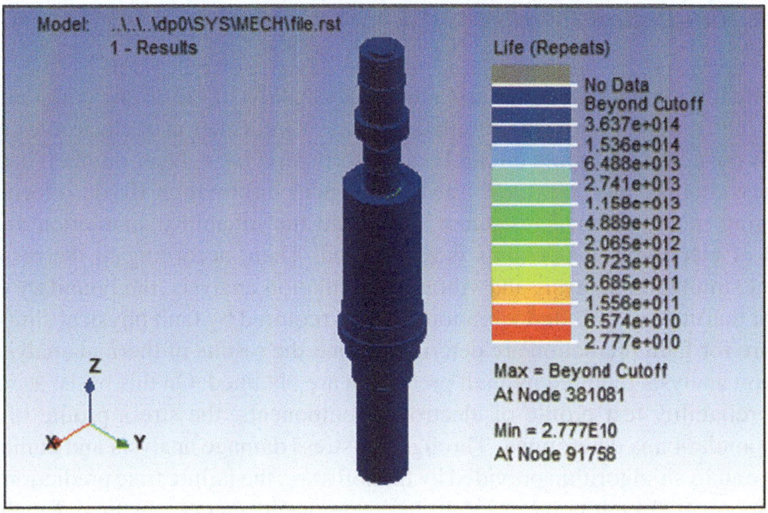

Fig. 5.29 Nephogram of fatigue life of transmission shaft

5.5 Simulation Calculation and Analysis of Reliability of Electronic Components

5.5.1 Purpose

By establishing the simulation model of electronic components on the fault physical simulation software, applying the load history (including temperature and vibration) of electronic components, and carrying out stress analysis and stress damage analysis, the life distribution of electronic components is obtained.

5.5.2 Introduction of Fault Physical Simulation Software

The commonly used fault physical simulation software is calcePWA software. CalcePWA is a reliability simulation software developed jointly by Calce (Computer Aided Life Cycle Engineering) Electronic Products and Systems Center and University of Maryland, which is used to carry out reliability simulation evaluation and fault prediction for printed assembly circuit boards. CalcePWA software includes three main modules: thermal analysis, vibration analysis and fault prediction. The algorithms come from classical reliability physics and published research papers on fault physics or related research projects within Calce Association.

5.5.3 *Simulation Process*

The reliability simulation calculation and analysis flow of electronic components is shown in Fig. 5.30. Firstly, the simulation analysis information of electronic components is collected, including circuit board information (size, layer number, material, thickness, copper clad ratio, etc.) and component information (basic information, packaging mode, thermal resistance, etc.), and the reliability simulation analysis model of electronic components is established. Then, according to the results of thermal simulation analysis and vibration simulation analysis, the boundary conditions of thermal analysis and vibration analysis required by fault physical simulation software for fault prediction are determined, and the results of thermal analysis and vibration analysis required by fault prediction are obtained. On this basis, according to the reliability test profile of electronic components, the stress profile of reliability simulation is determined. Through the stress damage analysis and cumulative damage analysis algorithm provided by the software, the failure time prediction value of each potential fault point in electronic components can be obtained. Finally, the failure time is fitted and analyzed, and the life distribution of electronic components is obtained.

5.5.4 *Monte Carlo Method*

5.5.4.1 Introduction to Monte Carlo

Monte Carlo Method is a method that sets stochastic process by computer, generates time series for target parameterism, determines target parameters by the length of time series, and then studies the distribution characteristics of things according to the parameters. Its basic idea is to first establish a probability model or stochastic process, and make its parameters be the required solution of the problem, and then calculate the statistical characteristics of the parameters by sampling experiments on the model, and solve the results.

5.5.4.2 Monte Carlo Thought

The basic idea of Monte Carlo method is to obtain a certain capacity of sample data for random variables of a known probability distribution (probability density function or probability distribution function), so that it has all the same statistical characteristics as the population of the distribution. The basic principle of this method is based on Bernoulli's law of large numbers in statistics. If random events x_i The probability of occurrence is $P\{x_i\}$, in progress N In the sub-independent sampling experiment, the frequency of events is $m/N(m$ For events x_i In N The number of times in the test), then for any given tiny positive number $\varepsilon > 0$, there are

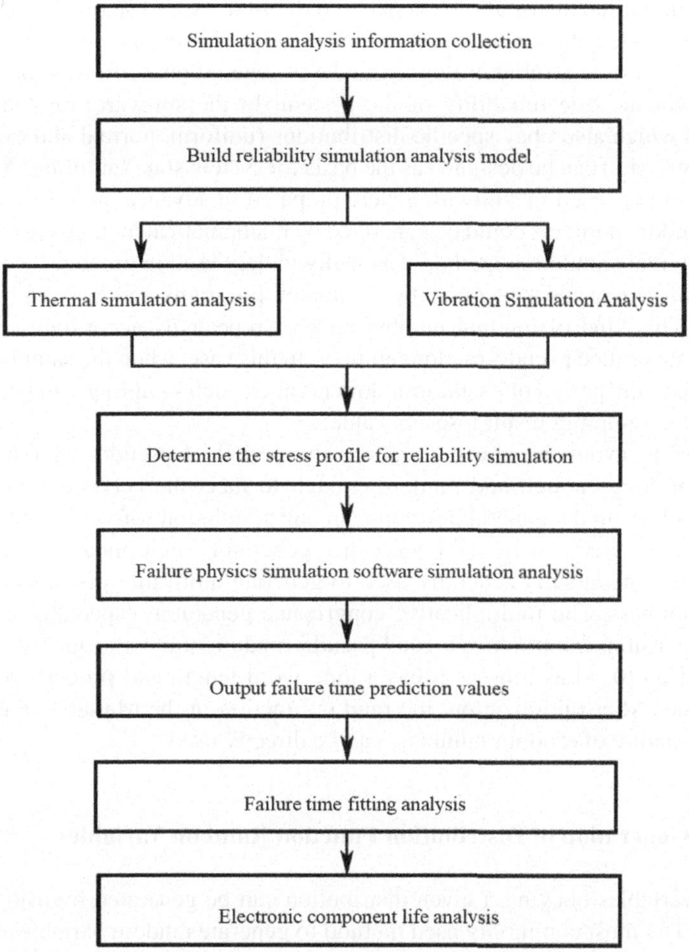

Fig. 5.30 Reliability simulation calculation and analysis process of electronic components

$$\lim_{N\to\infty} P\left\{\left|\frac{m}{N} - P\{x_i\}\right| < \varepsilon\right\} = 1 \tag{5.17}$$

That is to say, when the number of independent trials N is large enough, its frequency m / N will converge to its probability P{xi} with probability 1. Therefore, the probabilistic convergence of the simulation method is guaranteed.

5.5.4.3 Monte Carlo Principle for Generating Random Numbers

System failures are random and have great dispersion, but fundamentally speaking, they obey a certain probability distribution. Common distribution types are uniform distribution, normal distribution, exponential distribution and so on. A single failure state can not reflect the true reliability of the system. The mean value and probability distribution of system reliability index under a large number of different states can better reflect the true reliability of the system. In the software, random number sequences which also obey specific distributions (uniform, normal and exponential distributions, etc.) can be designed as the basis for system state sampling. At first, the random numbers used in simulation were prepared in advance, and it was not until pseudo-random numbers could be generated by mathematical methods in calculation technology that simulation method was really widely used in practice.

Random sequences generated by computer programs are not really random numbers. This kind of random number appears repeatedly according to a certain period, so it is called pseudo-random number. In this case, when the sampling period is the same as the period of pseudo-random number, each sampling will get the same result, so the sampling result loses its value.

In order to avoid the above situation, the period of pseudo-random numbers needs to be long enough and random enough to meet the needs of state simulation. Nowadays, in the general development and simulation software, multiplicative congruence generator or mixed congruence generator (multiplicative and additive congruence generator) is generally used to generate uniformly distributed pseudo-random numbers. The multiplicative congruence generator, especially in the case of one dimension, can produce a good pseudo-random number sequence uniformly distributed on [0, 1] as long as it has a long word length and properly selects the initial value. After optimization, the rand () function in the Matlab can produce a very good nature of random numbers, can be directly used.

5.5.4.4 Generation of Distribution Function Random Variables

Random variables obeying a given distribution can be generated by using random numbers. The most commonly used method to generate random variables is inverse function transformation.

If random variables U obeys the uniform distribution on [0,1], then the random variable $X = F^{-1}(U)$ is a continuous cumulative probability distribution function $F(X)$.

This proposition also applies to the case of discrete distribution, where the inverse function $F(X)$ can be defined as:

$$X = F^{-1}(U) = \min\{x : F(x) \geq U\}, (0 \leq U \leq 1) \tag{5.18}$$

The steps of generating random variables by inverse function method are as follows:

The first step is to generate a uniformly distributed random number sequence on [0, 1];

Step 2: Calculate the random variables of $F(X)$ that meet the requirement of cumulative probability distribution function according to $X = F^{-1}(U)$.

Taking exponential distribution as an example, random variables obeying exponential distribution are generated by inverse function transformation method, and the random variables satisfying exponential distribution include probability density function:

$$f(x) = \lambda e^{-\lambda x} \tag{5.19}$$

Its cumulative probability distribution function is:

$$F(x) = 1 - e^{-\lambda x} \tag{5.20}$$

According to the inverse transformation method:

$$U = F(x) = 1 - e^{-\lambda x} \tag{5.21}$$

Therefore:

$$X = F^{-1}(U) = -\frac{1}{\lambda}\ln(1 - U) \tag{5.22}$$

Among them, U is a random number sequence with uniform distribution; X is a random variable that obeys exponential distribution.

5.5.5 *Failure Time Fitting Analysis*

According to the analysis results of fault physical simulation software, the failure time data of each potential failure point of electronic components under a certain failure mechanism can be obtained. These failure data are fitted by statistical mathematics method to obtain the life distribution.

5.5.5.1 Single Point Life Distribution Fitting

The output results of the fault physical simulation software show that the failure of the device is caused by two fault mechanisms: vibration fatigue and thermal fatigue. For each fault mechanism, the life distribution function of the fault mechanism should be fitted first.

Fit the distribution of 1000 possible thermal fatigue failure times s… and 1000 possible vibration fatigue failure times t… for the i-th device separately.

5.5.5.2 Single Point of Failure Fusion

Distribution function of the device solder joint is obtained according to the life distribution function of the two failure mechanisms of the device solder joint. Its algorithm is as follows:

(1) For i the life distribution function of the device $F_i(x)$ and $G_i(x)$, use the Monte Carlo method to perform a sampling to obtain 2 random numbers $(t_{i1}, \ldots t_{i2})$;
(2) Arrange the two drawn random numbers $(t_{11}, \ldots t_{12})$ in ascending order, and take the smallest value among them as $t_{1\,\min}$;
(3) Take 2 more random numbers $(t_{21}, \ldots t_{22})$, and take the smallest one as $t_{2\,\min}$;
(4) Repeat the sampling 1000 times to obtain a set of sampling data $(t_{1\,\min}, t_{2\,\min}, \ldots, t_{1000\,\min})$, and use this set of sampling data to perform distribution fitting goodness test to obtain the life distribution function of the device.

Repeat (1)–(4) to get the lifetime distribution functions of all devices $H_i(t)$.

5.5.5.3 Life Distribution Fitting of Electronic Components

According to the life distribution function of the device, the life distribution function of the electronic component can be obtained. Its algorithm is as follows:

(1) Assuming there are K a total of devices, the life distribution functions corresponding to each device are respectively. $H_i(t)$, using the Monte Carlo method to perform K sub-sampling to obtain K a random number $(t_{11}, t_{12}, \ldots, t_{1K})$;
(2) Arrange the drawn K random numbers $(t_{11}, t_{12}, \ldots, t_{1K})$ in ascending order, and take the smallest value as $t_{1\,\min}$;
(3) Take K another random number $(t_{21}, t_{22}, \ldots, t_{2K})$, and take the smallest one as $t_{2\,\min}$;
(4) Repeat the sampling for 1000 times to obtain a set of sampling data $(t_{1\,\min}, t_{2\,\min}, \ldots, t_{1000\,\min})$, use this set of sampling data to test the distribution fit, and obtain the life distribution function of the electronic component $F(t)$.

Calculate the mean time between failures of electronic components according to the life distribution function of electronic components: $F(t)$

$$T = \int_0^{\infty} t f(t)\mathrm{d}t \tag{5.23}$$

5.5.6 Examples

The reliability simulation calculation and analysis of a certain electronic component are carried out. Using calcePWA software to carry out physical simulation analysis of faults, 1000 possible thermal fatigue failure times and vibration fatigue failure times of all components are obtained, as shown in Table 5.9.

The thermal fatigue failure time and vibration fatigue failure time were fitted for life distribution respectively, and the fitting results as shown in Table 5.10 were obtained.

Sampling, comparative analysis and fitting are carried out on the life distribution functions of thermal fatigue failure and vibration fatigue failure of each device, and the life distribution functions of each device are obtained in Table 5.11.

The life distribution function of each device is sampled, compared and fitted, and finally the life distribution function of electronic components is as follows:

$$F(t) = 1 - \exp\left(-\left(\frac{t}{109387.2}\right)^{5.46}\right) \tag{5.24}$$

The mean time between failure of this type of electronic components is:

Table 5.9 Thermal fatigue failure time and vibration fatigue failure time of devices

Serial number	Device 1		Device 2		–	Device *n*	
	Thermal fatigue failure time/h	Vibration fatigue failure time/h	Thermal fatigue failure time/h	Vibration fatigue failure time/h	–	Thermal fatigue failure time/h	Vibration fatigue failure time/h
1	86,078.9	83,509.0	71,608.4	145,762.6	...	83,367.7	59,015.7
2	113,795.9	124,365.9	128,127.9	167,207.7	...	100,592.4	114,009.3
3	107,040.1	106,727.2	85,054.2	155,659.7	...	99,358.9	107,319.1
4	66,950.8	116,319.3	107,450.4	162,312.6	...	79,134.6	73,907.9
5	143,964.8	135,180.6	127,511.7	152,757.3	...	129,060.8	126,718.5
6	61,333.4	107,604.2	116,571.3	131,326.1	...	68,434.0	60,974.8
7	125,528.2	122,714.6	109,215.8	157,432.9	...	88,639.4	110,510.5
8	69,172.3	102,856.8	86,125.6	133,401.9	...	83,252.2	80,698.9
9	119,405.5	120,431.4	81,170.5	145,058.2	...	103,852.6	103,368.9
10	100,746.5	138,517.8	91,998.3	90,450.8	...	81,960.7	75,562.3
11	124,222.5	127,747.5	93,967.3	126,049.3	...	90,868.7	88,105.9
12	119,689.2	111,646.9	103,797.6	150,654.9	...	107,815.9	109,059.6
–	–	–	–	–	–	–	–
999	97,478.3	119,212.7	136,793.9	109,926.0	...	85,419.9	98,473.6
1000	130,081.5	118,825.5	110,870.0	93,047.2	...	85,926.3	96,244.0

Table 5.10 Life distribution function of thermal fatigue failure time and vibration fatigue failure time of devices

Serial number	Device	Fault type	Life distribution function
1	Device 1	Thermal fatigue	$F_1(t) = 1 - \exp\left(-\left(\frac{t}{125683.5}\right)^{7.32}\right)$
		Vibration fatigue	$G_1(t) = \Phi\left(\frac{\ln t - 12.11}{0.168}\right)$
2	Device 2	Thermal fatigue	$F_2(t) = 1 - \exp\left(-\left(\frac{t}{124832.1}\right)^{5.39}\right)$
		Vibration fatigue	$G_2(t) = \Phi\left(\frac{\ln t - 12.32}{0.347}\right)$
–	–	–	–
N	Device n	Thermal fatigue	$F_n(t) = 1 - \exp\left(-\left(\frac{t}{132123.5}\right)^{4.83}\right)$
		Vibration fatigue	$G_n(t) = \Phi\left(\frac{\ln t - 11.94}{0.231}\right)$

Table 5.11 Lifetime distribution function of devices

Serial number	Device	Life distribution
1	Device 1	$H_1(t) = 1 - \exp\left(-\left(\frac{t}{113560.2}\right)^{6.28}\right)$
2	Device 2	$H_2(t) = 1 - \exp\left(-\left(\frac{t}{117345.2}\right)^{4.92}\right)$
–	–	–
N	Device n	$H_n(t) = \Phi\left(\frac{\ln t - 11.63}{0.451}\right)$

$$\text{MTBF} = 100944\text{h} \tag{5.25}$$

5.6 Simulation Calculation and Analysis of System Reliability

5.6.1 Purpose

Combined with the life distribution of each component of the system, Monte Carlo simulation calculation and analysis of the system are carried out to comprehensively evaluate the reliability index of the system.

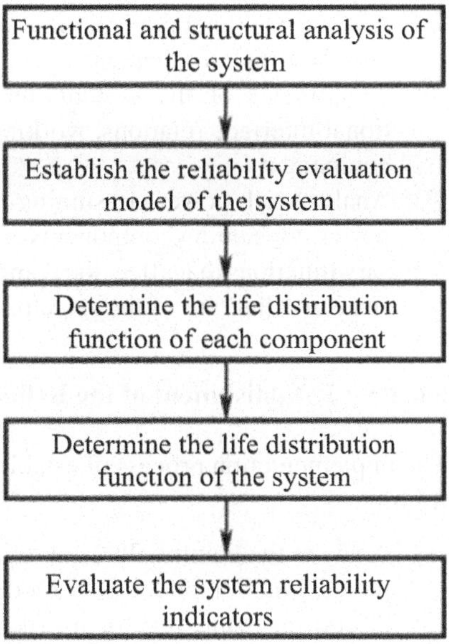

Fig. 5.31 Implementation flow of system reliability simulation calculation analysis

5.6.2 *Simulation Calculation Method*

5.6.2.1 Implementation Process

The implementation flow of system reliability simulation calculation and analysis is shown in Fig. 5.31. Firstly, the reliability evaluation model of the system is established by analyzing the function and structure of the system. Secondly, the reliability simulation results of power-consuming components, vibration-bearing components, power-consuming components and electronic components are collected, and the life distribution functions of all components of the system are obtained; Then, according to the life distribution function of components, Monte Carlo sampling simulation calculation and analysis are carried out to determine the failure time of the system, and the life distribution fitting is carried out to determine the life distribution function of the system; Finally, according to the life distribution function of the system, the reliability index of the system is evaluated.

5.6.2.2 Functional and Structural Analysis of the System

The implementation process of the system function and structure analysis method is as follows:

(1) Analyze the task process of the system, determine the system functions involved in the system task process, and clarify the necessary and unnecessary functions of the system;

(2) Analyze the functional relations among power consumption components, vibration bearing components, power consumption components and electronic components of the system, including functional hierarchy relations, functional interface relations, working modes and working time sequences of each component;
(3) Analyze all power-consuming components, vibration-bearing components, power-consuming components and electronic components involved in all necessary functions that affect the completion of system tasks, and form the functional structure diagram of the system.

5.6.2.3 Establishment of the Reliability Evaluation Model of the System

The implementation process of establishing system reliability evaluation model is as follows:

(1) Analyze the commonly used reliability models of the system, including series model, parallel model, K/N model, hybrid model and so on;
(2) According to the functional structure diagram of the system, the reliability block diagram or fault tree of the system is established;
(3) According to the reliability block diagram or fault tree of the system, the reliability evaluation model of the system is established.

5.6.2.4 Determining the Life Distribution Function of the Component

The implementation process of determining the component life distribution function is as follows:

(1) Collect the reliability simulation calculation and analysis results of power consumption components, vibration bearing components, power consumption components and electronic components, and obtain the failure time data of all components of the system by combining the development process data, reliability test data and actual use data of the system;
(2) Fitting the fault time data of a certain component;
(3) Through goodness-of-fit test and optimization, the optimal failure time distribution is obtained as the life distribution function of the component;
(4) Repeat steps (2) to (3) to obtain the life distribution function of all components of the system.

5.6.2.5 Determine the Life Distribution Function of the System

The implementation process for determining the system life distribution function is as follows:

(1) Assuming that the system is composed of n components, the life distribution function of each component is recorded as $F_i(t)$, in which i is taken from 1 to

n, and the Monte Carlo method can be used to perform a sampling to obtain n random number $t_{11}, t_{12}, \ldots, t_{1n}$;

(2) Referring to the reliability evaluation model of the system to analyze the extracted n random numbers to determine the failure time of the system t_1;

(3) After N times of sub-sampling, the failure time of a group of systems is obtained $t_1, t_2 \ldots, t_N$, and this group of sampling data is used for distribution fitting, goodness of fit inspection and optimization to obtain the life distribution function of the system.

5.6.2.6 System Reliability Evaluation

According to the life distribution function of the system, the reliability of the system is evaluated.

The calculation formula of system failure density function $f(t)$ is as follows:

$$f(t) = \frac{\mathrm{d}F(t)}{\mathrm{d}t} \tag{5.26}$$

The calculation formula of the system failure rate $\lambda(t)$ is as follows:

$$\lambda(t) = \frac{f(t)}{1 - F(t)} \tag{5.27}$$

The calculation formula of the system reliability $R(t)$ is as follows:

$$R(t) = \exp\,(-\int_0^t \lambda(t)\mathrm{d}t) \tag{5.28}$$

Mean time between failure of system MTBF The calculation formula of is as follows:

$$\mathrm{MTBF} = \int_0^\infty tf(t)\mathrm{d}t \tag{5.29}$$

5.6.3 *Failure Time Distribution Fitting*

5.6.3.1 Exponential Distribution Fitting

The probability density function and cumulative failure probability function of exponential distribution are as follows:

$$f(t) = \lambda \exp(-\lambda t), t > 0 \tag{5.30}$$

$$F(t) = 1 - e^{-\lambda t} \tag{5.31}$$

Among them, λ is the failure rate.

The least square method is used to estimate the unknown parameters of exponential distribution.

Make:

$$y = \ln \frac{1}{1 - F(t)} \tag{5.32}$$

$$x = t \tag{5.33}$$

The cumulative failure probability function is $F(t) = 1 - e^{-\lambda t}$ Transform to:

$$y = \lambda x \tag{5.34}$$

There are:

$$\hat{\lambda} = \frac{l_{xy}}{l_{xx}} \tag{5.35}$$

Among them:

$$l_{xx} = \sum_{i=1}^{n} (x_i - \overline{x})^2 = \sum_{i=1}^{n} x_i^2 - n\overline{x}^2 \tag{5.36}$$

$$l_{xy} = \sum_{i=1}^{n} (x_i - \overline{x})(y_i - \overline{y}) = \sum_{i=1}^{n} x_i y_i - n\overline{x}\overline{y} \tag{5.37}$$

5.6.3.2 Weibull Distribution Fitting Method

The probability density function and cumulative failure probability function of Weibull distribution are as follows:

$$f(t) = \begin{cases} \frac{\beta}{\alpha}\left(\frac{t}{\alpha}\right)^{\beta-1} \exp\left[-\left(\frac{t}{\alpha}\right)^{\beta}\right], & t \geq 0 \\ 0, & t < 0 \end{cases} \tag{5.38}$$

$$F(t) = 1 - \exp\left[-\left(\frac{t}{\alpha}\right)^{\beta}\right] \tag{5.39}$$

where:

α—Scale parameter;

β—Shape parameters.

The unknown parameters of Weibull distribution are estimated by least square method.

Make transformation of cumulative failure probability function $F(t) = 1 - \exp\left[-\left(\frac{t}{\alpha}\right)^{\beta}\right]$ to get:

$$\ln\ln\frac{1}{1-F(t)} = -\beta\ln a + \beta\ln t \tag{5.40}$$

If make:

$$y = \ln\ln\frac{1}{1-F(t)} \tag{5.41}$$

$$x = \ln t \tag{5.42}$$

$$A = -\beta\ln\alpha \tag{5.43}$$

$$B = \beta \tag{5.44}$$

There are:

$$\hat{B} = \frac{l_{xy}}{l_{xx}} \tag{5.45}$$

$$\hat{A} = \overline{y} - \hat{B}\overline{x} \tag{5.46}$$

Eventually:

$$\hat{\alpha} = \exp(-\hat{A}/\hat{B}) \tag{5.47}$$

$$\hat{\beta} = \hat{B} \tag{5.48}$$

5.6.3.3 Lognormal Distribution Fitting Method

The probability density function and cumulative failure probability function of lognormal distribution are as follows:

$$f(t) = \frac{1}{\sigma t\sqrt{2\pi}} \exp\left[-\frac{1}{2}\left(\frac{\ln(t) - \mu}{\sigma}\right)^2\right], t \geq 0 \tag{5.49}$$

$$F(t) = \int_0^t \frac{1}{\sigma t\sqrt{2\pi}} \exp\left[-\frac{1}{2}\left(\frac{\ln(t) - \mu}{\sigma}\right)^2\right] dt \tag{5.50}$$

where:

μ—Logarithmic mean;

σ—Logarithmic standard deviation.

Similarly, the least square method is used to estimate the unknown parameters of lognormal distribution.

The cumulative failure probability function is transformed to obtain:

$$F(t) = \int_{-\infty}^{\frac{\ln t - \mu}{\sigma}} \frac{1}{\sqrt{2\pi}} e^{-\frac{x^2}{2}} dx = \Phi\left(\frac{\ln t - \mu}{\sigma}\right) \tag{5.51}$$

Because of the standard normal distribution function $\Phi(x)$ is strictly monotonous rise, so there is an inverse function, and the inverse function is:

$$\Phi^{-1}[F(t)] = \frac{\ln t - \mu}{\sigma} \tag{5.52}$$

If make:

$$\Phi^{-1}[F(t)] = Y, X = \ln t \tag{5.53}$$

There are:

$$Y = \frac{1}{\sigma} X - \frac{\mu}{\sigma} \tag{5.54}$$

Eventually:

$$\hat{\sigma} = \frac{l_{xx}}{l_{xy}} \tag{5.55}$$

$$\hat{\mu} = \overline{x} - \hat{\sigma}\overline{y} \tag{5.56}$$

5.6.4 Test Method for Goodness of Fit of Failure Time Distribution

Kolmogorov–Smirnov test is used to test the goodness of fit of the system life distribution function. The test formula is:

$$D_n = \sup_{0 \le t < +\infty} |F_n(t) - F_0(t)| = \max\{d_i\} \le D_{n,\alpha} \tag{5.57}$$

where:

$F_n(t)$—Cumulative failure rate obtained by estimation method;
$F_0(t)$—Fitting the selected distribution model;
$D_{n,\alpha}$—Critical value;
α—Significant level;
n—Number of failures.

5.6.5 Optimization Method of Failure Time Distribution

The minimum distance sum method is used to optimize the life distribution function of the system. The optimal formula is:

$$d = \sum_{i=1}^{n} |F_n(t_i) - F_0(t_i)| \tag{5.58}$$

The sum of the absolute value of the difference between the distribution function of the statistical system and the distribution function selected for fitting, the smaller the statistical value obtained, the better the fitting result of the model.

5.6.6 Examples

A certain type of system is composed of power consumption components, vibration bearing components, power consumption components and electronic components. Through reliability simulation calculation and analysis of each component, the life distribution function is obtained as shown in Table 5.12.

Monte Carlo sampling is carried out by computer programming (in which, the sample size is 100,000), and the failure time of each component of the system is obtained, and the failure time of the system is analyzed, as shown in Table 5.13.

By fitting and optimizing the life distribution function of the system failure time, the optimal life distribution function of the system is obtained:

Table 5.12 Life distribution function of system components

Serial number	Sample name	Life distribution function
1	Power consumption component	$F = \Phi\left(\frac{\ln t - 12.03}{0.231}\right)$
2	Vibration bearing component	$F = \Phi\left(\frac{\ln t - 11.598}{0.081}\right)$
3	Wear-out parts	$F = 1 - \exp\left(-\left(\frac{t}{111975}\right)^{9.46}\right)$
4	Electronic components	$F = 1 - \exp\left(-\left(\frac{t}{139791.3}\right)^{5.61}\right)$

Table 5.13 Sampling of life distribution function of system components

Serial number	Failure of power consumption components Time/h	Failure time of vibration bearing components/h	Failure time of worn parts/h	Failure of electronic components Time/h	Failure life of system/h
1	76,365.2	97,345.3	74,270.3	147,758.8	74,270.3
2	112,739.2	112,883.9	123,686.3	162,703.3	112,739.2
3	103,345.0	118,440.2	97,274.5	160,071.3	97,274.5
4	83,065.9	118,627.1	107,792.2	157,720.5	83,065.9
5	132,351.2	126,098.7	124,566.6	156,315.7	124,566.6
6	67,832.3	125,882.3	116,248.8	134,317.9	67,832.3
7	108,595.0	110,391.5	105,078.6	150,049.6	105,078.6
8	87,625.4	110,551.3	75,173.2	132,075.6	75,173.2
9	123,674.4	117,268.2	92,830.2	141,909.0	92,830.2
10	112,890.0	120,273.7	90,990.0	102,483.4	90,990.0
11	119,179.1	116,950.3	97,910.1	133,591.4	97,910.1
12	112,974.0	114,100.2	104,069.9	144,448.4	104,069.9
–	–	–	–	–	–
99999	97,010.6	130,727.1	130,904.3	113,017.5	97,010.6
100000	118,757.1	124,850.0	113,117.8	89,733.1	89,733.1

$$F = 1 - \exp\left(-\left(\frac{t}{101246.7}\right)^{5.53}\right) \tag{5.59}$$

The mean time between failure of the system is:

$$\text{MTBF} = 93500\text{h} \tag{5.60}$$

5.7 Summary

This chapter focuses on reliability simulation analysis, and elaborates five kinds of simulation analysis methods in turn, such as thermal simulation of power consumption components, vibration simulation of vibration bearing components, durability life simulation of power consumption components, reliability simulation of electronic components and reliability simulation of whole machine system, which can be applied to objects with different characteristics at all levels of digital diagnosis and treatment equipment. Reliability simulation can use digital prototype to realize design improvement, the improvement opportunity is greatly advanced, the improvement does not need physical prototype reengineering, and the improvement difficulty and cost are greatly reduced. It is a very meaningful reliability design analysis method. However, readers may often be skeptical about the simulation results, and actually want the simulation results to be accurate: on the one hand, the modeling should be as reasonable as possible and the model simplification should be appropriate; On the other hand, simulation needs a lot of basic data support. In addition to data collection, each user needs to combine his own products for actual measurement, collect data suitable for himself, constantly adjust and optimize the data used in his own products, and achieve iterative improvement from simulation to test, so as to make the simulation results more accurate.

Chapter 6
Reliability Testing Technology of Digital Diagnosis and Treatment Equipment

6.1 Reliability Tests

6.1.1 Classification of Reliability Tests

At present, there is a lack of a set of systematic specifications and requirements in the field of reliability testing technology for digital diagnosis and treatment equipment, regardless of the whole machine or components. This chapter aims to study the reliability testing technology of digital diagnosis and treatment equipment.

According to the purpose and nature of the test, reliability test can be divided into engineering test and statistical test.

Reliability test that does not aim at quantitative evaluation of reliability indexes can be called reliability engineering test. Reliability engineering test includes reliability development test, environmental stress screening and reliability growth test. It should be noted that environmental stress screening does not belong to the category of environmental test, but belongs to the category of reliability test, and all kinds of engineering tests (including reliability enhancement test, reliability mapping test, etc.) can be included in the category of reliability development test.

Reliability tests that quantitatively evaluate reliability indexes or quantitatively determine reliability levels can be called reliability statistical tests. Reliability statistical test includes reliability appraisal test and reliability acceptance test in military field (appraisal and acceptance are important links in military product finalization), which must be carried out under controllable laboratory environment. In the field of civilian population, it is usually called reliability index verification. In order to reduce the cost of verification and take into account the relatively loose environmental conditions of civilian products, most industry standards tend to adopt on-site operation statistics for verification and evaluation, while a few industry standards include reliability tests conducted in laboratory controllable environment. In fact, laboratory verification and evaluation are often more rigorous, standardized and controllable,

X. Li et al., *Reliability Engineering Technology of Digital Diagnosis and Treatment Equipment*, https://doi.org/10.1007/978-981-99-5522-0_6

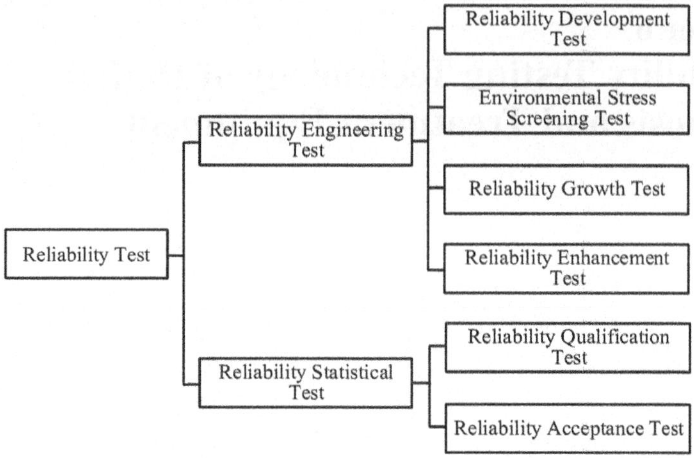

Fig. 6.1 Classification of reliability tests

so it is recommended to adopt laboratory reliability test with controllable environmental conditions when it is economically acceptable. Typical reliability indexes include Mean Time Between Failure (MTBF), reliability, success rate and so on. These indicators are usually agreed in advance and explicitly required. In addition, the reliability test for determining the reliability level of products, and the life test for testing or evaluating the service life are also statistical tests. The classification of reliability tests is shown in Fig. 6.1.

According to the stages of product life cycle, reliability test can be divided into reliability development test, finalized reliability verification test (such as military reliability appraisal test and civilian reliability index verification test), batch production reliability routine test (such as aging test and environmental stress screening), and statistical evaluation of service reliability. Major equipment will also involve life fixing and life extension verification.

6.1.2 Reliability Development Test

Reliability development test is a process of test-analysis-improvement. By applying proper environmental stress and working load to products, exposing product design defects and taking improvement measures, the inherent reliability level of products can be improved. Reliability development test is carried out in the development stage, covering a wide range, such as reliability mapping test for finding out the reliability of new products, reliability growth test for realizing reliability growth, reliability enhancement test for fully and quickly exposing defects, and reliability mapping growth test, etc.

In the past, the reliability development test was mainly to find out or control the newly developed prototype to reach a certain reliability level, which supported the newly developed prototype to pass the specified reliability index assessment. In recent years, the reliability development test is gradually developing towards fully and quickly exposing the defects of the newly developed prototype, mainly providing input for improvement, and rapidly improving the reliability of the newly developed prototype in a short time through improvement. With the deepening of understanding, reliability development test has been paid more and more attention, and the time of test development has moved forward more and more.

This chapter focuses on the reliability enhancement test of electronic control system of digital diagnosis and treatment equipment and the durability evaluation test of structural parts, which are the most general, efficient and effective reliability test means at present.

6.1.3 Reliability Verification Test

6.1.3.1 Purpose of Reliability Index Verification

The purpose of reliability index verification test is to check the reliability level of products under typical working environment conditions, verify whether products can meet the specified reliability index requirements, and use Failure Reporting, Analysis, and Corrective Action System (FRACAS) to return to zero management for failures, and provide reliability index qualification certificates.

6.1.3.2 Applicable Objects

Products with reliability index requirements (including complete equipment and core components) shall carry out reliability index verification test.

6.1.3.3 Time to Carry Out

According to the reliability index verification object, all planned tests and engineering tests (including environmental stress screening and reliability enhancement tests) should be completed in the test verification stage, and the responsible failures exposed in the test process should be returned to zero. After the technical state of the prototype is basically solidified and the environmental adaptability verification is completed, the reliability index verification can be carried out.

6.1.3.4 Statistical Test Scheme

According to the specific characteristics of the tested products, the statistical scheme of reliability verification test is selected, and the timed censoring statistical scheme is recommended. For newly developed products, it is recommended to adopt a lower risk statistical scheme; For improved and modified products, short-term and high-risk statistical schemes can be adopted.

Considering that the special reliability work of digital diagnosis and treatment equipment development is in the initial stage, the minimum acceptable value of reliability index (MTBF) (θ_1). No matter which reliability index verification method is adopted, it is necessary to select a certain statistical test scheme to determine the test time. Generally speaking, adopt a scheme with equal risks to the manufacturer and the user ($\alpha = \beta$), the required effective test time m (the multiple of θ_1) The number of liability failures decided is r. See Table 6.1 for commonly used reliability statistical test schemes.

For example: the lowest acceptable value of MTBF of a whole machine is $\theta_1 \geq 1000$ h, and if the high-risk statistical scheme 6 is selected for reliability index verification test, the required effective test time should be $1.2 \times 1000 = 1200$ h, and the allowable number of responsible failures is 0; If the medium risk statistical scheme 2 is selected, the effective test time is $2.99 \times 1000 = 2999$ h, and the allowable number of responsible failures is 1.

Whether single evaluation method, combined evaluation method or comprehensive evaluation method is adopted, the sum of effective test time of each part should not be less than $m \times \theta_1$. MTBF should be evaluated by lower confidence limit, and the bilateral confidence level selected C should not be less than 40% (unilateral confidence $C' = (1 + C)/2$ should not be less than 70%).

Table 6.1 Reliability statistical test scheme

Program number	Judgment risk		Discrimination ratio	Effective test time	Number of judgment liability failures r	
	Producer α (%)	User β (%)	$D = \theta 0/\theta 1$	m (Multiple of $\theta 1$)	Reject ($\geq r$+1)	Receive ($\leq r$)
1	20	20	3.0	4.3	3	2
2	20	20	3.63	2.99	2	1
3	20	20	7.22	1.61	1	0
4	30	30	1.89	3.62	3	2
5	30	30	2.22	2.44	2	1
6	30	30	3.37	1.2	1	0

6.1.3.5 Verification Method Selection

According to the type of digital diagnosis and treatment equipment, its own characteristics and index characteristics, the reliability index verification should be carried out by laboratory reliability test, on-site reliability statistics, reliability evaluation combined with internal and external fields, reliability comprehensive evaluation based on development process information and accelerated reliability test. No matter which method is adopted for reliability index verification, the reliability index verification test outline should be compiled, and the reliability information should be strictly managed to ensure the integrity, truthfulness and accuracy of the information.

(1) Laboratory reliability test: simulating the typical use environment conditions of products in the laboratory, and carrying out reliability index verification in this environment, which is suitable for digital diagnosis and treatment equipment with appropriate volume and low index and can be tested in the laboratory reliability test system. When conditions are met, laboratory reliability test methods should be given priority.
(2) Reliability statistics for field use: reliability verification is carried out in combination with field use such as test, operation, joint test and trial, which is suitable for products with huge volume and no laboratory test conditions at all, or digital diagnosis and treatment equipment with very valuable and precise, good use environment and no relevant reliability information data.
(3) Reliability evaluation of combination of internal and external fields: combining laboratory test with field use to evaluate reliability, it is suitable for digital diagnosis and treatment equipment which requires long laboratory test time due to high index and small number of prototypes, or has special field use conditions and cannot completely rely on laboratory test for index evaluation.
(4) Comprehensive evaluation of reliability based on development process information: the complete set of digital diagnosis and treatment equipment is divided into three states according to development characteristics: use, improvement and new research. By using historical use or development process information, the reliability of each component of the prototype is comprehensively evaluated by means of statistical evaluation, analysis evaluation and experimental verification, and the conclusion whether the reliability of the complete set of digital diagnosis and treatment equipment meets the requirements is obtained. It is suitable for large-scale, complex, high index requirements, few prototypes but related reliability information data.
(5) Accelerated reliability test: for digital diagnosis and treatment equipment or key components with particularly high reliability index, such as the stress value (environmental stress, electrical stress, etc.) that can bear higher than the conventional laboratory environment, the stress can be increased, and accelerated reliability test is used to evaluate reliability.

6.1.3.6 Determination Method of Reliability Index

6.1.4 Ideas on Reliability Index Demonstration

The first step to obtain reliable products is to put forward and determine the reliability quantitative index requirements. Only when the reliability quantitative index requirements are put forward and determined can we have a definite object in view, carry out reliability design analysis, management control, verification test, improvement and optimization to obtain products that meet the proposed reliability quantitative index requirements, and realize the equal treatment of reliability, performance and cost. Therefore, in the early stage of research and development of digital diagnosis and treatment equipment, it is very important to clarify the requirements of quantitative indicators of reliability.

The most commonly used quantitative index of reliability is Mean Time Between Failure (MTBF) for repairable products and Mean Time To Failure (MTTF) for irreparable products, which can also be called service life. Of course, there is also basic/mission reliability (R), failure/fault rate (λ), Mean Time Between Critical Failure (MTBCF), intrinsic/operative availability (A), mission success probability (P) and other indicators.

This chapter selects the most used reliability index-Mean Time Between Failure (MTBF) as the focus. This index can be used as the evaluation index of the whole machine and repairable parts. In addition, in order to meet the examination and verification of some consumable core components in digital diagnosis and treatment equipment, the service life index is also selected for explanation.

The determination of reliability quantitative index should go through the demonstration process from initial determination to determination, and from use requirement to contract requirement. The general demonstration process is as follows:

(1) In the demonstration process of research and development of digital diagnosis and treatment equipment, preliminary requirements for the use of reliability indicators should be put forward;
(2) The reliability index should be weighed, coordinated and adjusted to match the capacity status, strategic objectives and resource constraints;
(3) Before the end of the program phase, the target value and threshold value of reliability use requirements shall be determined and converted into the specified value and minimum acceptable value in the contract.

In a project, reliability index demonstration usually needs to complete two aspects:

(1) Determine the overall reliability index requirements of digital diagnosis and treatment equipment. In the demonstration stage, the reliability index requirements of digital diagnosis and treatment equipment should be determined. In the contract management with the constraint relationship between Party A and Party B, the reliability index of digital diagnosis and treatment equipment should often be included in the development contract or task book and assessed at the time of acceptance. Therefore, once the reliability index of the whole machine is

determined, it cannot be changed, otherwise it will mean that the development contract or task book will be changed, and a series of change processes and procedures will be needed.

Considering that when determining the reliability index of digital diagnosis and treatment equipment, the reliability index of each component is often not determined, and finally the whole component index should be decomposed into components, therefore, in the demonstration stage, each component development unit should cooperate with the overall research and development unit of the whole machine to achieve the reliability index of the whole machine and obey the reliability distribution results of components.

(2) The reliability index requirement of the whole machine is reasonably distributed to each component. The reliability index of the whole machine is assigned to the lower product level as the initial basis of product reliability design. After completing the preliminary reliability allocation, the reliability level that the whole machine can achieve should be preliminarily predicted by using the reliability data of low-level products and compared with the required value through reliability modeling prediction. If the required value is not met, the reliability index of individual components should be adjusted moderately, and the above allocation and prediction should be repeated until a reasonable allocation value is obtained.

6.1.5 Demonstration of Reliability Index of Whole Machine

In the digital diagnosis and treatment equipment project, we summarized a set of factors that should be considered in determining the reliability index of the whole machine:

(1) When determining the reliability index, factors such as use requirements, cost, schedule, technical level and reliability of similar products should be fully considered;
(2) When choosing reliability parameters, the factors such as mission, type characteristics, complexity and whether the parameters can be measured or not should be considered comprehensively;
(3) On the premise of satisfying the requirements of system integrity and task success, the number of selected reliability parameters should be as minimum as possible and the parameters should be coordinated with each other;
(4) The basic reliability requirements should be derived from the system integrity requirements. According to the provisions of GJB 3872 and GJB 1909, the requirements of reliability, maintainability, support system and its resources should be coordinated and weighed to meet the system integrity requirements;
(5) The mission reliability requirement should be derived from the mission success requirement of equipment;

(6) In the process of determining the reliability requirements, the basic reliability and task reliability requirements should be fully weighed to finally meet the requirements of system integrity and task success;
(7) When determining reliability requirements, failure criteria and verification methods must be clearly defined at the same time;
(8) The ordering party can put forward the reliability requirements of the equipment separately, and the reliability requirements of the lower-level products that the ordering party does not specify are determined by the undertaker through the method of reliability distribution.

In addition, it is worth paying attention to the following points:

(1) The reliability index is progressive for itself: the design of new products must make efforts to ensure and improve the reliability. Therefore, designers should avoid the solidified thinking of "only reaching this level now is set at this level", otherwise, there will be no chance to improve the reliability of products ideologically.
(2) The reliability index should reflect the strategic goal of the enterprise: the reliability index should not only meet the needs of users, but also be comparable or even surpassed with competitors. Digital diagnosis and treatment equipment is expensive and scarce for a single user, and it is usually used frequently, so reliability is extremely important. It is of great significance for equipment R&D enterprises to bring reliability indicators into strategic objectives for sustainable development of enterprises.

For example, for a PET-CT device, how to improve the reliability index? If users can accept two failures in one year, how much should the reliability index be raised? In order to solve this problem, we need to start from the typical use scenarios of PET-CT. In hospitals, PET-CT works for about 8 h every day, and about 25 patients are examined every day. Each patient's detector works for about 12 min, that is to say, the detector works for about 5 h every day. Generally speaking, a PET-CT equipment works for about 250 days a year, so it can be calculated that the typical working hours of PET-CT are 2000 h/year on power and 1250 h/year on high voltage. According to two failures in one year, the Mean Time Between Failures MTBF is: 1000 h/year under power-on state; 625 h/year under high pressure. Therefore, the reliability index of PET-CT should be raised to MTBF $\geq$ 1000 h (power on), MTBF $\geq$ 625 h (high pressure); Or MTBF $\geq$ 1000 h (power-on), requiring 62.5% of the power-on time to turn on high voltage.

6.1.6 Allocation Method of Component Reliability Index

The reliability index of the whole machine is reasonably decomposed into various components. As a target and assessment index of component research and development, all components meet the requirements of reliability index, that is, the realization of reliability index of the whole machine is guaranteed.

Usually, the reliability index allocation method can be used to decompose the whole machine index, and the reliability index allocation is carried out layer by layer from top to bottom. In fact, the process of index allocation is the process of responsibility decomposition.

6.1.6.1 Purpose of Work

Through appropriate models and considerations, the overall reliability index of the complete set of digital diagnosis and treatment equipment is distributed to all levels of products from top to bottom, and the distribution results are taken as the main basis for the reliability requirements of components.

6.1.6.2 Applicable Objects

The overall R&D unit of the whole machine shall organize the distribution of reliability index, and distribute the reliability index to each component R&D unit. Component R&D units can also carry out reliability index allocation according to the situation, and determine the reliability index of R&D units and various departments within the unit responsible for R&D.

6.1.6.3 Time to Carry Out

In the programming stage, the reliability index distribution should be carried out as soon as possible, and the reliability index should be determined for each research unit as soon as possible. When the index conflicts, coordination and redistribution should be carried out.

6.1.6.4 Implementation Process

The implementation process of reliability index allocation is shown in Fig. 6.2.

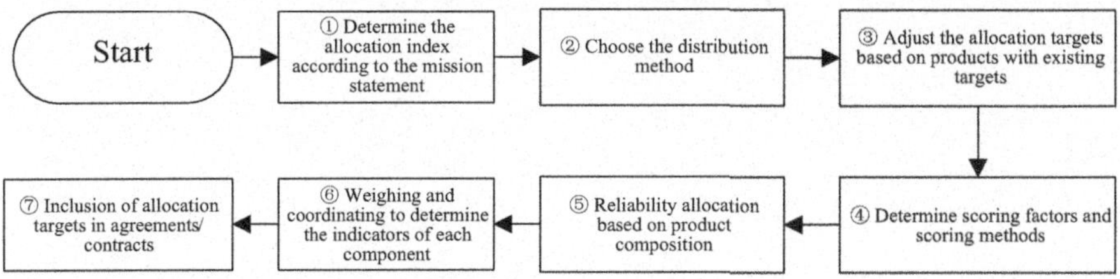

Fig. 6.2 Implementation process of reliability index allocation

Table 6.2 Commonly used reliability index allocation method

Development stage		Scheme design	Prototype development	Scope of application
Allocation method	Proportional distribution method	Applicable	Applicable	Basic reliability allocation
	Expert scoring method	Applicable	Applicable	Basic reliability allocation
	Similar product distribution method	Applicable	Not applicable	Basic reliability allocation

6.1.6.5 Indicator Allocation Method

Commonly used are liability index allocation methods include proportional allocation method, expert scoring method, similar product allocation method, etc. See Table 6.2 for details.

6.1.6.6 Work Requirements

Reliability index allocation requirements are as follows:

(1) The product level which needs to control reliability should be clearly defined, and the method and depth of reliability index distribution should be determined;
(2) Components that do not care about reliability can be treated as a whole when distributing reliability index;
(3) Reliability index allocation and reliability modeling prediction can be carried out together to guide the design work more effectively.

6.1.6.7 Output

Reliability index allocation generally outputs the following results:

(1) Project reliability index demonstration and distribution report;
(2) Task reliability index responsibility (reflected in the task book or agreement).

6.2 Verification Method of Reliability Index of Whole Machine or Component

6.2.1 Key Elements of Reliability Index Verification Method

6.2.1.1 MTBF Indicator Determination

Before the test, the minimum acceptable value of Mean Time Between Failure (MTBF) of the whole digital diagnosis and treatment equipment should be confirmed (θ_1).

During the test, the MTBF index requirements (θ_1) determined before the test should not be changed.

6.2.1.2 Selection of Statistical Schemes

In order to determine the Mean Time Between Failure verification scheme, the statistical scheme should be selected first, which includes the following five parameters:

(1) Producer risk (α): it refers to the risk that the batch quality meets the requirements but is rejected, which is recorded as α. When the true value of MTBF of the tested prototype is greater than the upper limit of inspection, $Theta_0$The true value of MTBF is determined to be less than the upper limit of test Theta_0The maximum probability of.
(2) User risk (β): it refers to the risk that the batch quality does not meet the requirements but is accepted, which is recorded as β. When the true value of MTBF of the tested prototype is less than the lower limit of inspected θ_1, the true value of MTBF is judged to be higher than the maximum probability of the lower limit of inspected $\theta_{1.}$
(3) Lower limit of MTBF test (θ_1): If the true value of MTBF of the tested prototype is not higher than the lower limit of inspected θ_1, then the probability that the device will be accepted is up to 100β %. The lower limit of MTBF test (θ_1) is the lowest acceptable value for Mean Time Between Failure (MTBF).
(4) The upper limit of MTBF test (θ_0): If the true value of MTBF of the tested prototype is not less than the upper limit of inspected θ_0, then the probability of acceptance of the prototype under test is at least 100 $(1 - \alpha)$%.
(5) Discrimination ratio (D): $D = \theta_0/\theta_1$ (θ_0 is the upper limit of MTBF test, and θ_1 is the lower limit of MTBF test)

According to factors such as product quality, risk tolerance and verification cost, it is recommended to select the timed censoring statistical scheme according to Table 6.3.

Table 6.3 Statistical scheme of timing censoring

Scheme serial number	Characteristics of the scheme			Censoring time T (Multiple m of θ_1)	Decided number of failures r	
	Nominal value of risk (%)		Discrimination ratio $D = \theta_0/\theta_1$		Rejected (≥)	Received (≤)
	Producer risk α	User risk β				
1	30	30	3.37	1.20	1	0
2	30	30	2.22	2.44	2	1
3	30	30	2.00	3.70	3	2
4	20	20	7.22	1.61	1	0
5	20	20	3.63	2.99	2	1
6	20	20	3.00	4.30	3	2
7	10	10	21.85	2.30	1	0
8	10	10	7.32	3.89	2	1
9	10	10	4.83	5.32	3	2

Based on the selected statistical scheme, the total time requirement for verification (θ_1 multiplies m) and the corresponding number of allowed judgment failures r can be determined.

6.2.1.3 Calculation of Effective Test Time

1. **Total Valid Verification Time Requirements**

According to the selected statistical scheme, the total effective verification time can be obtained by checking Table 6.3 as m times of the average failure interval θ_1, i.e.:

$$T = \theta_1 \times m \tag{6.1}$$

where:
T—Total valid verification time (h);
θ_1—The lowest acceptable value of MTBF (h);
m—The multiple of θ_1.

2. **Valid Verification Time of Single Unit Plan**

Determine the number of prototypes tested (n), the average valid verification time plan per set can be obtained according to Eq. (6.2):

$$t = T/n = \theta_1 \times m/n \tag{6.2}$$

In the formula:

t—The average effective verification time of each prototype, in h;
T—Total effective verification time, in h;
m—The multiple of θ_1;
n—The number of test machines.

Under the premise of ensuring that the cumulative effective verification time of each prototype reaches the total effective verification time requirement, the actual effective verification time of each sample machine can be adjusted due to the failure of the prototype in verification.

6.2.1.4 Verification Method

Referring to Sect. 4.3.2 of GB/T 5080.1–2012, one of the following three methods can be adopted for the MTBF verification of the sample machine:

(1) On-site use reliability statistics (no environmental condition control);
(2) Laboratory reliability test (environmental condition control);
(3) Combined reliability assessment of internal and external fields.

6.2.1.5 Indicator Verification Environmental Conditions

(1) **Classification of Environmental Conditions**

Three basic categories according to the conditions of use and transportation and circulation:

Class I: Used in a good environment, usually refers to the equipment used in a controlled environment with air conditioning and other equipment;

Class II: used in general environment, usually refers to the equipment used in an environment with heating and ventilation;

Class III: Used in harsh environments, usually refers to the use of equipment in environments without thermal insulation, heating and ventilation, and similar outdoor environments.

The recommended environmental conditions for each category are shown in Table 6.4.

(2) **On-Site Operating Environment Conditions**

In the evaluation of the Mean Time Between Failures of the on-site operation, the environmental conditions of the on-site operation should meet the requirements specified by the product of the sample machine.

The field operation assessment using MTBF is recommended only for the large, single set of digital diagnosis and treatment equipment belonging to Class I.

Table 6.4 Classification of environmental conditions for digital medical equipment (recommended values)

Category	Non-working low temperature limit/°C	Working low temperature limit/°C	Non-operating high temperature limit/°C	Working high temperature limit/°C
Class I	/	20	/	25
Class II	−20	5	+55	35
Class III	−40	−10	+70	55

(3) **Laboratory Tests to Verify Environmental Conditions**

If there is no other requirement, the laboratory test verification should be carried out under the combined action of temperature, humidity, electrical stress and other possible stresses in actual use.

The laboratory test verification environment conditions corresponding to the digital diagnosis and treatment equipment are as follows:

(1) Digital diagnosis and treatment equipment used under Class I environmental conditions

MTBF verification in a temperature-controlled and humidity-controlled laboratory. The temperature range is controlled within the range of 20–25 °C or within the temperature range specified by the product.

(2) Digital diagnosis and treatment equipment used under Class II environmental conditions

It is recommended to adopt the test cycle diagram in Fig. 6.3 to place the sample machine in the test equipment in the laboratory for verification of the Mean Time Between Failures. The verification time corresponding to the typical room temperature of 25 °C can be carried out in a temperature-controlled laboratory.

(3) Digital diagnosis and treatment equipment used under Class III environmental conditions

For digital diagnosis and treatment equipment used under Class III (no vibration) environmental conditions, it is recommended to adopt the test cycle diagram in Fig. 6.4 to place the sample machine in the test equipment in the laboratory for verification of the Mean Time Between Failures.

For digital diagnosis and treatment equipment used in Class III (with vibration) environmental conditions, it is recommended to adopt the test cycle diagram in Fig. 6.5 to install the sample machine in the test equipment in the laboratory for the verification of the Mean Time Between Failures. The vibration spectrum shown in Fig. 6.5 is a typical transportation vibration spectrum. When the actual measurement conditions are available, the actual measurement results are preferred to apply the vibration spectrum.

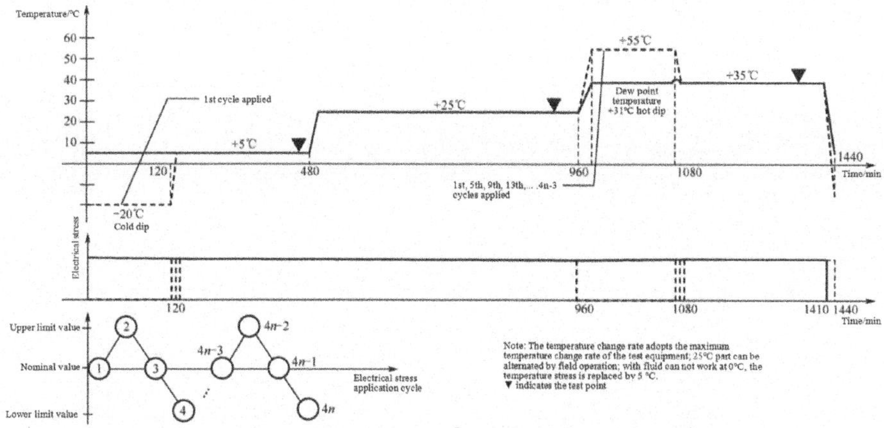

Fig. 6.3 Laboratory MTBF verification test cycle for digital diagnosis and treatment equipment used under class II environmental conditions

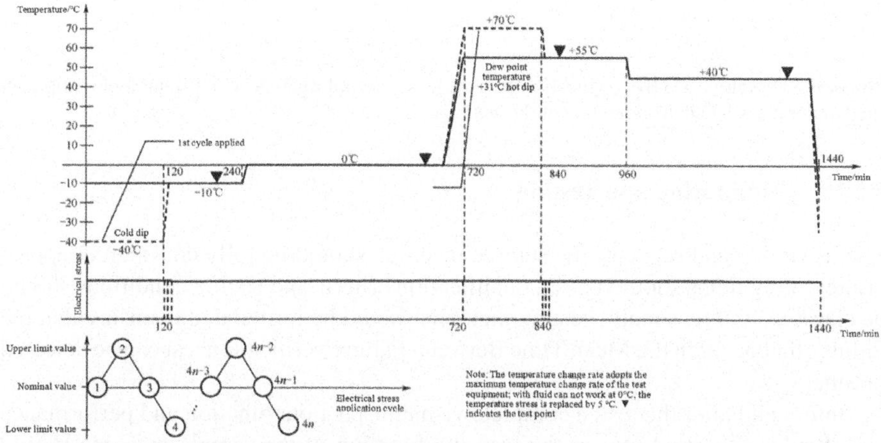

Fig. 6.4 Laboratory MTBF verification test cycle for digital diagnosis and treatment equipment installed and used under class II environmental conditions

6.2.1.6 Prototype Operating Conditions

During the Mean Time Between Failure verification test, the actual operating conditions and scenarios of the sample machine should be combined to simulate various typical operation and working modes of the sample machine synchronously. When there are multiple working conditions, various Combination and matching of operating conditions and applied stresses.

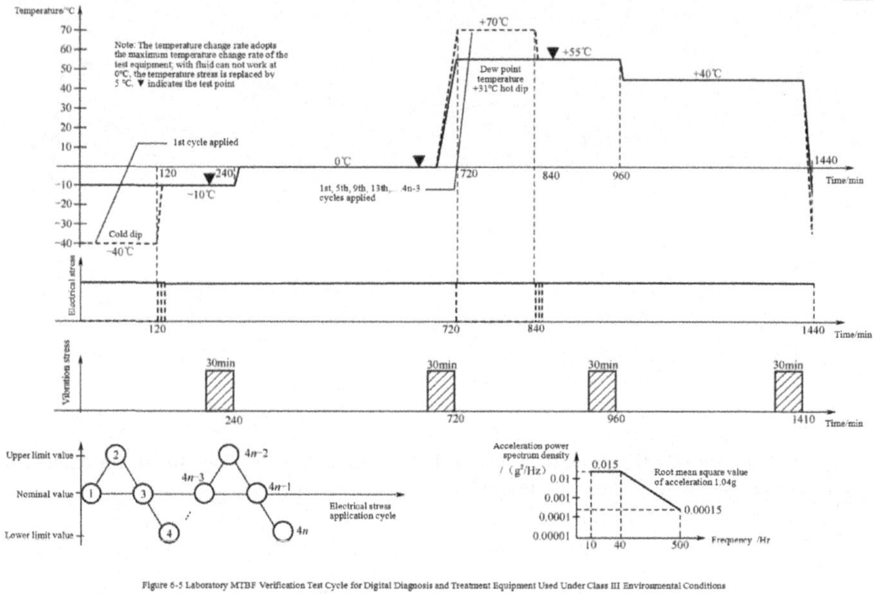

Fig. 6.5 Laboratory MTBF verification test cycle for digital diagnosis and treatment equipment used under class III environmental conditions

6.2.1.7 Monitoring and Testing

The use mode and scene of the sample machine should be fully considered, appropriate testing items should be set, qualification criteria and testing conditions should be clarified, and reasonable testing methods should be formulated to ensure that the failures that occur in the Mean Time Between Failure verification test can be detected in time.

Before and after the test, a complete visual inspection, function and performance test should be carried out; in the test, the function of the sample machine should be monitored during the power-on operation of the sample machine, and the test point should be selected as harsh as possible when the stress is comprehensively applied., the test items should be as complete as possible, but at least include the main functions and performance, and the reasons for the cut-off test items in the test should be explained.

6.2.1.8 Maintenance

The sample machine should be maintained according to the specified maintenance requirements, and any maintenance work other than the specified ones is not allowed during the test.

6.2.1.9 Failure Criteria and Classifications

1. **Failure Criteria**

If the following conditions occur during the Mean Time Between Failure verification test of the sample machine, it can be considered to be failure:

(1) Any function of the sample machine is abnormal or lost;
(2) The performance parameters of the sample machine are out of tolerance;
(3) Cracks, breaks or damage to mechanical parts, structural parts or components that affect the function, performance and structural integrity of the test machine.

2. **Classification of Failure Consequences**

Serious failure: The failure of the sample machine to complete the specified tasks due to the direct loss of all or part of the functions of the sample machine, or the out-of-tolerance of some performance indicators of the sample machine is judged as a serious failure. Serious failures include, but are not limited to:

(1) The subject machine cannot be powered on or used;
(2) All or part of the function of the sample machine is lost, and the technical index exceeds the standard, which makes the sample machine unusable;
(3) The standard sample test results or data processing results of the sample machine are inaccurate;
(4) Protection, protection, interlocking switches, buttons, and devices fail;
(5) The keys or buttons, display, and software of the sample machine fail to operate;
(6) During the same test period, the fuse of the same sample machine was blown 3 times or more;
(7) In the same test cycle, the same action device of the same sample machine mis-operates 3 times or more without external causes;
(8) During the whole test process, the same intermittent failure occurs 5 times or more.

General failure: Although it does not affect the final completion of the specified tasks of the sample machine, the failure that affects the normal use or efficiency of the prototype is recorded as a general failure. General failures include but are not limited to:

(1) Some functions of the sample machine are lost and the technical indicators are out of tolerance, but the sample machine can be used normally;
(2) Failure of test components, redundant components, auxiliary indicating and displaying components does not affect normal operation;
(3) The failure of general switches and buttons will not lead to the inability to complete the specified functions;
(4) Defects or deficiencies found during the user's operation, such as slight scratches on the appearance, minor defects of parts (such as looseness, drift, noise, leakage, etc.), but do not cause loss of function, can be repaired on site and recorded as general failure;

(5) Other failures that do not affect the completion of the main functions of the sample machine.

3. **Classification of Failure Characteristics**

Responsible failure: During the test, the associated independent failure caused by the defect of the sample machine itself and the resulting subordinate failure are counted as a responsible failure, and the responsible failure usually requires failure resetting and improvement measures. Liability failures include, but are not limited to:

(1) Failures caused by design defects, process defects or poor manufacturing;
(2) Failures caused by latent defects in parts and components;
(3) failures caused by software errors;
(4) failures caused by obvious improper operation, maintenance and repair procedures;
(5) Unconfirmed failures (refers to failures that cannot be reproduced or whose causes have not been identified).

Non-responsible failures: Non-responsible failures are usually not related to the product itself, and it is not required to take failure reset and improvement measures for non-responsible failures of the prototype. Non-liability failures include but are not limited to:

(1) Failures caused by failures of test equipment and testing instruments;
(2) The failure of the sample machine caused by the application of test stress and working conditions beyond the specified ones;
(3) The failure of the sample machine caused by improper operation, maintenance and repair;
(4) The overdue use of life parts and components, the failure of the overdue parts and components and the subordinate failures caused by them.

4. **Statistical Principles of Judgment Failures**

Judgment failures should be counted according to the following principles:

(1) According to the definition of serious failure, a responsible failure with serious consequences will be recorded as a judgment failure;
(2) 5 or more general liability failures caused by the same reason will be counted as a judgment failure;
(3) For every 5 kinds of general liability failures, it will be recorded as a judgment failure;
(4) Non-responsible failures are not included in judgment failures.

During the verification process, the failure location, analysis, and treatment should be completed as soon as possible for the failures that occur, the classification of failure consequences and failure characteristics should be clarified, and the number of failures should be counted and judged in time to avoid the situation that the verification that should be terminated is still going on.

5. **Troubleshooting**

When failures are found during the pre-verification test, during the verification test, after the verification test and at any time, the failure handling shall be carried out according to the following regulations:

(1) Confirmation and location of failures;
(2) Handling of failures and tests;
(3) Failure mechanism analysis;
(4) Failure records.

6.2.1.10 Valid Verification Time Statistics

The effective verification time of a single sample machine is the sum of its determinable uptime.

When performing reliability evaluation, the effective verification time of each sample machine shall be accumulated as the total effective verification time.

The effective verification time statistics principles are as follows:

(1) If no failure occurs during the test of the sample machine, the entire test time is valid verification time;
(2) If the machine under test fails during the test, the time spent running with the failure cannot be used as the valid verification time;
(3) When a failure of a sample machine is found in the verification test, the invalid verification time is between the end time of the test corresponding to the normal test result of the failure sample machine last time and the start time of the test corresponding to the failure found in this test time.

6.2.1.11 Determination of Test Interruption, Termination and End Conditions

Test interruption: During the verification process, if the prototype fails, the verification should be interrupted, the failure location and treatment should be carried out, and the verification should be continued after the failure treatment is completed (the laboratory verification should continue the test from the test interruption point).

Termination of the test: During the verification process, if the prototype fails, and the number of failures judged by statistics exceeds the number of failures allowed by the statistical plan, the verification should be terminated.

End of test: On the premise that the test is not terminated, if the total cumulative effective verification time of the prototype reaches the required verification time, the verification will end normally.

6.2.1.12 Verification Index Evaluation Method

When the verification is passed according to the statistical scheme, under the confidence level C, the lower confidence limit of MTBF $\theta_{L,C}$ is:

$$\theta_{L,C} = \frac{2T}{\chi_{\beta}^{2}(2r+2)} \tag{6.3}$$

In the formula:
T—Cumulative effective test time;
r—The number of judgment failures;
β—The risk of the user in the statistical scheme, usually 10%, 20%, 30%;
C—Confidence degree $C = 1 - \beta$, usually corresponding to 90%, 80%, 70%;
$\chi_{\beta}^{2}(2r+2)$—Chi-square distribution, $2r+2$ is its degree of freedom.

When the verification fails according to the statistical scheme, under the confidence level C, the lower confidence limit of MTBF is:

$$\theta_{L,C} = \frac{2T}{\chi_{\beta}^{2}(2r)} \tag{6.4}$$

In the formula:
$\theta_{L,C}$—MTBF one-sided lower confidence limit (C) assessment results;
T—Cumulative effective test time;
r—The number of judgment failures;
β—The risk of the user in the statistical scheme, usually 10%, 20%, 30%;
C—Lower confidence limit, $C = 1 - \beta$, usually corresponding to 90%, 80%, 70%;
$\chi_{\beta}^{2}(2r)$—Chi-square distribution, 2r is its degree of freedom.

6.2.1.13 Verification Conclusion

1. **Pass**

When the verification work is completed (the cumulative effective verification time reaches the time specified in the statistical plan), and the cumulative number of judged failures of the sample machine before, during and after the test does not exceed the number of received failures allowed by the statistical plan, the verification conclusion is that the verification is passed.

2. **Fail**

When any of the following situations occurs, the verification conclusion is that the verification fails:

(1) During the verification period, if the number of failures judged by the sample machine exceeds the number of receiving failures allowed by the statistical plan, the test is terminated in advance;

(2) After the verification work (including the post-verification test) is completed, the accumulative number of judged failures of the sample machine before, during and after the test exceeds the number of received failures allowed by the statistical plan.

When the verification fails, the submitting party shall complete failure reset and rectification, and re-send samples for verification test.

6.2.1.14 Typical Test Process Chart

The typical test process chart of the reliability index is shown in Fig. 6.6.

6.2.1.15 Monitoring and Recording Requirements During the Test

The inspection requirements of the tested product and the monitoring requirements of the test facilities during the test shall be specified, and corresponding record forms shall be given at the same time.

6.2.1.16 Failure Reporting and Handling Requirements

It should be clear how to report when a failure occurs during the test, which records should be filled in and the handling procedure for the failure.

6.2.1.17 Explanation of Relevant Issues

Matters that are not clear in other chapters of the test program should be specified to ensure the integrity and rigor of the test program. For example, the replacement requirements of life parts in the tested product, etc.

6.2.2 Development of the Test Plan

According to the requirements of the research and development of digital medical equipment, the reliability appraisal test plan should be prepared according to the situation, which is used to explain the overall planning of the reliability appraisal test, and outline the required reliability appraisal test products, sample quantity, statistical plan, Comprehensive environmental conditions, test parties, schedules, etc., provide guidance for subsequent reliability identification tests.

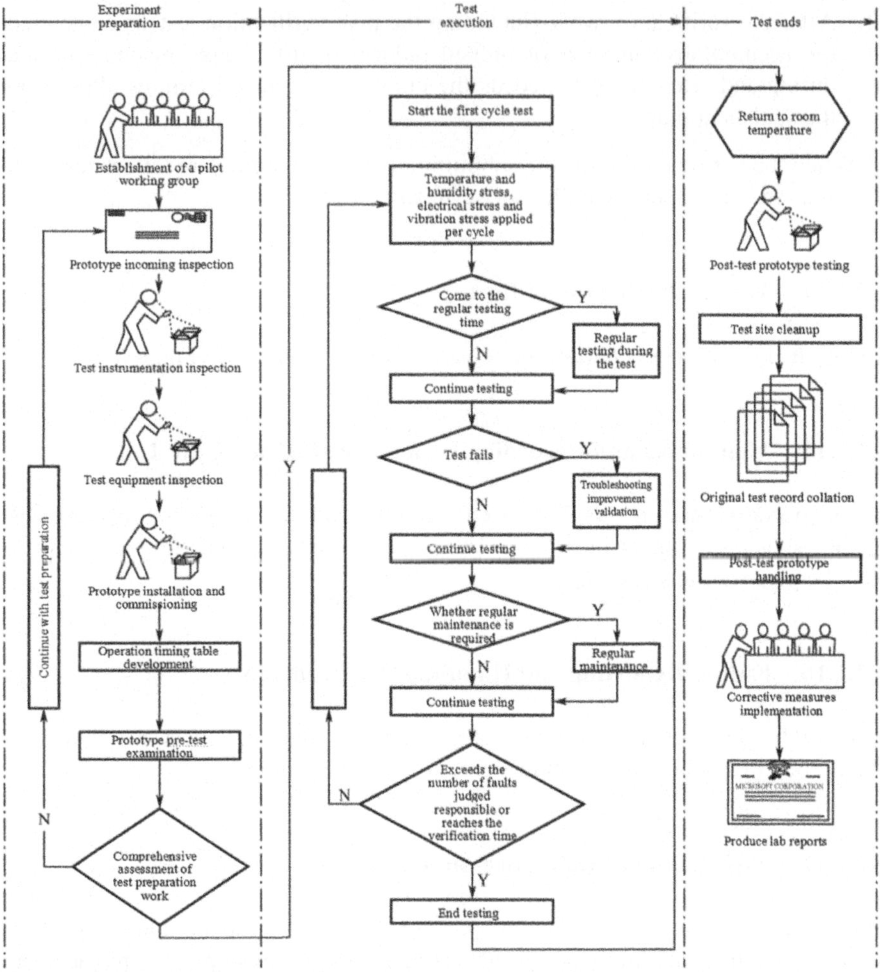

Fig. 6.6 Typical test process chart of reliability index

6.2.2.1 Determination of the Tested Product

In principle, reliability identification tests should be carried out for products with reliability index requirements. Generally, the products that can be tested for reliability identification according to the system combination should be tested according to the system combination. When the reliability qualification test is only carried out on a part of the system, the verification test shall be carried out according to the new reliability index formed by the reliability index of the tested part.

When determining the product to be tested, the quantity of the product to be tested should be determined, and information such as the size, weight, power supply, and installation requirements of the sample machine to be tested should be provided.

6.2.2.2 Determination of the Statistical Scheme

Select a statistical plan to clarify the total test time and the number of allowable failures. According to the number of prototypes, the average test time of each prototype can be calculated. According to the test time of each cycle in the test profile, the number of planned test cycles can be further calculated.

6.2.2.3 Determination of Comprehensive Environmental Conditions

According to the actual use environment of the whole machine and core components of digital medical equipment, determine the comprehensive environmental conditions for its reliability verification. It usually includes typical high and low temperature, humid heat and its comprehensive environment, and individual samples also have vibration or other special environments. The selection of environmental conditions and test equipment is often mutually restrictive. The reliability verification test usually selects the actual typical environment. Most equipment can apply typical environmental parameters, and special environmental parameters often require specific equipment to apply.

6.2.2.4 Put Forward Work Progress Requirements

In the reliability appraisal test plan, key nodes such as the review of the test plan, the review of the test program, the arrival of the tested product at the test site, and the review of the completion of the test should be clearly defined.

6.2.2.5 Determination of the Test Undertaker

The reliability identification test should be carried out in a laboratory that is independent of the research and development unit, has obtained the CNAS qualification certificate, and has reliability test qualifications.

6.2.2.6 Other Requirements

Requirements such as organization and management of the test, technical status of the product under test, status of the test facility, and status of the test equipment should also be put forward in the reliability qualification test plan.

6.2.3 Preparation of Test Outline

The test undertaker shall formulate a reliability identification test outline. The reliability qualification test outline mainly includes test purpose and scope of application, reference standards and documents, test product description and requirements, test statistical plan, comprehensive environmental conditions, test facilities and test equipment requirements, test product test items and qualification criteria, failure statistics principles, relevant work before the test, monitoring and recording requirements during the test, failure reporting and handling requirements, and descriptions of related issues, etc.

6.2.3.1 Test Purpose and Scope of Application

Clarify the purpose and object of the test, as well as the reliability index of the test verification.

6.2.3.2 References to Standards and Documents

List all the standards and related documents for test execution, and pay special attention to citing technical documents such as general requirements for research and development including technical indicators and qualification criteria, and technical agreements for finished products.

6.2.3.3 Test Product Description and Requirements

Explain the function and use, composition, installation and use environment, technical status and quantity of the tested product.

6.2.3.4 Test Statistical Scheme

Describe the statistical scheme and related parameters used in the experiment.

6.2.3.5 Comprehensive Environmental Conditions

According to the installation and use environment of the tested product, specify the comprehensive environmental conditions and working conditions used in the test. Describe the comprehensive environmental conditions, specify the application method and timing of each test stress.

6.2.3.6 Test Facility and Equipment Requirements

Clarify the capability, accuracy and testing requirements of test facilities and test equipment.

If necessary, provide a schematic diagram of the connection of the test facility, explain the model, manufacturer, capacity, verification period and validity period of the test facility and test equipment used in the test.

6.2.3.7 Testing Items and Qualification Criteria of the Tested Product

Clarify the testing requirements of the product during the test.

Including testing content, testing method, testing timing and qualification criteria, etc. The general testing content should be able to cover the general requirements for product development or the main performance requirements of the product in use in the finished product technical agreement.

For items that cannot be tested under comprehensive environmental conditions, a certain stress or comprehensive stress of the test should be suspended before testing, and even under the supervision of the test undertaker and the orderer, the test product can be returned to the research and development unit for testing. However, when carrying out the reliability identification test, the number of inspections should be greater than the maximum number of failures allowed under the receiving conditions in the test plan.

6.2.3.8 Failure Criteria, Classification and Statistical Principles

1. **Failure Criteria**

During the test, if any of the following states occurs, it should be determined that the product under test has failed.

(1) Under the specified conditions, the product under test cannot work;
(2) Under the specified conditions, the performance test results of the tested product do not meet the specified requirements;
(3) During the test, the mechanical, structural parts or components of the tested product are loosened, cracked, broken or damaged.

2. **Failure Classification**

The failures that occur during the reliability test can be divided into associated failures and non-associated failures, and associated failures should be further divided into responsible failures and non-responsible failures.

(1) Non-responsible failures: During the test, only the following situations can be judged as non-responsible failures:

- Failure of the product under test due to misuse;
- The failure of the product under test caused by the failure of the test device and the test instrument;
- Failure of the product under test due to environmental conditions and operating conditions that exceed the operating limits of the product;
- Failures introduced during the repair process.

(2) Responsibility failures: except those that can be judged as non-responsible failures, all other failures are judged as responsible failures, such as:

- Failures due to design defects or poor manufacturing processes;
- Failures caused by component failure due to latent defects of components;
- Intermittent failure;
- Adjustments outside the normal range of technical specifications;
- All failure symptoms caused by non-dependent failure causes during the test (not exceeding the performance limit);
- Unverifiable exception.

(3) Principle of failurc statistics: during the test, only responsible failures can be used as the basis for judging whether the tested product is qualified or not. Responsible failures can be counted according to the following principles:

- When it can be proved that multiple failure modes are caused by the same cause, the entire event is recorded as one failure;
- When multiple components fail at the same time during the test, if it cannot be proved that the failure of one component caused the failure of others, the failure of each component is recorded as an independent failure; if it can be proved that the failure of one component When other failures are caused by other failures, the failures of all components are recorded as one failure;
- It can be proved that the intermittent failure is caused by the same reason. If the corrective measures are verified to be effective after analysis and confirmation, and the failure will no longer occur, multiple failures will be counted as one failure;
- Verified to be effective after analysis and confirmation, and the failure will no longer occur, the multiple failures will be collectively recorded as one failure;
- Already reported by the same cause of failure, due to the failure to truly eliminate and reappear, and the original reported failure should be recorded together as a failure;
- During the failure detection and repair period, if it is found that there are other failures in the tested product and cannot be determined to be caused by the original failure, it should be regarded as a separate responsible failure for statistics.

6.2.3.9 Relevant Work Before the Test

Before the test, the work content that should be completed by the test undertaker, the research and development unit, and the purchaser should be clearly defined, including the test items that should be completed before this, the organizational structure that should be established, the test documents that should be prepared, the test facility capability investigation, The installation and testing requirements of the product under test and the pre-test preparation review requirements, etc.

6.2.4 Preparations Before Starting the Test

6.2.4.1 Establishment of a Verification Working Group

In order to strengthen the management and monitoring of verification, a verification working group should be established before verification. The verification working group has five roles: group leader, deputy group leader, person in charge of prototype technology, person in charge of condition assurance, and members of the verification working group.

When the test is carried out in a third-party laboratory, the team leader is the person in charge of the laboratory test of the third-party testing institution; when there is no supervision party, the deputy team leader is responsible for the quality of the site by the sending party, and when there is supervision party, the deputy team leader will be the supervision party; the person in charge of condition guarantee shall be the person in charge of condition guarantee in the laboratory of the third-party testing organization; the person in charge of prototype technology shall be the technician at the test site who is familiar with the sample machine; other participants of the parties in this test are members of the validation working group.

When the verification is carried out by the sending party, the team leader shall be the person in charge of the laboratory test of the sending party; when there is no supervisory party, the deputy team leader shall be the person in charge of on-site quality; when there is a supervisory party, the deputy team leader shall be the supervisor The person in charge of condition assurance shall be the person in charge of condition assurance in the laboratory of the submitting party; the person in charge of prototype technology shall be the technician at the test site who is familiar with the sample machine of the submitting party; other personnel participating in this test shall be members of the verification working group.

6.2.4.2 Preparation by the Developer Before Entering the Site

For developers who have no test experience, they often do not know what preparations to make before the test, and there are usually negligent or insufficient preparations. Before entering the site, the developer should prepare prototypes, installation fixtures, test instruments, connecting cables, spare parts and spare cables. wait. The verifier shall confirm that the test equipment can meet the requirements imposed by the test conditions.

Capability investigation of test facilities: Before the installation of the tested products, carry out a capability investigation on the test facilities to ensure that the test facilities used can meet the test requirements.

Fixture fabrication and vibration measurement: If special fixtures are required for the test to install the product under test, the developer should make relevant fixtures and perform vibration measurements on the fixtures used. It is recommended to use the sinusoidal scanning method. Only when it is confirmed that the used fixture has no resonance or resonance has no effect on the test, and the transfer rate meets the requirements, and does not affect the inherent characteristics of the product under test and the stress it bears, can the fixture be considered usable.

Test instruments and special devices: Test instruments and meters should be within the validity period of measurement and calibration, and special devices should be able to prove their usability and accuracy. In order to improve the detection efficiency and reduce errors in the test process, it is best to use test fixtures to facilitate cable connection and channel switching, etc., and use software tools to simplify, standardize and automate test operations.

6.2.4.3 The Inspection of the Sample Machine Entering the Site

When the sample machine arrives at the site or laboratory, the verification working group should carry out the inspection of the sample machine:

(1) Before unpacking, check whether the appearance and structure of the outer packaging are damaged;
(2) After unpacking the outer packaging, check the inner packaging for appearance and structural damage;
(3) After taking the prototype out of the package, check the prototype for appearance and structural damage;
(4) Check the conformity of technical status information such as prototype appearance, composition integrity, software version, size and weight with the outline;
(5) Connect the prototype to the power supply, test equipment, load, etc.;
(6) Power on to check whether the function and performance of the prototype are normal;

(7) Record the results of the on-site inspection (including outer packaging, inner packaging, appearance and structure of the prototype, and functional performance).

If problems are found during the on-site inspection, the failure resetting management method should be adopted to deal with the problem, and the failure report form, failure analysis and corrective measure form should be filled out in detail, and the corrective measures should be implemented in documents, drawings and objects.

6.2.4.4 Test Instruments and Gauges Status Inspection

Before the verification, the verification working group checks the measurement certificates and technical specifications of all test instruments and meters used in this test to confirm that the test instruments and meters are within the valid period of measurement qualification and meet the following allowable error regulations:

(1) Its accuracy should be at least one-third of the tolerance of the measured parameter;
(2) Its calibration should be traceable to the highest national measurement standard.

6.2.4.5 Test Equipment Status Inspection

When the laboratory test method is adopted, before the test, the person in charge of condition assurance shall set the temperature, humidity, vibration, and electrical stress control procedures according to the test profile and test operation schedule, and trial run the test equipment to be used in this test. It can generate and maintain the test conditions required for the test to ensure that the test equipment can meet the control accuracy requirements:

(1) Temperature: up to $\pm$ 2 °C after the temperature stabilizes;
(2) Relative humidity: up to $\pm$ 5% after the humidity is stable;
(3) Vibration: The power spectral density of random vibration does not exceed $\pm$ 3 dB.

The verification working group checks the measurement certificates, technical specifications, test run curves and other related operation records of all test equipment used in this test to confirm that the test equipment is within the validity period of measurement and qualification.

6.2.4.6 Formulation of Operation Schedule

According to the sequence diagram of the test profile, the person in charge of the laboratory test is responsible for formulating the operation schedule, coordinating and reasonably arranging the start time of the test, determining the daily operating

Table 6.5 Example of operating time table

1st cycle				
Profile point	Intervals	Section stress	Operational matters	Operating time
0 min	0:00:00	−20 °C	Cool down to −20° C, the cycle begins	8:00:00
120 min	2:00:00	−20 °C	Check if the temperature starts to rise automatically (maximum rate) − 20 °C → +5 °C	10:00:00
150 min	0:30:00	+5 °C	Adjust the voltage, power on and start three times, check whether the temperature reaches +5 °C	10:30:00
480 min	5:30:00	+5 °C	Test 1, check temperature stress +5 °C	16:00:00
510 min	0:30:00	+25 °C	Check if it starts to heat up automatically (maximum rate) +5 °C→ +25 °C	16:30:00
960 min	7:30:00	+25 °C	Test 2, check if the temperature reaches +25 °C, power off	00:00:00
990 min	0:30:00	+55 °C	Check if it starts to heat up automatically (maximum rate) +25 °C → +55 °C	00:30:00
1080 min	1:30:00	+55 °C	Check temperature +55 °C (dew point temperature 28 °C)	2:00:00
1110 min	0:30:00	+35 °C	Power on and start three times, check whether it starts to automatically cool down (maximum rate) +55 °C→ +35 °C	2:30:00
1410 min	5:00:00	+35 °C	Test 3, check temperature +35 °C	7:30:00
1440 min	0:30:00	-20 °C	Check if automatic cooling starts (maximum rate) +35 °C → − 20 °C	8:00:00

time during the test, and checking the temperature and humidity environmental stress, adjusting the electrical stress and energizing for the test implementation. And power off, vibration on and off, prototype test provide clear time requirements. See Table 6.5 for an example of an operating schedule (following the test profile shown in Fig. 6.3).

6.2.4.7 Test Stress Setting

When the laboratory test method is adopted, the person in charge of the test is responsible for organizing the test personnel to set the test stress according to the test profile and operation schedule. The test personnel should check the consistency between the test profile diagram and the operation schedule and give feedback to the test leader. The person in charge of the test should check the test stress set by the test personnel to ensure that it is consistent with the test profile and operation schedule.

Specific requirements are as follows:

(1) Temperature and humidity environmental stress setting: on the temperature and humidity comprehensive stress box controller, set the temperature and humidity stress curve according to the test profile, and save and download it;
(2) Electrical stress adjustment: adjust the power supply voltage of the sample machine to the specified value of this cycle according to the time sequence of the test section (*N* represents the *Nth* large electrical stress cycle, including 4 temperature and humidity cycles, and the electrical stresses are 4*N*-3 Nominal, 4*N*-2 Lower Limit, 4*N*-1 Nominal, 4*N* Upper Limit);
(3) Vibration stress setting: If there is vibration stress, set and store the vibration spectrum pattern on the control computer of the vibration table, and confirm that the vibration table has the test capability according to the parameters of the vibration table, prototype and fixture;
(4) Check the test profile setting: check that the temperature and humidity stress curve, electrical stress and vibration spectrum pattern are consistent with the specified test profile.

6.2.4.8 Installation and Trial Operation of the Sample Machine

After the inspection of the sample machine is completed, the party sending the inspection is responsible for installing the sample machine and trial operation:

(1) Fix or install the sample machine according to the following methods:

- When the on-site operation verification method is adopted, the sample machine is fixed on the site according to the fixing/installation direction during actual use or installed on a place that meets the requirements or on the corresponding bench;
- Place the sample machine in the test box according to the fixed/installation direction in actual use, and keep the space distance between the sample machine and the test box;
- When the laboratory test verification method is adopted and there is vibration stress, the sample machine is installed on the vibrating table of the test box according to the installation direction of the actual use, and the ambient air flow around the sample machine simulates the predetermined working conditions of the sample machine. The center of gravity of the prototype and the fixture should be adjusted to a proper position to ensure the reasonable application of the vibration stress. Select the vibration control point on the vibration table and install the acceleration sensor. The best number is 3. The three-point average control method is adopted to ensure The safety of vibration control should avoid unnecessary damage to the vibration table and control system that may be caused by loose control of a single sensor;
- After the product under test is installed in accordance with the provisions of the test procedure, a small amount of pre-vibration is performed on it to check the compatibility between the test facility, the fixture and the product

under test. For the selection of vibration control points, in principle, it should be able to make the vibration stress of the product under test as uniform as possible, close to the test conditions.

(2) Connect the sample machine to the power supply, load, test cables, test instruments, testing equipment, etc., and seal the wire holes of the test box so that the sample machine can be completely in a state of real or simulated operation.
(3) After completing all the installation work, test run the sample machine and conduct a preliminary self-examination of its functional performance to confirm that it is installed in place, connected correctly, and in normal condition.

6.2.4.9 Prototype Testing Before Verification

The person in charge of the test organizes the verification working group to carry out a comprehensive appearance inspection and functional performance test on the sample machine before the verification, to confirm that the appearance of the prototype machine is normal before the test, and the function and performance meet the requirements.

If a failure is found in the pre-verification inspection, the failure resetting management method should be adopted to deal with the problem, and the failure report form, analysis and corrective action form should be filled out in detail, and the corrective measures should be implemented in documents, drawings and objects.

6.2.4.10 Verification Readiness Assessment

Checks the preparations for the sample machine, test equipment, test instruments and meters, test participants, logistics support, etc., and confirms that:

(1) Whether the test program is detailed, clear and operable;
(2) Test results and status of special test equipment and test facilities;
(3) Whether the quality control and guarantee measures are perfect;
(4) Summary and resetting of problems and failures found before the test;
(5) The readiness of the failure reporting, analysis and corrective action system;
(6) Whether the technical status of the tested product and the related work completed meet the requirements of the reliability appraisal test.

After passing the inspection, freeze the technical status of the sample machine. The verification working group combines the verification operation schedule to determine a reasonable verification start time and issue instructions to start the test.

6.2.5 *Operation of Reliability Qualification Test*

6.2.5.1 Application of Test Stress

During the test, the comprehensive environmental stress specified in the test program is applied according to the test procedure.

6.2.5.2 Testing and Monitoring During the Test

During the test, the performance test of the product under test shall be carried out according to the requirements of the test procedure, and the test results shall be recorded. During the detection process, if a failure is found in this detection and the specific time of the failure cannot be judged, the time of the failure occurrence is considered to be the last detection time.

During the testing process of the reliability qualification test, the test undertaker and the ordering party shall conduct the testing together with the test personnel of the research and development unit, and sign the test results.

During the test, the test undertaker shall continuously monitor the test facilities to ensure that the electrical stress, temperature stress, humidity stress and vibration stress are within the specified tolerance range, and continuously record the monitoring results.

6.2.5.3 Troubleshooting Procedure During the Test

1. **Failure Report**

During the test, when the abnormal phenomenon of the tested product is judged to be a failure, the "reliability identification test failure report form" should be filled in according to the requirements of FRACAS, and the failure phenomenon, the environmental conditions when the failure was found, and the failure when the failure occurred should be recorded in detail. The test time and energization time of the product. If multiple pieces of testing are used, the cumulative test time and energization time of all tested products should be recorded.

In the column of failure phenomenon description, the on-site staff should describe the abnormal phenomena seen in detail as much as possible, such as the indicator light is off, the display screen shows "surface display failure", current indication value, voltage indication value, and oscilloscope display content. Record the operation content in detail, such as which buttons are pressed, which parameters are adjusted, etc., so that product designers and experts can perform failure location and failure cause analysis based on this.

2. **Failure Analysis**

The research and development unit conducts failure analysis on the failed products, and fills in the "reliability identification test failure analysis report form" according to the requirements of FRACAS.

The failure mode column should specify the failure device, the failure cause column should describe the cause of the failure in detail, and the analysis description column should analyze the failure mechanism, and attach the failure mechanism analysis report, DPA report and other documents if necessary.

3. **Troubleshooting**

Correct failures and verify corrective actions as required. The R&D unit shall fill in the corrective measures in the "reliability identification test failure corrective measure report form" according to the requirements of FRACAS.

The column of corrective measures should describe in detail the content of the measures taken, including the content and steps of changing the design. The effect column should describe in detail the situation of corrective action verification.

After verifying that the measures taken are effective and the failure has been reset to zero, classify the failure according to the relevant regulations.

6.2.5.4 Preventive Maintenance During the Test

During the reliability identification test, only the preventive maintenance specified during the service period of the product and included in the test program shall be carried out. Except for those specially approved by the purchaser, no other precautions shall be taken during the reliability identification test or during the repair process. maintenance measures.

6.2.5.5 End of the Test

When the number of responsible failures during the test exceeds the number of receiving failures specified in the statistical plan, a rejection judgment can be made, and the reliability appraisal test is over.

When the cumulative test time reaches the test time specified in the statistical plan, and the number of responsible failures of the tested product is less than the number of rejected failures specified in the statistical plan, an acceptance decision can be made. For multiple product tests, as long as the cumulative test time of one product is less than half of the average test time of all tested products, a qualified judgment should not be made.

6.2.6 Work After Reliability Qualification Test

6.2.6.1 Failure Reset

For responsible failures that occur during the reliability appraisal test, the research and development unit should complete the resetting work and form a resetting report.

The main content of the failure reset report is as follows:

(1) Failure timing and environmental conditions, including cumulative test time, cumulative energized working time, temperature conditions, humidity conditions, vibration conditions and electrical stress in the comprehensive environment;
(2) Failure phenomenon. The condition of the product at the time of the discovery of the failure;
(3) Cause of failure. The specific reasons and principles leading to the failure phenomena should generally be analyzed by failure tree and a report should be issued;
(4) Failure recurrence situation. In order to confirm the accuracy of the cause of the failure, the failure recurrence should be conducted if necessary;
(5) Taking corrective actions, including design and management corrective actions;
(6) The effectiveness verification work of corrective measures;
(7) Drawing inferences about the work situation;
(8) Managing the resetting situations;
(9) Summary of materials such as reports and minutes formed during the resetting process;
(10) Other related content.

6.2.6.2 Reliability Index Evaluation

Whether the test is qualified or not shall be judged according to the total effective test time of the sample machine and the total number of responsible failures. When the sample machine reaches the cumulative total effective test time T, if the number of responsible failures is less than or equal to the number of responsible failure judgments (r_0), it is judged as qualified; within the cumulative total effective test time T, if the number of responsible failures is greater than the number number (r_0), it is judged as unqualified.

The timed censored test scheme adopted in this project, the point estimation of MTBF observation value is:

$$\widehat{\theta} = \frac{T}{r} \tag{6.5}$$

In the formula:
T—Cumulative total effective test time;
r—The number of responsible failures observed in the test.

The timed censored test scheme adopted in this project, the lower confidence limit of the MTBF observation value is estimated as:

$$\theta_L = \begin{cases} \frac{2T}{\chi^2_{\left(\frac{1-c}{2},2r+2\right)}} \text{ When receiving} \\ \frac{2T}{\chi^2_{\left(\frac{1-c}{2},2r\right)}} \text{ When rejecting} \end{cases} \tag{6.6}$$

Among them, C is the two-sided confidence level. Generally speaking, for the timed censoring scheme, $C = 1 - 2\beta$; when the timed censoring scheme is not used, the value of C should not be lower than 0.4 (that is, one-sided The confidence level is not less than 70%).

6.2.6.3 Compiling Test Report

After completing the reliability qualification test, the test undertaker shall prepare a reliability qualification test report. The main contents of the reliability appraisal test report are as follows:

(1) Test content, purpose and conclusion;
(2) Test basis;
(3) Test time, place and test participants;
(4) Description of the product under test;
(5) Test statistics plan;
(6) Description of comprehensive environmental conditions and stress application methods;
(7) Conditions of test facilities and instruments;
(8) Preparatory work before the test;
(9) Description of the test process;
(10) The number of failures, failure classification and failure handling during the test;
(11) Reliability assessment conclusion;
(12) Existing problems and suggestions;
(13) Other relevant matters that need to be explained.

6.2.6.4 Test Completion Inspection

When necessary, the test results should be inspected after the test to assess whether the test results meet the requirements of the contract, product specifications and test program. The completion of the test should mainly check the following contents:

(1) Integrity of test records and reports, including test logs, test facility monitoring records, test product test records, failure reset reports, reliability identification test reports, and test summary reports;
(2) Whether the failure handling method and failure diagnosis during the test are correct, and whether the measures taken are effective;
(3) The rationality of the test result analysis, if the test is terminated early, whether the basis is sufficient;
(4) Unresolved problems and failures and expected improvement measures;
(5) Completion of the work items specified according to the preliminary review results.

6.3 Electrical Equipment Reliability Enhancement Test Technology

6.3.1 Intensive Test Introduction

With the development of science and technology, the complexity of digital diagnosis and treatment equipment is getting higher and higher, and the traditional reliability environment simulation test can no longer meet the development requirements. Due to the shortcomings of long cycle, low efficiency and high cost in environmental simulation tests, a new type of reliability test technology—reliability enhancement test has been born. Its biggest advantage is that it is efficient, economical and thorough in exposing problems.

The proposal of the reliability enhancement test solution first comes from the requirements of aviation airborne equipment. Therefore, the typical reliability enhancement test stress mainly applies the typical use stress types with the best effect on the exposure of airborne equipment- high temperature, low temperature, rapid temperature Change, vibration and its comprehensive stress.

The generalized reliability enhancement test can select various stresses that can most effectively stimulate the failure of the product under test and have good consistency with the failure mode that occurs in the actual use of the product, and is not limited to the existing typical reliability enhancement test equipment and its applied stress.

For ease of understanding, we mainly elaborate on the existing typical reliability enhancement test ideas and methods, and other stress reliability enhancement tests can be designed with reference to typical reliability enhancement tests.

The reliability enhancement test adopts the method of systematically applying step stress to the sample, allowing the sample to withstand gradually increasing environmental stress (mainly temperature, temperature change, vibration and comprehensive), additional stress (power cycle on and off, voltage bias and frequency Pull deviation, etc.) and working load (such as speed, torque, etc.), stimulate product defects, expose weak links, determine the working limit and damage limit of the product, and provide information for product improvement design in a short period of time. In order to quickly and fully stimulate defects, the stress imposed by the reliability enhancement test can greatly exceed the limit of the technical specification, but the failure mechanism of the product should not be changed, causing the failures exposed in the test to be irrelevant to the actual field use.

If the number of failures exposed by the test per unit time is measured, a large amount of engineering experience shows that the efficiency of the reliability enhancement test is dozens or even hundreds of times that of the traditional reliability test. Therefore, reliability enhancement test technology has been widely recognized and widely used by international equipment manufacturing giants.

6.3.1.1 Commonly Used Terms

Step Stress Test: In order to explore, determine, and improve the working limit or damage limit of the sample machine, a multi-step, gradually increasing stress test is adopted. Usually includes low temperature step test, high temperature step test, vibration step test. For other test stresses, step stress tests may also be adopted when the bearing capacity of the test machine is uncertain.

Working Limit: Under a certain stress condition of the step test, the sample machine no longer meets the requirements of the technical conditions, but after the test stress is stopped, the test sample can still return to the normal working state. The stress condition of the step test It is the stress working limit of the test machine.

Destruction Limit: Under a certain stress condition of the step test, the sample machine no longer meets the technical requirements, and after the test stress is stopped, the test sample machine can no longer return to the normal working state. The stress condition of the step test It is the stress failure limit of the test machine.

Micro-flutter Vibration: In order to prevent the high vibration value from covering up the failure point that has been excited in the electrical system, the vibration value is reduced to a low level to detect whether the failure occurs.

Comprehensive Stress Test: a test in which two or more (including two) test stresses are applied simultaneously. Usually includes rapid temperature change—vibration comprehensive stress test, temperature and humidity comprehensive stress test, temperature and humidity—vibration comprehensive stress test.

Regression Verification: After the reliability enhancement test of the sample machine, corrective measures have been taken to improve it. In order to verify the effectiveness of the corrective measures and evaluate the possible negative impact of the corrective measures on the sample machine, the improved sample is used Carry out the reliability enhancement test again.

6.3.1.2 Development History and Application Status

In some industrially developed countries abroad, especially the United States, reliability enhancement tests have been widely accepted and widely used by a large number of international manufacturing companies.

As early as the 1970s, many products on equipment exposed a large number of problems. The United States set up an expert group to conduct research. At that time, it was found that a large number of problems could be stimulated by rapid temperature changes and random vibrations, so environmental stress screening was proposed for the first time. Screening is classified as impact test, the earliest representative of provocative test, since there is no special accelerated test in the design stage, it is used in the early design to stimulate possible problems.

In the 1990s, some test procedures have been formed to determine the reliability enhancement test. The reliability enhancement test is a test method for design quality verification and manufacturing quality verification extended by the US military, and has now become the standard digital diagnostic equipment in the US electronics industry. Verification methods, such as GE, HP, IBM and other international equipment manufacturing giants use a large number of reliability enhancement tests. After applying this method, the new product reliability test, which originally took six months to one year, can now be completed in only one week, and the problems found in the digital diagnosis and treatment equipment products during this week are almost the same as those found in the actual application of customers Therefore, the reliability enhancement test method has become a test that new digital medical equipment must pass before it goes on the market.

According to the figures released by Hobbs Engineering Company of the United States in 1988, after adopting the reliability enhancement test for printers, the MTBF increased by 838 times, and the MTBF of other computer peripheral equipment increased by 4.7 times; for the power supply equipment that has been produced for 4 years, only press IEC guidelines for temperature screening, the effectiveness of use is 94%, and the effectiveness of the reliability enhancement test is 99.6%, reaching 99.7% within the first two months of production, and the MTBF of field use is greater than 64,000 h. The effectiveness of various power supplies of his company increased from 67% to 99.5% after the reliability enhancement test was applied.

The reliability enhancement test is a means, it will not improve the reliability of the product, only by analyzing and improving the problems it stimulates, and expanding the environmental resistance, the reliability of the product can be improved, so the experience of failure analysis is very important for product improvement has a very large effect. A large number of European and American companies have already used reliability enhancement testing as one of the R&D and production assessment tests. Absorbing and adopting the reliability enhancement testing enterprise specifications of international companies can help us accumulate experience in reliability enhancement testing program design and engineering implementation.

6.3.1.3 Principle of Reliability Enhancement Test

The reliability enhancement test is different from the traditional reliability test, it belongs to the excitation test, its test conditions are not simulated the real environment, but the targeted application of stress to achieve the purpose of rapid excitation failure. The comparison between the traditional reliability test and the enhancement test is shown in Table 6.6. For the comparison between the traditional reliability test and the enhancement test, see Table 6.6. By applying step-by-step stress, the potential defects of the product are continuously stimulated, and the improvement and verification are carried out, so that the reliability of the product is continuously improved. Reliability enhancement test is a kind of test of development nature, not for the purpose of assessing the reliability level of products, but for failure and failure as the main research object. Quickly stimulate product defects and expose weak links in product design by applying environmental stress higher than the product specification, find and improve the working limit and damage limit of the product, and at the same time, through the mechanism analysis of failures and failures during the test, Take improvement measures to achieve the purpose of finding and correcting defects as early as possible.

The principle of enhanced reliability test can be explained by the simplest stress intensity interference model. The strength of the product is assumed to obey a certain distribution, but in actual use there will be an environmental stress, which may be temperature, vibration or humidity, and its strength is also a distribution. It is assumed that once the product strength is less than the environmental stress product, failure will occur. Then the larger the overlapping portion (shaded area) of stress and strength, the higher the probability of failure. Figure 6.7 shows the stress intensity distribution model for product failure.

Table 6.6 Comparison of traditional reliability test and enhanced test

Content	Traditional reliability test	Enhanced reliability test
Test purposes	Assess the reliability level of the product	Quickly expose potential defects in the product
Test type	Environmental simulation test	challenge test
Test stress	Simulates typical environmental conditions experienced by the product in actual use	Gradually increase the test stress value from small to large, which may exceed the product stress limit, which is more severe than the actual environmental conditions of the product
The basis for determining the test plan	Determined according to statistical principles	According to the failure mechanism of the product and the results of failure physical analysis

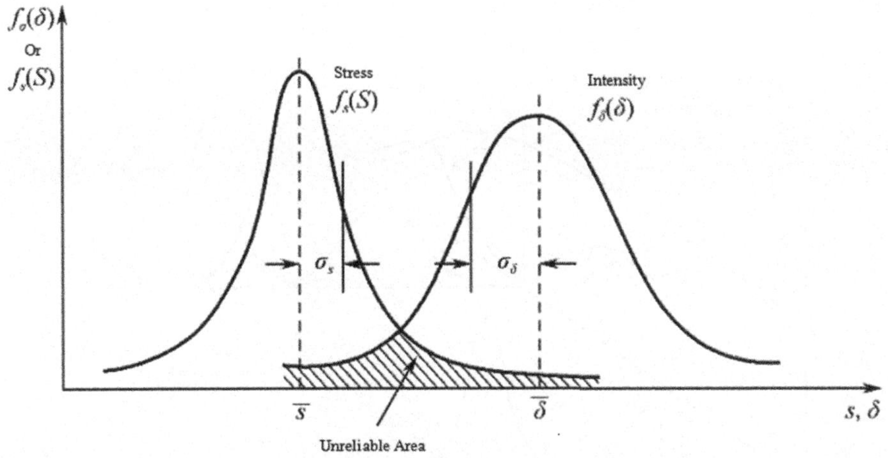

Fig. 6.7 Stress intensity distribution model for product failure

The environmental stress remains constant over time, but the strength of the product will gradually weaken, and the overlap between stress and strength will become larger and larger, as shown in Fig. 6.8. To improve this situation, one is to reduce environmental stress, and the other is to increase product strength. However, the environmental stress is generally constant during the use of the product, so the greater the design margin for the strength of the product, the higher the reliability of the product. If the initial strength of the product is high enough, it will maintain a high level even if it degrades over time.

In the design stage of the product, the use of intensive testing means and the way of applying strong stress can expose the failures in the product life cycle in advance, find out the weak points in the design, and make preventive improvements, thereby improving the robustness of the product. According to a large number of research reports in the United States, 80% of external field problems can be exposed through rapid temperature changes followed by random vibration tests.

After the product is designed, theoretically, it should go through simulation analysis, and then strengthen the test after improvement, that is to say, the reliability enhancement test should be carried out at the beginning of the sample, so that the cost-effectiveness ratio is the highest. There are two contributions of the intensified test: first, the reliability test is very useful for process design defects that fail early; second, the useful end of the bottom of the pre-stored curve minimizes its failure rate, so it mainly affects the front Two phases, namely intensive test accelerated life test, high accelerated stress screening. These three tests add up to the latest accelerated stress test system that is more popular in the world. The position of reliability enhancement test in the product design and production cycle of digital medical equipment is shown in Fig. 6.9.

The relationship between the reliability enhancement test method and the corresponding reliability pot-shaped curve is shown in Fig. 6.10.

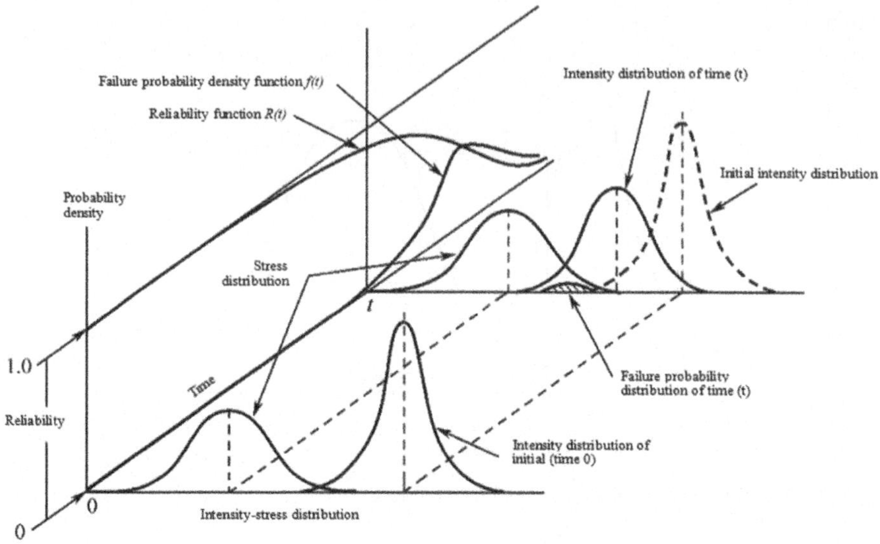

Fig. 6.8 Schematic diagram of the relationship between strength—stress distribution and failure time mode

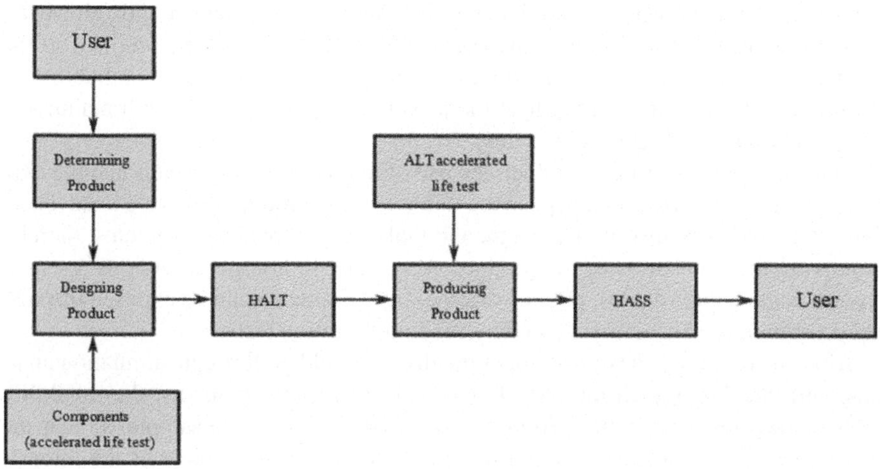

Fig. 6.9 The position of reliability enhancement test in the product design and production cycle of digital medical equipment

Through the intensive test, two kinds of limits of the product can be obtained. One is called the working limit of the product. After the limit is exceeded, the product will not work normally. When the stress is below the working limit, the product will return to normal. There is also a damage limit. After reaching this limit, the product is completely destroyed and cannot be restored to normal. By widening the working

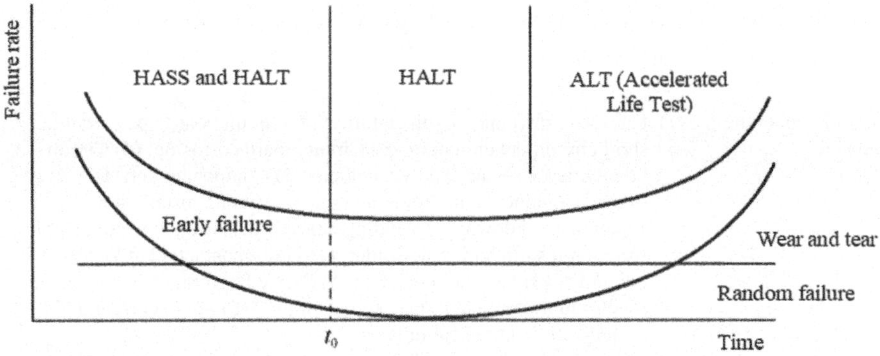

Fig. 6.10 The relationship between the reliability enhancement test method and the corresponding reliability pot-shaped curve

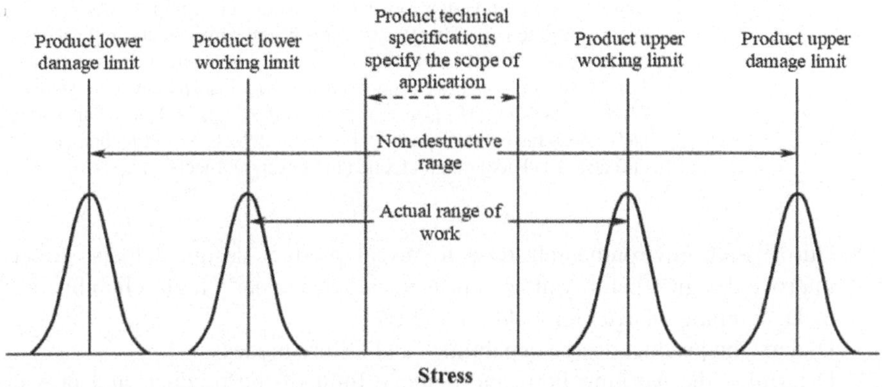

Fig. 6.11 Broaden the working limit and improve environmental resistance

limit, the ability to withstand the environment can be improved, thereby improving the reliability of the product, as shown in Fig. 6.11.

6.3.1.4 Various Environmental Stress Intensification Effects

See Table 6.7 for the failure modes that can be induced by the environmental stress that is often applied in the reliability enhancement test under normal conditions.

6.3.1.5 Function of Reliability Enhancement Test

The functions of the reliability enhancement test are as follows:

Table 6.7 Environmental stresses and correspondingly excited failure modes

Environmental stress	Trigger failure mode
Rapid temperature change	(1) Parameter drift and circuit stability; (2) Circuit board open circuit, short circuit, delamination; (3) Circuit board corrosion; (4) Circuit board cracks, surface and via defects; (5) Component defects; (6) Loose components, improper assembly or wrong installation; (7) Junction breakdown; (8) Welding defects such as open welding, cold welding, insufficient or no solder; (10) Poor contact; (11) Weak bonding; (12) Fastener defects; (13) Brittle fracture; (14) Electromigration; (15) Thermal matching; (16) Surge current; (17) Metallization; (18) Seal failure
Humidity	(1) Electrical short circuit; (2) Active components stuck; (3) Circuit board corrosion; (4) Surface layer damage; (5) Performance degradation of insulating materials, etc.
Vibration	(1) The circuit board is open or short−circuited; (2) The components are improperly assembled or loose; (3) The adjacent components are short−circuited; (4) The pins or wires of the components are broken or defective; (5) The IC socket is defective; (6) Welding defects such as virtual welding, open welding, cold welding, insufficient or no solder; (7) Weak bonding; (8) Loose or poor connection; (9) Loose hardware; (10) Loose fasteners or pads; (11) crystal defects; (12) Mechanical defects; (13) Packaging defects; (14) Foreign objects, etc.

(1) Utilize high environmental stress to reveal product design defects, greatly improve design reliability after improvement, ensure early high reliability, and make equipment have high field reliability;
(2) Understand product design capabilities and failure modes;
(3) Determine the working limit and damage limit of the product, and provide reference for the design of test conditions for other tests;
(4) Quickly find out the flaws in the product development process, and greatly reduce the failures in the identification test;
(5) Increase product reliability and reduce maintenance costs;
(6) Establish a product design capability database as a basis for research and development and shorten design and manufacturing time.

6.3.2 General Requirements for Reliability Enhancement Test

6.3.2.1 Connotation of Reliability Enhancement Test

Reliability enhancement test is to quickly stimulate product defects and expose product weak links by applying stress higher than the product specification, and find the working limit and damage limit of the product; at the same time, through the positioning analysis and failure mechanism of the failures that occur during the test

Analyze and take improvement measures to improve the working limit and damage limit of the product, and realize the improvement of product reliability.

The reliability enhancement test belongs to the development test and engineering test. It is not aimed at assessing and verifying product reliability indicators. It is mainly to quickly stimulate and fully expose failures, provide input for product improvement, improve product environmental resistance and robustness, and improve product maturity. Accuracy and reliability, shorten product development cycle and speed up product launch.

6.3.2.2 Selection of the Timing of Tests

For users with a good reliability work foundation, the reliability enhancement test is recommended to be carried out before the end of the initial sample stage of the sample machine. After the functional performance verification of the initial sample is completed, the reliability enhancement test can be carried out to fully expose the potential defects of the prototype as soon as possible. Implement improvement and verification as early as possible to reduce quality loss time and economic costs.

For users with weak reliability work foundation, it is recommended to carry out the reliability enhancement test before the end of the prototype phase of the sample machine. After the functional performance verification and routine test tests are completed on the prototype, the reliability enhancement test is carried out to further expose the potential defects of the prototype., to achieve a rapid and significant improvement in the reliability of the prototype.

6.3.2.3 Stress of Reliability Enhancement Test

Stresses that can fully and quickly expose failures can be used as reliability enhancement test stresses, which may include high temperature, low temperature, rapid temperature changes and their combination, and may also include alternating damp heat, electrical stress pull, increased power, and increased working load, working frequency acceleration, etc., the selection mainly considers the typical environmental stress types in actual use, the effectiveness of stimulating failures, and the consistency between the stimulated failure mode and the actual use of the entire life cycle.

6.3.2.4 Equipment for Reliability Enhancement Test

Common reliability enhancement test equipment is comprehensive environmental stress reliability enhancement test system, including air hammer three-axis six-degree-of-freedom ultra-Gaussian random vibration test bench and rapid temperature change test chamber. The stresses that can be applied mainly include low temperature, high temperature, rapid Temperature change, three-axis six-degree-of-freedom vibration and its comprehensive stress.

Considering the typical temperature and humidity working environment and effects of the core components of digital medical equipment, a temperature—humidity—vibration comprehensive environmental stress reliability test chamber can also be used to implement reliability enhancement tests. The stresses that can be applied mainly include low temperature, high temperature, and high temperature—high Humidity, rapid temperature change, uniaxial random vibration and its combined stress.

For some core components of digital medical equipment, which may be mechanical products or electromechanical products, the working load is the main stress that leads to their failure. Large working load stress, increased electrical stress (voltage, current or power consumption, etc.), etc.

For the core components of some digital diagnostic equipment, which may be metal structural parts, corrosion is the main failure mode during long-term use. The reliability enhancement test can use a composite salt spray test chamber to enhance the temperature, salt spray concentration and comprehensive stress, and quickly expose Corrosion defects of metal material structural parts; it may be polymer material parts, and aging is its main failure mode during long-term use. The reliability enhancement test can use xenon lamp aging test chamber to increase temperature, light intensity and comprehensive stress, and quickly expose high Aging defects in molecular material pieces.

6.3.2.5 Determination Principles of Working Limit and Damage Limit

The function and performance of the test machine at this temperature step can meet the product technical conditions requirements, this temperature step is not used as the temperature working limit or temperature damage limit, and so on. Until the failure of a certain temperature step can no longer be improved with the existing technology, the temperature step will be used as the high (low) temperature working limit or high (low) temperature damage limit of the sample machine (if the sample machine is directly found The high (low) temperature damage limit, then the high (low) temperature damage limit is taken as the high (low) temperature working limit). In principle, if a certain part of the sample machine can take protective measures (local temperature protection or isolation outside the test chamber, etc.) The temperature working limit or temperature damage limit of the non-protected part of the prototype.

6.3.2.6 Determination Principles of Vibration Working Limit and Vibration Damage Limit

In the stage of vibration step stress test, when the test machine fails on a certain vibration platform, if it can be improved or repaired, the test can be continued, and the function and performance of the test machine on this vibration platform meet the product technical requirements. If conditions require, this vibration step will not be used as the vibration working limit or vibration damage limit, and so on. Until the failure of a certain vibration step can no longer be improved with the existing technology, the vibration step is used as the vibration work limit or vibration damage limit of the sample machine (if the vibration damage limit of the sample machine is directly found, the vibration damage The upper limit is taken as the vibration working limit). In principle, if a certain part of the subject machine can take protective measures (isolation outside the test chamber, etc.) to continue the test, it can be determined that the subject machine is not protected Part of the vibration work limit or vibration damage limit.

6.3.2.7 Determination Principles of Other Stress Working Limit and Failure Limit

Generally speaking, electrical stress (power, voltage, current, etc.), mechanical load (rotational speed, load, etc.) and other stress types have working limits and damage limits. The method of finding limit values for these stresses is similar to vibration and temperature stress.

For temperature and humidity stress, the humidity range is limited, usually between 0 and 98%RH, and temperature and humidity tests are often carried out according to equipment capabilities. The limit of high temperature and high humidity conditions of the temperature and humidity test chamber is roughly (95 °C, 95%RH).

6.3.3 Preparations Before the Test

Before carrying out the reliability enhancement test, the developer should complete the following preparatory work:

(1) Technical information (development mission statement or technical requirements, product manual, electrical system test rules, test outline, etc.);
(2) Subject sample machine (clear composition, technical status, size, weight, quantity, etc.);
(3) Chassis (shell) of the test machine;
(4) Equipment and water, electricity and water facilities for reliability enhancement tests that can meet the test requirements;
(5) Fixtures, test fixtures and their connecting cables (used for installation and testing of the sample machine);
(6) Guarantee equipment and load devices (power supply, computer, simulated load, etc. required for the normal operation of the sample machine);
(7) Instruments and meters for testing and monitoring (within the validity period of measurement and calibration);
(8) Troubleshooting, maintenance tools and spare parts;
(9) Prototype technical support team (including testing, troubleshooting and maintenance).

6.3.3.1 Technical Data Requirements

Before the reliability enhancement test, the following information should be completed as much as possible:

(1) Relevant technical information: development mission statement or technical requirements, product instructions, etc., to ensure the reasonable formulation of the test program;
(2) Test rules: specify all test items, qualification criteria, test conditions and test methods of the prototype, and give suggestions for test items before, during and after verification;
(3) Operation and maintenance instructions: clarify the requirements for the operating conditions of the prototype (power supply, air source, cooling, load, etc.), typical operating conditions and their operating ratios, and maintenance requirements;
(4) Component list and FME (C) A review: the development unit shall provide the component information sheet of the tested product, the FME (C) A analysis report and the failure summary table found in the process of production, test and inspection, test We should focus on weak links such as components and parts with lower quality grades and weaker temperature and vibration resistance;
(5) Outline of Reliability Enhancement Test: Specify the purpose of the test, reference standards and documents, requirements of the sample machine, test conditions and methods, test items and qualification criteria, test equipment and test instruments, etc., to ensure that the test work meets the requirements of the outline.

6.3.3.2 Preparation of the Sample Machine

1. **Technical Status Requirements**

(1) Electrical equipment should be debugged and optimized, functional performance tested, meet the technical requirements, and the functional performance is basically stable;
(2) The function of the test sample represents the expected function and performance design indicators of the product, the quality of components and materials, and the level of manufacturing technology;
(3) (If any) Prototype environmental test and environmental stress screening should be arranged before the reliability enhancement test, and it is ensured that corrective measures have been taken for the problems in the above tests and the failure reset has been completed.

2. **Clear Quantity Requirements**

The number of sample machines for electrical equipment used for reliability enhancement tests is generally 2 to 4 (sets). The maximum number of samples can be determined according to the number of prototypes that can be installed on the vibration table of the reliability enhancement test, so as to ensure that the prototypes can be tested in batches.

3. **Clear Prototype Information**

Before the test, it is necessary to clearly provide information such as the composition, function, size, weight, installation requirements, power supply requirements and operating conditions of the prototype.

6.3.3.3 The Shell (Chasis) of the Test Machine

In order to allow the enhancement stress to quickly penetrate into the prototype and quickly achieve stability, the shell (chassis) with better sealing performance of the prototype can be removed, or the hollow shell (chassis) can be specially processed for testing.

When designing the casing (chassis), it should be considered to take necessary protective measures to prevent water accumulation inside the electrical system, and to avoid abnormal damage to the prototype caused by abnormal condensation and frosting of the electrical system.

6.3.3.4 Support Equipment and Load Devices

The protection equipment is mainly to provide the power supply, signal and gas source required for the electrical system to work.

The load device is mainly to provide protection for the electrical system to perform the control function.

The operation of the protection equipment and the load device should be safe and convenient, and the connection with the prototype of the electrical system should be firm and reliable. The cables required to connect with the prototype should be consistent with those actually used, and the influence of signal attenuation caused by the length of the connecting cable should be considered and corresponding compensation measures.

6.3.3.5 Fixtures and Test Fixtures

1. **Fixtures**

Fixtures are mainly used for installation and fixing of electrical systems, and should be consistent with the actual vibration environment of electrical systems in digital medical equipment. Fixtures should have good vibration transmission characteristics, sufficient rigidity, strength and durability to ensure that the stress can quickly penetrate into the electrical system and quickly reach stability, and ensure that the prototype is firmly and reliably installed and fixed under high-intensity test conditions. At the same time, the fixture should be as convenient as possible for prototype testing and improve testing efficiency, avoiding the need for out-of-box testing during testing. During the reliability enhancement test of the core components of digital medical equipment, in order to achieve the purpose of quickly penetrating the stress into the product and quickly achieving stability, for the test samples with a better sealing shell (chassis), the shell can be removed or the shell can be used. Hollow out the casing (chassis), and at the same time, raise the bottom of the sample machine as high as possible, and place it on a fixture (bracket) with large holes. At the same time, it should be considered that there may be abnormal conditions of condensation and frosting inside the product during the experiment, and necessary protective measures should be taken to prevent water accumulation inside the product and avoid abnormal damage to the prototype. When the sample machine is subjected to a vibration stress test or a comprehensive environmental stress test with vibration, the sample machine should be rigidly installed on the vibration table as directly as possible (or with a clamp). If the sample machine is equipped with an external shock absorber, the test shall be performed after the external shock absorber is removed.

2. **Test Fixtures and Connecting Cables**

Test fixtures and connecting cables are mainly used for testing electrical systems to improve test efficiency and reliability. The test fixture can efficiently connect cables, signal lines, data lines, etc. through test adapters and other equipment; connect buttons, switches and other hardware operating components to the adapter outside the test box to avoid the need to enter the box during the test.

6.3.3.6 Instruments and Gauges for Testing and Monitoring

The instruments and gauges used for testing and monitoring shall meet the test requirements of prototype functional performance indicators and meet the following requirements:

(1) It should have a measurement certificate issued by an accreditation agency and be within the valid period of measurement qualification;
(2) The accuracy should be at least one-third of the tolerance of the measured parameter;
(3) Able to adapt to the measured environmental conditions.

In order to strengthen the monitoring of the status of the prototype during the test, the main functions and performance parameters of the prototype can be monitored through the monitoring system. In order to reduce the monitoring burden of personnel, the monitoring system can be equipped with automatic testing functions and data storage functions.

6.3.3.7 Troubleshooting, Repair Tools and Spare Parts

Troubleshooting and maintenance tools usually include soldering iron, solder, etc., and prepare a certain number of spare parts that are expected to fail.

6.3.3.8 Test Equipment

In order to fully apply various stresses in a typical service environment, the number of required test equipment should be reduced as much as possible according to the capability of the test equipment, and the comprehensive stress reliability enhancement test should be applied after the step test. In the case of being limited by the type of stress applied by the test equipment, multiple test equipment may be used in the reliability enhancement test, and multiple equipment may be used in series to apply the required enhancement stress.

The equipment for the reliability enhancement test shall meet the following capability requirements:

(1) The test temperature capability range is not less than –70 °C–+150 °C;
(2) It has the ability of rapid temperature rise and fall, and the maximum temperature change rate is not less than 5 °C/minute;
(3) The vibration stress application capability of the equipment shall meet one of the following two conditions:

- With a three-axis six-degree-of-freedom vibration table, the vibration bandwidth is not less than 5-5000 Hz, and the vibration stress range requires that the *Z* -axis should not be less than $60g_{rms}$, and *the X*- axis and *Y*- axis should not be less than $30g_{rms}$;
- Equipped with an electromagnetic vibrating table, which meets the GJB 1032 vibration spectrum type diagram, the vibration bandwidth is not less than 5-2000 Hz, the root mean square acceleration ($G_{rms} \geq 13.56g_{rms}$) or power spectral density ($W \geq 0.20$ g ^{2}/Hz) of the vibration stress range, GJB 1032 random vibration reference spectrum is shown in Fig. 6.12.

(4) When other special stresses are used to carry out reliability enhancement tests, the test equipment should meet the requirements for applying relevant stresses.

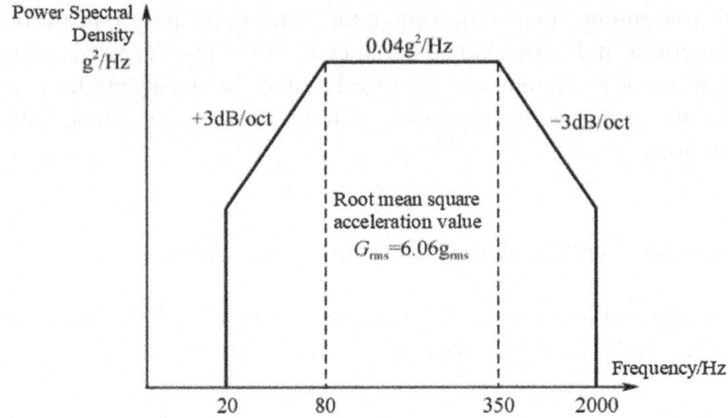

Fig. 6.12 GJB 1032 random vibration reference spectrum

6.3.3.9 Testing and Technical Support Team

In order to ensure the progress of the reliability enhancement test and improve the efficiency of failure analysis and location during the test process, the test support team should guarantee the test organization and implementation and the test duty arrangement, and the prototype technical support team should guarantee the prototype functional performance test, failure analysis and location, maintenance and improvement work.

6.3.3.10 Test Program

The reliability enhancement test program is the basis for the reliability enhancement test of the tested product. In combination with the specific situation of the product, the reliability enhancement test program generally includes the following contents:

(1) Purpose of the test;
(2) Scope of application;
(3) Reference standards and documents;
(4) Description of the product under test (including product composition, function, performance, technical status, quantity, etc.);
(5) Description and requirements of test equipment and testing instruments;
(6) Test plan;
(7) Test conditions;
(8) Testing requirements for performance and functions (including testing items, content, methods, etc., which can reflect the main functions and performance of the working status of the product under test);
(9) Failure criterion, failure classification and failure statistics;
(10) Troubleshooting;

(11) Regression verification;
(12) Implementation of corrective measures;
(13) Requirements for collection, recording and processing of test data;
(14) Regulations on organizational structure and test management;
(15) Others.

6.3.3.11 Temperature Inspection

Before carrying out the reliability enhancement test, an infrared thermal imager should be used to conduct a non-contact temperature survey of the product under test or a temperature patrol instrument should be used to conduct a contact temperature survey of the product under test, so as to understand the thermal distribution and temperature of the product under test. It provides a reference for the arrangement of the temperature sensor in the test. In principle, the temperature sensor should be arranged at the heat concentration point of the circuit board of the product under test, or the part that the designer pays attention to.

6.3.3.12 Vibration Inspection

Before carrying out the reliability enhancement test, conduct a vibration response survey on the product under test to get a preliminary understanding of the vibration response characteristics of the product under test. In order to obtain the vibration value of the test point, it can provide reference for troubleshooting in the test.

6.3.3.13 Pre-test Examination

After the preparatory work before each test is completed, the test working group holds a pre-test examination meeting to review the technical status of the tested product, test equipment, test instruments, product installation, temperature investigation, vibration investigation and related technical information. Check to determine whether the relevant provisions of the test program are met.

6.3.4 Intensive Test Implementation

6.3.4.1 Test Organization Management

For the management and monitoring of the test. The test party is fully responsible for the test work, including formulating relevant rules and regulations, comprehensively arranging the implementation of the test, troubleshooting and handling of emergencies, etc. The research and development unit participates in the test working group as a member, and is responsible for technical support such as function and performance detection of the tested product, failure analysis and improvement work during the test. The purchaser is responsible for monitoring the whole process of the test, including the performance test and function check of the tested product, checking and signing various test records.

6.3.4.2 Workflow and Implementation Points

Reliability enhancement tests generally include: pre-test preparation, single-stress step-by-step, multi-stress synthesis, and regression verification. At the same time, failures are processed, analyzed, and corrected during the entire test process.

For the reliability enhancement test of single stress, the steps that can usually be taken are: step stress (feel out the ultimate stress), ultimate stress (short-time) operation, constant value—limit alternating operation or extreme alternating operation at both ends; at the same time Accompanied by the repeated process of stress application—stop, the start-up state of the prototype is assessed.

For the temperature and humidity—vibration stress reliability enhancement test, the following steps can usually be used: constant temperature and humidity step (feel out the working limit), vibration step (feel out the vibration limit), constant temperature and humidity—vibration working limit (short-term) Operation, constant temperature and humidity vibration comprehensive stress test.

In addition to the prototype, spare parts, maintenance tools and consumables, test instruments, test equipment, documents and personnel (usually including test, maintenance, design, process professionals), the preparation before the test mainly investigates and tests the stress to be applied by the test. Clear sensitive stress points so that monitoring points can be arranged during the test and necessary local stress protection measures can be taken. When simplifying the implementation of reliability enhancement experiments, stress investigation work can also be exempted.

After the prototype has undergone the reliability enhancement test, based on the preliminary corrective measures taken on site, further thorough corrective measures will be taken for the failures in the test, and the management of failure reset will be supplemented and perfected. After the prototype is improved, the reliability enhancement test will be carried out again verify. Generally speaking, the final step of the comprehensive stress test is used for verification, and the comprehensive test verification can also be carried out in strict accordance with the previous steps of the reliability enhancement test, which may further discover the problems of the prototype and increase the stress resistance limit.

6.3.4.3 Classical Reliability Enhancement Test Process

For the most typical rapid temperature change—vibration stress reliability enhancement test, the steps are usually as follows: (1) preparation before the test; (2) low

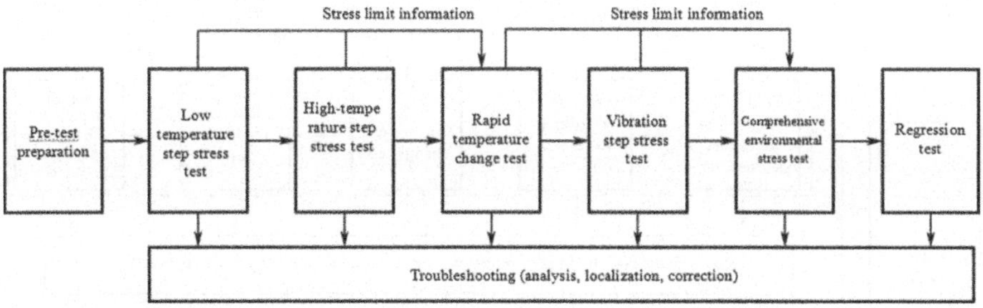

Fig. 6.13 General steps of reliability enhancement test

temperature step stress test; (3) high temperature step stress test; (4) rapid temperature change (5) Vibration step stress test; (6) Comprehensive environmental stress test; (7) Regression verification and other stages. The general steps of the reliability enhancement test are shown in Fig. 6.13. Among them, steps (2) to (6) are typical 5 steps of reliability enhancement test.

6.3.4.4 Implementation Process of Enhanced Reliability Test

According to the typical characteristics of the use environment of electrical equipment, the reliability enhancement test can take low temperature step, high temperature step, rapid temperature change, temperature and humidity integrated, vibration step, rapid temperature change—vibration integrated, temperature and humidity—vibration integrated and other typical stress test items.

In order to shorten the test cycle, the research and development party can divide the electrical equipment prototype into two groups (group A and group B), and carry out rapid temperature change—vibration stress reliability enhancement test and temperature humidity—vibration stress reliability enhancement test respectively. Reliability enhancement test The implementation process is shown in Fig. 6.14.

Group A rapid temperature change—vibration stress reliability enhancement test steps are as follows: (1) Low temperature step stress test; (2) High temperature step stress test; (3) Rapid temperature change test; (4) Vibration step stress test; (5) Rapid temperature change—vibration comprehensive environmental stress test.

Group B temperature and humidity—vibration stress reliability enhancement test steps are as follows: (1) 40 °C constant damp heat test; (2) 55 °C constant damp heat test; (3) 30–60 °C alternating damp heat test; (4) temperature and humidity–Vibration comprehensive stress test.

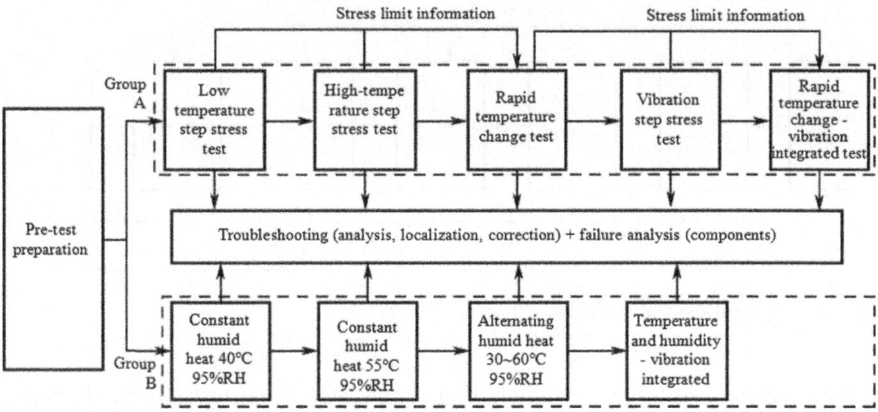

Fig. 6.14 Reliability enhancement test implementation process

The research and development party can choose to carry out some test items according to the composition characteristics of the test object and the ability of the test equipment, and can also adjust the test condition parameter settings in the test items, such as temperature change rate, temperature holding time, etc., to encourage the research and development party to maximize the application of The technical method quickly and fully exposes the failure of the developed electrical equipment. See Table 6.8 for reliability enhancement test items and tailoring requirements.

Table 6.8 Reliability enhancement test items and cutting requirements

Serial number	Reliability enhancement test items	Whether to choose	Test conditions and time	Tailoring requirements
A1	Low temperature step			
A2	High temperature step			
A3	Rapid temperature change			
A4	Vibration step			
A5	Rapid temperature change—vibration synthesis			
B1	Constant Damp Heat Step Test			
B2	Constant damp heat limit test			
B3	Alternating damp heat test			

6.3.4.5 Pre-test

After the product under test is installed on the test equipment, a comprehensive function and performance test should be carried out first to ensure that the product is intact before the test stress is applied. Before the formal test, a short-term small-scale vibration pre-test is required to confirm that the tested sample is firmly installed on the table and can effectively transmit energy.

6.3.4.6 Test Implementation

Conduct the test according to the pre-set test profile, and strictly follow the test plan to test, record the test stress data and all information of the tested product.

If a failure occurs during the test, stop the test, record the failure mode and stress level, and locate the failure, and then analyze the cause of the failure. For failures that cannot be analyzed temporarily, they can be left for further analysis and continue to other test steps to find other failures.

6.3.5 Implementation Process of Classical Intensive Test

6.3.5.1 Low Temperature Step Test

In addition to the use of special reliability enhancement test chambers, high temperature chambers, high and low temperature humid heat chambers, rapid temperature change chambers, temperature shock chambers, temperature and humidity comprehensive stress chambers, etc. can be used to carry out low temperature step tests. The test process is as follows:

(1) Refer to Fig. 6.15 for the stress application of the low temperature step test (low temperature step test profile (example));
(2) During the low-temperature step-by-step test, try to remove the sealing cover or shell of the sample machine without affecting the function and performance of the sample machine;
(3) Starting temperature: when the electrical system has not yet experienced the environmental test, take 5 °C as the starting temperature of the low temperature step test; when the electrical system has undergone the environmental test, take the lowest working temperature of the environmental test plus 10 °C as the low temperature The starting temperature of the step test;
(4) Step length condition: –10 °C or –5 °C can be selected as the step length for each step according to the tolerance capacity and test efficiency of the sample machine;

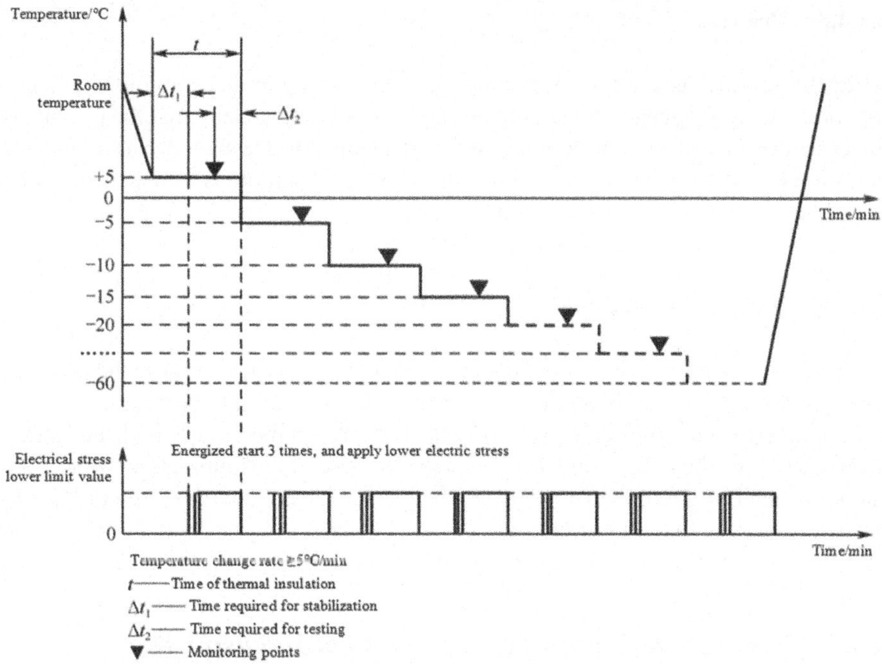

Fig. 6.15 Low temperature step test profile (example)

(5) Holding time: The holding time of each temperature step, *t* minutes, should not be less than the sum of the time required for the sample machine to reach stable temperature and the time required for testing;

(6) Start-up and power-on: After the time required for the sample machine to stabilize at each temperature step t_1 (t_1 should not be less than 10 min), to adjust the electromechanical stress of the sample to the lower limit and carry out 3 start-up tests to assess its start-up ability under low temperature conditions, and then keep the power on until the end of the heat preservation of the step;

(7) Temperature change rate: it should not be lower than 5 °C/min, and a larger temperature change rate can be adopted according to the actual temperature change capability of the test chamber;

(8) Prototype inspection: Before the end of each temperature step, complete the functional performance inspection specified by the sample machine;

(9) Termination condition: In the test planning stage, the minimum operating temperature specified by the sample machine minus 30 °C is the end temperature of the low temperature step stress test. In the test implementation stage, the low temperature step stress test can be carried out as planned or beyond the plan, until it can no longer be stopped when temporary improvement and protection measures on site can no longer be taken.

6.3.5.2 High Temperature Step Test

In addition to special reliability enhancement test chambers, high temperature step tests can be carried out in high temperature chambers, high and low temperature humidity chambers, rapid temperature change chambers, temperature shock chambers, and temperature and humidity comprehensive stress chambers. The test process is as follows:

(1) The stress application of the high temperature step test is shown in Fig. 6.16.
(2) During the step-by-step test at high temperature, try to remove the sealing cover or shell of the sample machine without affecting the function and performance of the sample machine;
(3) Starting temperature: When the electrical system has not yet experienced the environmental test, take 40 °C as the starting temperature of the high temperature step test; when the electrical system has experienced the environmental test, take the maximum operating temperature of the environmental test minus 10 °C as the high temperature The starting temperature of the step test;
(4) Step length conditions: according to the tolerance and test efficiency of the test machine, select + 10 °C or + 5 °C as the step size for each step;
(5) Holding time: the holding time of each temperature step (*t* minutes) should not be less than the sum of the time required for the sample machine to reach stable temperature and the time required for testing;

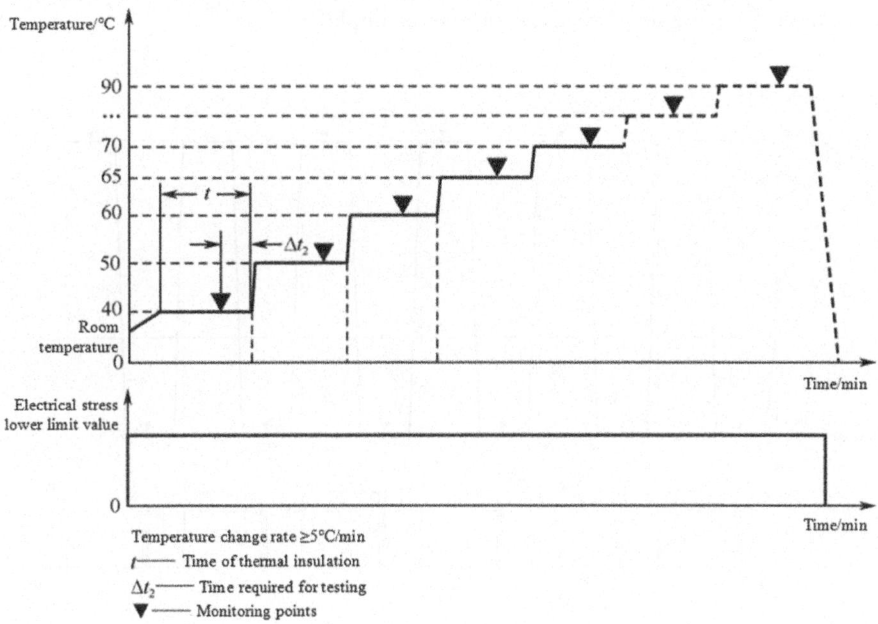

Fig. 6.16 High temperature step test profile (example)

(6) Startup and energization: before the start of the test, adjust the electromechanical stress of the sample to the upper limit, and keep the sample machine energized during the entire high-temperature step test;
(7) Temperature change rate: it should not be lower than 5 °C/min, and a larger temperature change rate can be adopted according to the actual temperature change capability of the test chamber;
(8) Prototype inspection: Before the end of each temperature step, complete the functional performance test specified by the sample machine;
(9) Termination condition: In the stage of test planning, the maximum working temperature specified by the sample machine plus 30 °C can be used as the end temperature of the high temperature step stress test. In the test implementation stage, the high temperature step stress test can be carried out as planned or beyond the plan, until it can no longer be stopped when temporary improvement and protection measures on site can no longer be taken.

6.3.5.3 Rapid Temperature Change Test

In addition to the special reliability enhancement test chamber, the rapid temperature change test can be carried out by using the rapid temperature change chamber, temperature shock chamber, and temperature and humidity comprehensive stress chamber. The test process is as follows:

(1) The stress application of the rapid temperature change test refers to Fig. 6.17 (rapid temperature change test profile (example));

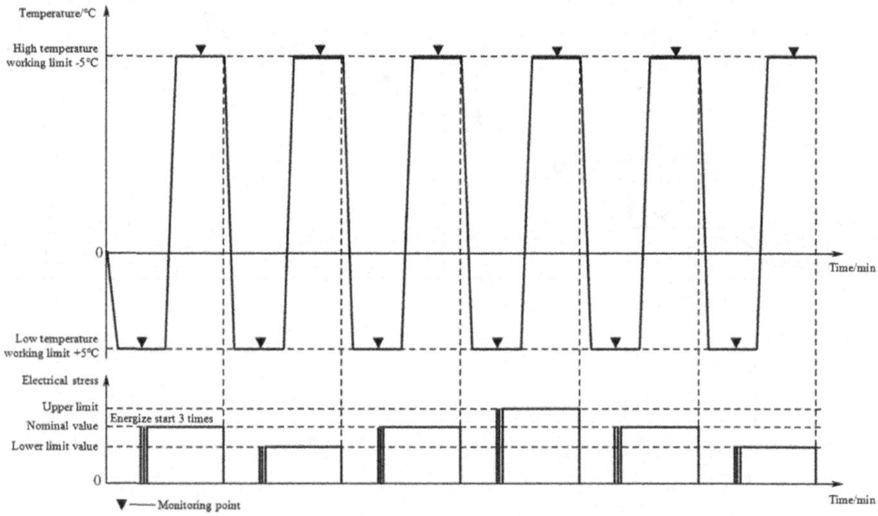

Fig. 6.17 Rapid temperature change test profile (example)

(2) During the rapid temperature change test, try to remove the sealing cover or shell of the sample machine without affecting the function and performance of the sample machine;
(3) Temperature range: the low temperature value is set to increase the low temperature working limit temperature (or the lowest test working temperature) by 5 to 10 °C, and the high temperature value is set to increase the high temperature working limit temperature (or the highest test working temperature) by 5 to 10 °C. The rapid temperature change test starts from the low temperature stage and ends at the high temperature stage;
(4) Holding time: the holding time in the low-temperature stage and high-temperature stage of each cycle should not be less than the sum of the time required for the sample machine to reach temperature stability and the time required for testing;
(5) Start-up and power-on: 3 times of start-up detection after the holding time of 10 min in the low-temperature holding stage of each cycle to assess the start-up ability of the sample machine under rapid temperature changes, and then continue to energize it until the end of the high-temperature holding stage power off;
(6) Number of cycles: no less than 6 cycles;
(7) Electrical stress conditions: During the rapid temperature change process, the electrical stress of the sample machine is applied in the order of "nominal value—lower limit value—nominal value—upper limit value".
(8) Temperature change rate: it should not be lower than 5 °C/min, and a larger temperature change rate can be adopted according to the actual temperature change capability of the test chamber;
(9) Prototype inspection: complete the functional performance test of the prototype before the end of each temperature step;

6.3.5.4 Vibration Step Test

When the air hammer type three-axis six-degree-of-freedom ultra-Gaussian random vibration table is available, the test process is as follows:

(1) For the stress application of the vibration step test, refer to Fig. 6.18 (the section of the three-axis six-degree-of-freedom pneumatic hammer vibration step test (example));
(2) Initial condition: 5 *g*;
(3) Step length condition: 5 *g*;
(4) Holding time: the duration *t* of each vibration level should not be less than 10 min, and the test should be carried out at each vibration step;
(5) Startup and energization: before the start of the test, adjust the electromechanical stress of the sample to the nominal value, and keep the sample machine energized throughout the vibration step test;

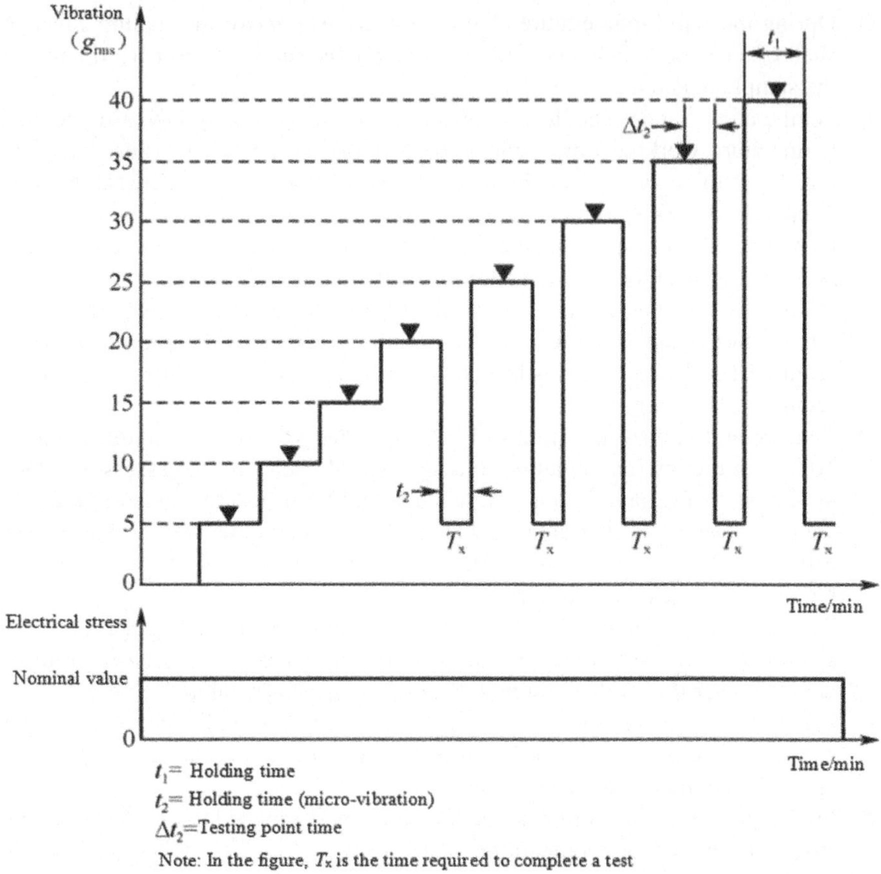

Fig. 6.18 Three-axis six-degree-of-freedom pneumatic hammer vibration step test section (example)

(6) Micro-flutter vibration: When the vibration value exceeds 20 g_{rms}, reduce the vibration value to 5 g_{rms} after the end of each vibration level step, and the vibration duration is generally sufficient to complete the specified test prevail;
(7) Prototype inspection: complete the appearance inspection and functional performance test of the prototype during the application of high-level vibration stress for each vibration, and continue to observe whether the prototype is normal during the application of low-level micro-vibration vibration;
(8) Termination condition: In the test planning stage, it is recommended that the termination condition of the vibration step test should not be lower than 40 g_{rms}. During the implementation stage of the test, the test can be carried out according to the plan or beyond the plan, until it can no longer be stopped when temporary improvement and protection measures on site cannot be taken.

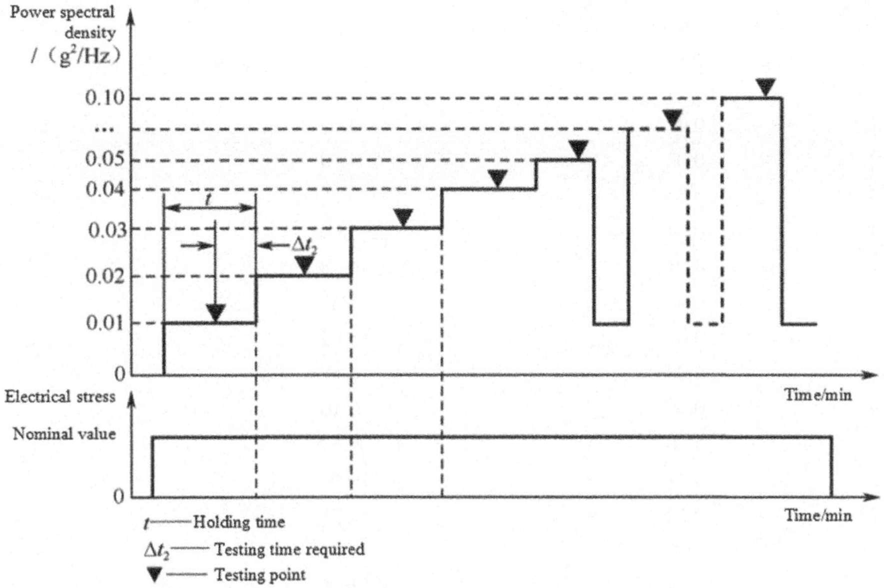

Fig. 6.19 Uniaxial random vibration step test profile (example)

When a (uniaxial) random vibration table is used, the test procedure is as follows:

1. Refer to Fig. 6.18 for the stress application of the vibration step test;
2. Refer to Fig. 6.19 for the random vibration spectrum (single-axis random vibration stepping test profile (example)), frequency range: 20-2000 Hz, using Z -axis random vibration;
3. Initial condition: 0.01 g^2/Hz;
4. Step condition: 0.01 g^2/Hz, see Table 6.9 for details;
5. Holding time: The holding time t of each vibration level should not be less than 10 min, and the test needs to be carried out at each vibration step;
6. Start-up and energization: Before the test starts, adjust the electromechanical stress of the sample to the nominal value, and keep the sample machine energized during the entire vibration step test;
7. Prototype inspection: Complete the prototype appearance inspection and functional performance test before the end of each applied vibration;
8. Termination condition: In the test planning stage, it is recommended that the termination condition of the vibration step test should not be lower than 0.1 g^2/Hz (corresponding to 9.59 g_{rms}). During the implementation stage of the test, the test can be carried out according to the plan or beyond the plan, until it can no longer be stopped when temporary improvement and protection measures on site cannot be taken.

Table 6.9 Random vibration step test conditions

Serial number	Power spectral density (*g* 2/Hz)	Root mean square acceleration value (grms)
1	0.01	3.03
2	0.02	4.29
3	0.03	5.25
4	0.04	6.06
5	0.05	6.78
6	0.06	7.43
7	0.07	8.02
8	0.08	8.58
9	0.09	9.10
10	0.10	9.59
11	0.11	10.06
12	0.12	10.51
13	0.13	10.93
14	0.14	11.35
15	0.15	11.75
16	0.16	12.13
17	0.17	12.50
18	0.18	12.87
19	0.19	13.22
20	0.20	13.56

6.3.5.5 Rapid Temperature Change—Vibration Comprehensive Stress Test

The comprehensive stress test system combined with a special reliability enhancement test box, a rapid temperature change box and a shaking table can carry out a rapid temperature change—vibration comprehensive stress enhancement test. The test process is as follows:

(1) The stress application of the rapid temperature change—vibration comprehensive test refers to Fig. 6.20 (rapid temperature change—vibration comprehensive stress test profile (example));
(2) Rapid temperature change: The stress applied by the rapid temperature change of the sample machine is consistent with the steps in Sect. 6.4.5.3;
(3) Vibration stress: The sample machine is lowered by 1 to 2 orders of magnitude steps on the basis of the working limit of the vibration step stress test, and the corresponding vibration magnitude 10 is applied 15 min before the end of each

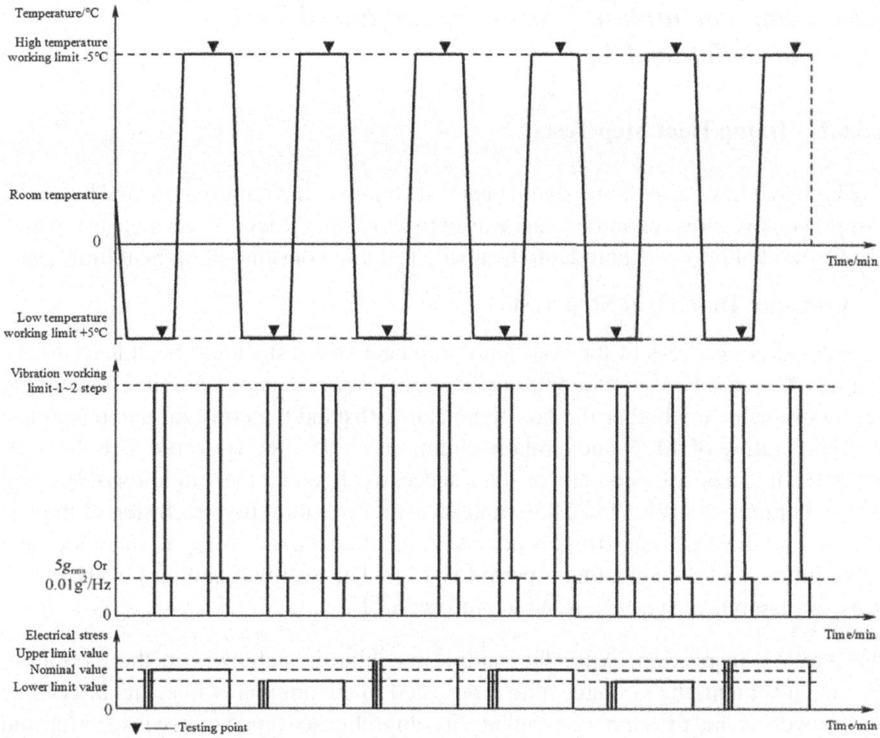

Fig. 6.20 Rapid temperature change—vibration comprehensive stress test profile (example)

rapid temperature-changing heat preservation stage. Minutes, then reduce the vibration level to 5 g $_{rms}$ (air hammer shaker) or 0.01 g ^{2}/Hz (random shaker) for 5 min;

(4) Electrical stress: During the rapid temperature change process, the electromechanical stress applied to the sample is consistent with the steps in 6.4.5.3;

(5) Number of cycles: rapid temperature change—vibration comprehensive stress requires no less than 6 cycles;

(6) Prototype inspection: complete the appearance inspection and functional performance test of the prototype during the application of high-level vibration stress for each vibration, and continue to observe whether the prototype is normal during the application of micro-vibration vibration.

6.3.6 Implementation Process of Enhanced Type of Enhanced Test

6.3.6.1 Damp Heat Step Test

The high and low temperature damp heat test chamber and temperature and humidity comprehensive stress chamber can be used to carry out the damp heat step test, which can be divided into constant damp heat step test and constant damp heat limit test.

1. **Constant Dam Heat Step Test**

The temperature stress of the constant damp heat step test should be at least 40 °C, and 40 °C is used as an example to illustrate. When it is not possible to directly accept or evaluate whether the prototype can withstand the constant damp heat test at a temperature of 40 °C and a relative humidity of 95%RH (referred to as 40 °C & 95%RH), it can be applied in three steps successively under the condition of keeping the temperature at 40 °C 75%, 85% and 95% relative humidity; each step of the test is 24 h, and the electrical stress is adjusted and changed according to the upper and lower limits, and the adjustment period is 12 h. The profile (example) of the 40 °C constant damp heat step test is shown in Fig. 6.21.

(1) Pre-test inspection: After the sample machine is stabilized in the laboratory environment, the voltage value is adjusted to the nominal value, and after three power-on and off-start assessments, a comprehensive appearance inspection and functional performance test are performed, and recorded raw data;
(2) Temperature and humidity stress: keep 75%RH, 85%RH, and 95%RH for 24 h at a constant humidity of 40 °C;

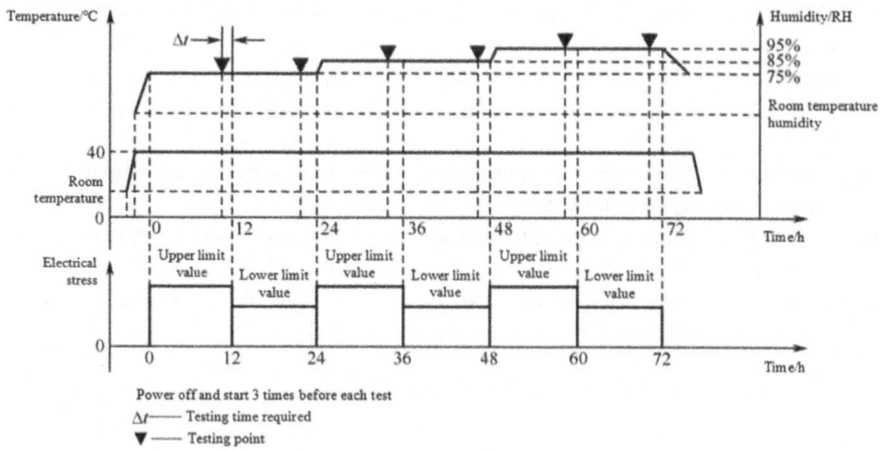

Fig. 6.21 40 °C constant damp heat step test profile (example)

(3) Temperature change rate: it should not be lower than 5 °C/min, and a larger temperature change rate can be adopted according to the actual temperature change capability of the test chamber;
(4) Electrical stress bias: at each humidity step, the upper limit of electrical stress is applied for the first 12 h, and the lower limit of electrical stress is applied for the next 12 h;
(5) Detection during the test: Δtt *hours* before the end of each electrical stress step (the time required for detection), after 3 power-on and power-off start-up assessments, conduct a comprehensive functional performance test and record the original data;
(6) Inspection after the test: After the sample machine is stabilized in the laboratory environment, adjust the voltage value to the nominal value, and conduct a comprehensive appearance inspection and functional performance test after three power-on and off-start assessments, and record Raw data.

2. **Constant Damp Heat Limit Test**

The temperature and stress of the constant humidity and heat limit test can be selected according to the specific conditions of the sample machine, and 40 °C & 95%RH is used as an example to illustrate. When the acceptable or evaluation prototype can withstand 40 °C & 95%RH constant damp heat test, under the condition of keeping the temperature 40 °C constant, 95%RH relative damp heat can be directly applied; the test is 24 h, and the electrical stress is adjusted according to the upper and lower limits, the adjustment period is 12 h. 40 °C & 95%RH constant damp heat limit stress test profile (example) is shown in Fig. 6.22.

(1) Pre-test inspection: After the sample machine is stabilized in the laboratory environment, the voltage value is adjusted to the nominal value, and after three power-on and off-start assessments, a comprehensive appearance inspection and functional performance test are performed, and recorded raw data;
(2) Temperature and humidity stress: constant damp heat 40 °C & 95%RH-24 h;
(3) Temperature change rate: According to the actual temperature change capability of the test chamber, the maximum temperature change rate is adopted, and the temperature change rate should not be lower than 5 °C/ minute;
(4) Electric stress pulling deviation: the upper limit of electrical stress is applied in the first half of the time, and the lower limit of electrical stress is applied in the second half of the time;
(5) Detection during the test: Δt time before the end of each electrical stress step (the time required for detection), after 3 power-on and power-off start-up assessments, a comprehensive functional performance test is carried out, and the original data is recorded.
(6) Inspection after the test: After the sample machine is stabilized in the laboratory environment, adjust the voltage value to the nominal value, and conduct a comprehensive appearance inspection and functional performance test after three power-on and off-start assessments, and record Raw data.

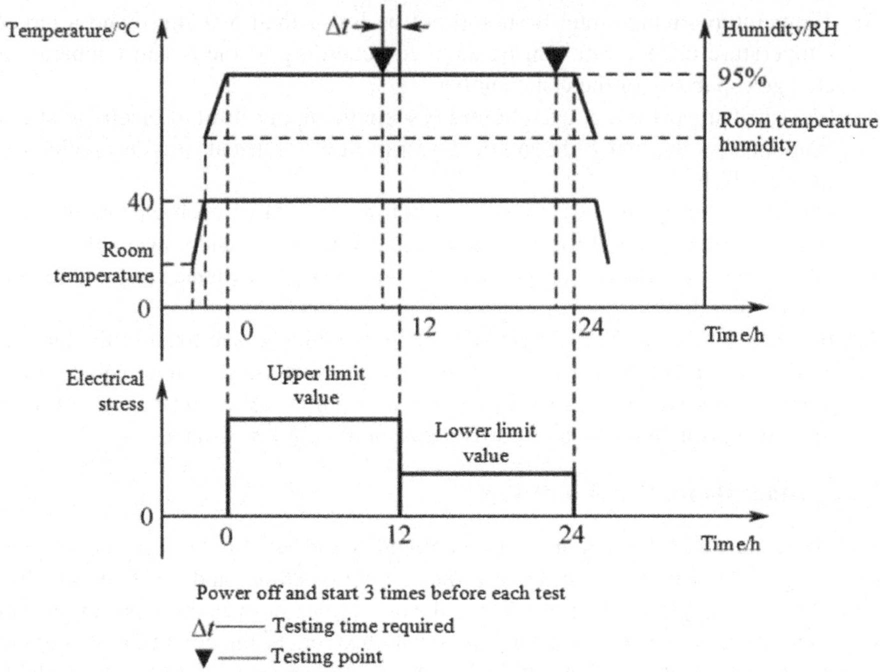

Fig. 6.22 40 °C & 95%RH constant humidity heat limit stress test profile (example)

6.3.6.2 Alternating Damp Heat Test

The temperature and stress of the alternating damp heat test can be selected according to the specific conditions of the sample machine, taking 30–60 °C, 95%RH as an example. The test lasted 96 h and was divided into 8 cycles.

The temperature and humidity alternating stress test section is shown in Fig. 6.23.

(1) Detection before the test: the detection after the constant damp heat (55 °C & 95%RH) test can be used as the detection before the test;
(2) Temperature and humidity stress: alternating humid heat 30–60 °C & 95% RH-12 h, in each cycle, 60 °C & 95% RH for 8 h, 30 °C & 95% RH for 3 h, a total of 8 cycles;
(3) Temperature change rate: it should not be lower than 5 °C/min, and a larger temperature change rate can be adopted according to the actual temperature change capacity of the test chamber:
(4) Electric stress pulling bias: each temperature and humidity alternating cycle changes alternately according to the upper limit value—lower limit value, and the electric stress adjustment cycle is 12 h;
(5) Detection during the test: Δt *t hours* before the end of each cycle (the time required for detection), conduct a comprehensive functional performance test

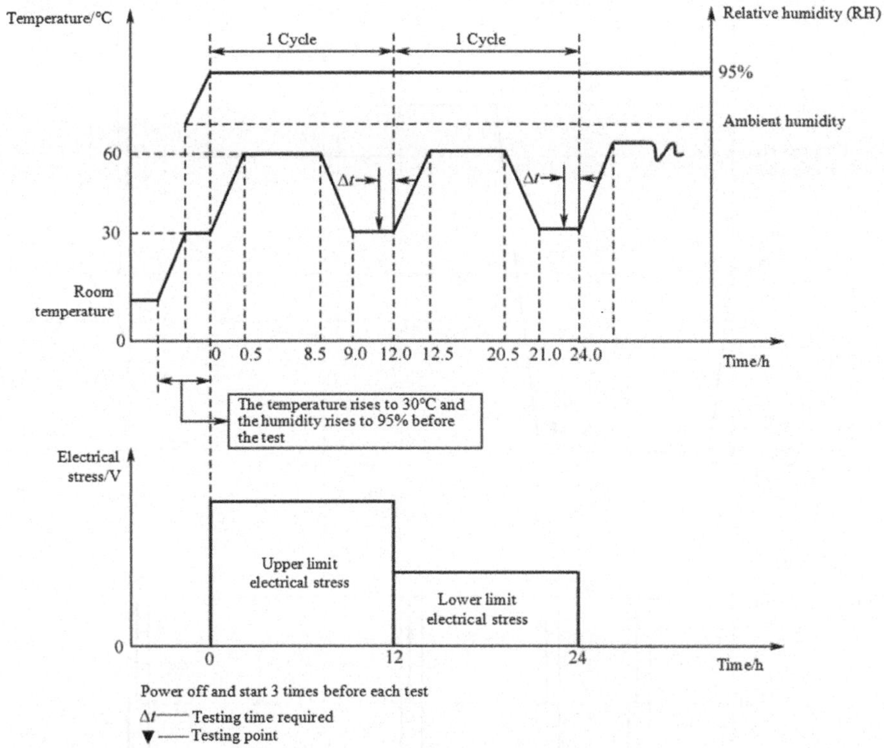

Fig. 6.23 Temperature and humidity alternating stress test profile (example)

after 3 times of power-on and power-off start-up assessments, and record the original data;

(6) Inspection after the test: After the sample machine is stabilized in the laboratory environment, the voltage value is adjusted to the nominal value, and after 3 power-on and power-off start-up assessments, a comprehensive appearance inspection and functional performance test are performed, and recorded Raw data.

6.3.6.3 Temperature Humidity—Vibration Comprehensive Stress Test

The temperature-humidity—vibration comprehensive stress intensification test can be carried out by using the temperature-humidity—vibration comprehensive stress chamber. The temperature and humidity—vibration comprehensive stress enhancement test process is as follows:

(1) Refer to Fig. 6.24 for the stress application of the comprehensive environmental stress test (the profile of the temperature and humidity—vibration comprehensive stress test (example));

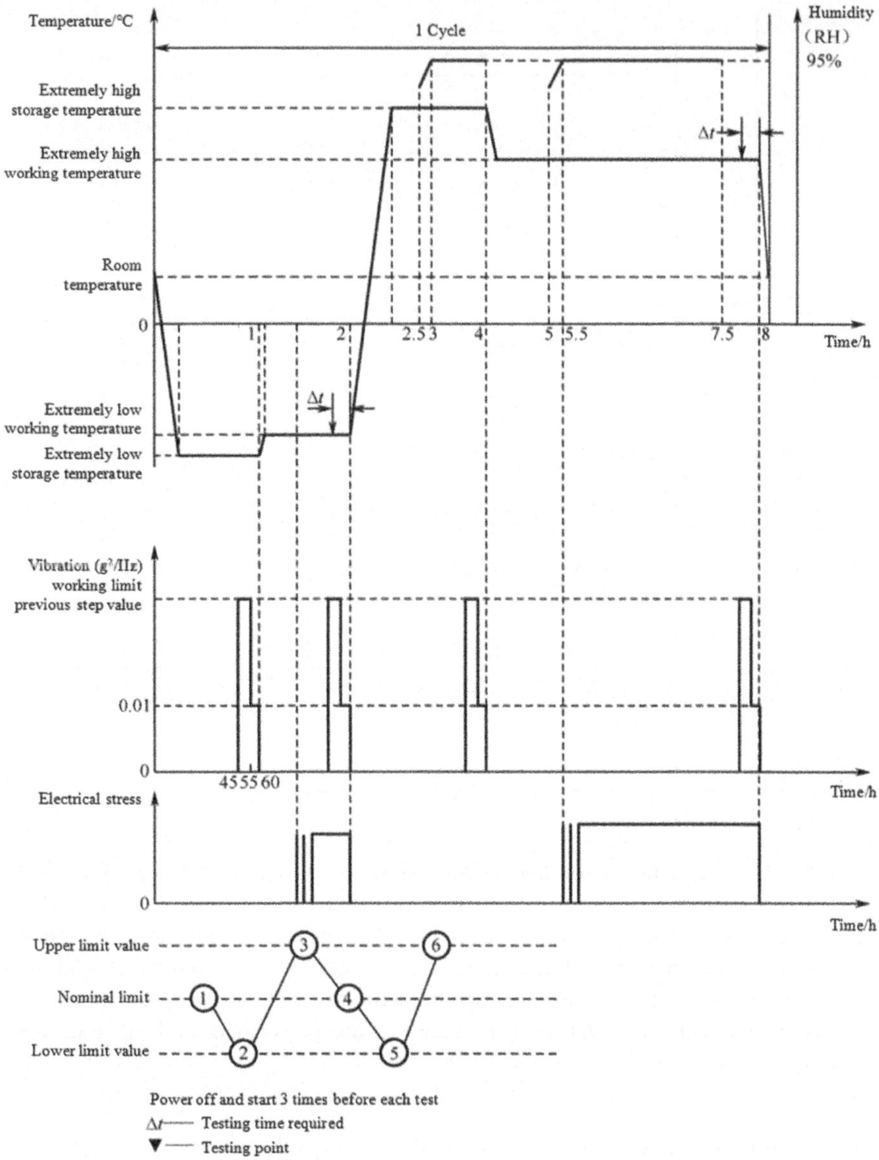

Fig. 6.24 Temperature humidity—vibration comprehensive stress test test profile (example)

(2) Number of cycles: no less than 6 cycles are required;
(3) Temperature and humidity stress: minimum storage temperature (1 h)—minimum working temperature (1 h)—maximum storage temperature (2 h, humidify for 1 h after keeping for 30 min)—maximum working temperature (4 h, humidify for 2 h after keeping for 1 h);

(4) Temperature change rate: it should not be lower than 5 °C/min, and a larger temperature change rate can be adopted according to the actual temperature change capability of the test chamber;
(5) Humidity stress: After the temperature rises to the specified temperature, the humidity stress is humidified to the specified humidity within 30 min;
(6) Electrical stress adjustment: each temperature cycle is subjected to the electrical stress of the sample machine in the order of "nominal value—lower limit value—upper limit value—nominal value—lower limit value—upper limit value";
(7) Start-up and power-on: In each temperature cycle, do not power-on in the low-temperature storage stage until it enters the extreme low-temperature working stage and keep it for 30 min, then start it 3 times in a row to observe whether the prototype is normal, and then keep energizing until the end of the extreme low-temperature working stage.;In the extreme high temperature storage stage, do not turn on the power until it enters the extreme high temperature working stage and keep it for 30 min, then start it 3 times in a row to observe whether the prototype is normal, and then keep the power on until the end of the extreme high temperature working stage;
(8) Vibration stress: the subject machine is lowered by 1–2 orders of magnitude steps on the basis of the working limit of the vibration step stress test, and the limit is 15 min before the end of the extreme low temperature storage stage and the extreme low temperature working stage of each cycle. 15 min before the end of humidification in the high-temperature storage stage and extreme high-temperature working stage, apply the corresponding vibration level for 10 min, and then reduce the vibration level to 0.01 g^2/Hz (random vibration table) for 5 min;
(9) Prototype inspection: Complete the functional performance test of the prototype during the high-level vibration stress applied to each vibration, and continue to observe whether the prototype is normal during the low-level vibration stress.

6.3.7 Implementation Process of Durability Enhancement Test

6.3.7.1 Alternating Damp Heat Endurance Test

When the durability life is considered, and the main typical use environment of the sample machine is a hot and humid environment, please refer to Sect. 6.4.6.2 to carry out the alternating damp heat enhancement test in a hot and humid environment. The recommended environmental stress is 30–60 °C & 95% RH; recommended The time is 240 h, 480 h, 720 h, 960 h, 1200 h; the test time required for the corresponding durability life can also be determined based on the accelerated test model and method.

6.3.7.2 Rapid Temperature Change—Vibration Comprehensive Stress Endurance Test

When the durability life is considered, and the main typical use environment of the sample machine is the environment of rapid temperature change and vibration comprehensive stress, refer to Sect. 6.4.5.5 to conduct the rapid temperature change-vibration comprehensive stress durability enhancement test, and the recommended time is 100 cycles, 200 cycles, 500 cycles, 800 cycles, 1000 cycles; it can also be based on the accelerated test model and method to determine the test time required for the corresponding durability life.

6.3.7.3 Temperature and Humidity—Vibration Comprehensive Stress Endurance Test

When the durability life is considered, and the main typical use environment of the sample machine is the comprehensive stress environment of temperature, humidity and vibration, please refer to Sect. 6.4.6.3 to carry out the durability enhancement test of the comprehensive stress of temperature, humidity and vibration. The recommended time is 25 cycles, 50 cycles, 75 cycles, 100 cycles, 125 cycles; the test time required for the corresponding durability life can also be determined based on the accelerated test model and method.

6.3.8 Test Report

After the end of the test, the test summary should be carried out immediately, and the test report should be written. The test report shall record in detail the description of all failures found in the test, stress level, failure location information, failure cause analysis and improvement measures.

6.3.9 Verification of Improvement Measures

After the improvement measures are implemented, reliability enhancement tests should be continued on the improved products to confirm the effectiveness of the improvement measures and whether the adopted improvement measures introduce new problems. Continuing to carry out the reliability enhancement test does not necessarily have to be carried out completely according to the test profile, and the steps before the failure can be omitted. If new problems arise, failure analysis should be carried out in accordance with the formal test procedures, and improvement measures should be taken, and then the test section can be redesigned to continue the test verification as needed. Repeat the process of test—analysis—improvement—retest until the product reliability level meets the requirements.

6.3.10 Precautions

6.3.10.1 Failure Analysis Requirements

The purpose of the intensive test is to improve product reliability. The test itself can only find defects. To improve product reliability, analyze all the failures that occur as much as possible, take improvement measures and verify them.

6.3.10.2 Teamwork Requirements

During the test, it is necessary to cooperate with all personnel in the test, design and manufacture, jointly design the test, conduct failure analysis, discuss whether improvement measures need to be taken and how to determine the improvement measures.

6.3.10.3 Failure Rectification Requirements

There may be many failures in the test, and paying attention to all failures does not mean taking improvement measures for all failures. If it is confirmed that the failure in the test is unlikely to occur in the product, there is no need to make improvements, or the stress level of the failure is much higher than the product design specification, that is, the product has sufficient safety margin, and no improvement measures can be taken. While not all failures require corrective action, all contributing causes should be clear and documented.

6.3.10.4 Prototype Disposal After Test

Prototypes that have undergone reliability enhancement tests are subjected to stress beyond the specifications during the test process, which may cause unknown damage or even destruction. Considering that most of the core components of digital diagnosis and treatment equipment are critical parts, and the consequences of failure are severe, especially the core components with wear characteristics of electromechanical and mechanical, after undergoing reliability enhancement tests, it is recommended not to sell them for use, but they can be retained. For personal use.

6.4 Accelerated Test and Rapid Evaluation Technology for Electrical Equipment

6.4.1 Definition of Accelerated Test Terms

Accelerated test: In order to shorten the test time and (or) improve the test effect, increase the stress value or frequency of the product. Accelerated tests usually include qualitative accelerated tests and quantitative accelerated tests. Qualitative accelerated tests are usually aimed at fully and quickly exposing product defects or failures, the most typical ones are reliability enhancement tests, highly accelerated life (HALT)/highly accelerated stress screening (HASS). Quantitative accelerated tests are usually for the purpose of quantitatively and quickly evaluating reliability index requirements, including accelerated life tests (based on failure as the criterion) and accelerated degradation tests (based on performance degradation as the criterion). Accelerated tests can usually be achieved through time compression, event compression (accelerating action frequency), and stress enhancement (increasing environmental stress and working load).

Benchmark conditions: The environmental conditions for normal storage, use, and testing of products are relative to the accelerated test conditions, and are the benchmarks for calculating and determining the acceleration factor.

Accelerated test conditions: In order to shorten the test time of the product, the stress value applied to the product is significantly increased. This type of stress is often the typical stress of normal storage, use, and testing of products, and it is also the main (sensitive) stress that causes product failure in reality. The stress value should not be too large, as it will cause changes in the failure mechanism of the product; the stress value should not be too small, as the acceleration factor will be too small if it is too small, making it difficult to significantly shorten the test time.

Acceleration factor: The ratio of the failure distribution characteristics (or reliability level) of the product under high stress conditions to that under reference conditions. For tests with acceleration effects, the acceleration factor is greater than 1. The acceleration factor can usually be expressed by the ratio of the time required to reach the same cumulative failure probability under the reference conditions and the accelerated stress conditions for two groups of test machines respectively.

Acceleration model: The mathematical model used in the acceleration test usually reflects the functional relationship between the rate or life characteristic value and stress, and reflects the influence of model-related stress on life.

Activation energy (E_a): An empirical coefficient used to evaluate the ability to accelerate from a change in absolute temperature. The unit of activation energy is eV/K; activation energy is the energy required for the atoms on the lattice lattice in the crystal to move to another lattice or gap position, and it is an indicator reflecting the influence of temperature stress on product life. For matter, there is a potential barrier in the transition process from the normal unfailed state to the failed state, which is the activation energy. The smaller the activation energy, the easier it is for the physical process of failure to proceed. The greater the activation energy, the greater the acceleration coefficient, and the easier it is to be accelerated and fail. In the accelerated test, the statistical significance of the activation energy varies with the definition of the failure judgment basis. During the accelerated life test, when all the failures of the test object are combined and counted, the activation energy in the accelerated model is The activation energy of the object; when the failure mechanism of the test object is classified and counted, the activation energy in the accelerated model solved is the activation energy of the failure mechanism of the object. In the accelerated degradation test, when the degradation of a certain performance parameter of the test object is predicted and judged, the activation energy of the accelerated model solved is the activation energy of the parameter of the object.

6.4.2 Accelerated Test Model Method

6.4.2.1 Acceleration Factor Measurement and Acquisition Method

Acceleration factor measurement methods usually include:

(1) The ratio of the time used for normal tests to the time used for accelerated tests when the same cumulative failure probability is reached;
(2) The ratio of the reaction rate under accelerated test conditions to the reaction rate under normal conditions.

According to the measurement method of the acceleration factor, the methods for obtaining the acceleration factor usually include:

(1) By carrying out accelerated tests under multiple sets of stresses, the reliability characteristic values under each set of stresses are obtained, and the acceleration factor can be obtained by extrapolating the stress intensity model;
(2) On the premise of knowing the base conditions and acceleration conditions, by using the empirical model and empirical parameters, the acceleration factor of a single object can be obtained, and even the acceleration factor of higher-level products can be obtained through modeling.

6.4.2.2 Life Distribution Model and Acceleration Factor

1. **Exponential Distribution Models and Acceleration Factors**

Exponential distribution is one of the life distributions commonly used in products, and is widely used in life distribution models of electronic products.

See formula (6.7) for the single-parameter exponential distribution reliability function:

$$R(t) = e^{-\lambda t} \tag{6.7}$$

In the formula:

λ—Failure rate;

$R\ (t)$—Reliability of the product at time t.

t when the corresponding reliability value of the product is R is shown in formula (6.8):

$$\begin{aligned} t &= \frac{-\ln R}{\lambda} \\ &= \frac{-\ln(1-F)}{\lambda} \end{aligned} \tag{6.8}$$

In the formula:

F—Cumulative failure probability, $F = 1 - R$.

The failure distribution function of components under $F_0(t_u)$ normal stress level is S_u, the failure rate λ_u is the time t_u to reach the failure probability F_0. Assume that the failure distribution function of $F_a(t_a)$ the single body under the accelerated stress level is S_a, and the failure rate is λ_a the time when t_a the failure probability reaches F_0.

According to the definition of acceleration factor, the product acceleration factor AF is shown in formula (6.9):

$$\begin{aligned} \mathrm{AF} &= \frac{t_u}{t_a} \\ &= \frac{\lambda_a}{\lambda_u} \end{aligned} \tag{6.9}$$

In the formula:

λ_u—The failure rate of the product under normal test or service conditions;

λ_a—The failure rate of the product under accelerated test conditions;

AF—The acceleration factor of accelerated test conditions relative to conventional test or service conditions.

If the failure rate λ_u and acceleration factor AF of a product under conventional conditions are known, its failure rate λ_a under accelerated stress conditions S_a can be derived in formula (6.10):

$$\lambda_a = \mathrm{AF} \cdot \lambda_u \tag{6.10}$$

The service life of a complete machine obeys the exponential distribution and is m composed of similar components. The i-th type of components has N_i a failure rate λ_i and an acceleration factor of AF_i. According to the basic reliability model, the failure rate of the complete machine λ_s can be expressed as formula (6.11):

$$\lambda_s = \sum_{i=1}^{m} N_i \lambda_i \tag{6.11}$$

In the formula:

m—The number of types of components included in the whole machine;

N_i—The quantity of the i-th type components, $i = 1, 2, \ldots, m$;

λ_i—Failure rate of the i-*th* type components;

λ_s—The failure rate of the whole machine.

Combined with the definition of acceleration factor and the basic reliability model of the whole machine, the acceleration factor of the whole machine can be obtained AF_s as shown in formula (6.12):

$$\begin{aligned} AF_s &= \frac{\lambda_{sa}}{\lambda_{su}} \\ &= \frac{\sum_{i=1}^{m} N_i AF_i \lambda_{iu}}{\sum_{i=1}^{m} N_i \lambda_{iu}} \end{aligned} \tag{6.12}$$

In the formula:

λ_{iu}—Failure rate of class i-th type components under normal test and service conditions;

AF_i—The acceleration factor of the i-th type components under the accelerated test conditions relative to the normal use or test conditions;

AF_s—The acceleration factor of the whole machine under accelerated test conditions relative to that under normal use or test conditions.

It can be seen that for electrical equipment, the acceleration factor of the complete electrical equipment can be obtained by modeling on the premise of knowing the type, quantity, and activation energy of the components.

2. **Weibull Distribution Model**

Weibull distribution is a relatively complex distribution commonly used in reliability research, and is widely used in the life distribution model of complex electromechanical products. See formula (6.13) for the reliability function of Weibull distribution:

$$R(t) = \exp\left[-\left(\frac{t-\gamma}{\eta}\right)^m\right] \tag{6.13}$$

In the formula:

η—This is the scale parameter;

m—This is the shape parameter;

γ—This is a positional parameter.

When the position parameter $\gamma=0$, the reliability function of the two-parameter Weibull distribution is shown in formula (6.14):

$$R(t) = \exp\left[-\left(\frac{t}{\eta}\right)^m\right] \quad (6.14)$$

Assuming that the failure distribution function of components under $F_0(t_u)$ normal stress level is S_u, the shape parameter is m, the scale parameter is η_u, and is the time t_u when the failure probability reaches F_0. Assume that the failure distribution function of $F_a(t_a)$ the single body at the accelerated stress level is S_a, the shape parameter is kept as m, the scale parameter is η_a, and its time is t_a when the failure probability reaches F_0.

According to the definition of acceleration factor, the single individual acceleration factor AF is shown in formula (6.15):

$$\mathrm{AF} = \frac{t_u}{t_a} = \frac{\eta_a}{\eta_u} \quad (6.15)$$

In the formula:

η_a—Scale parameters under accelerated test conditions;

η_u—Dimensional parameters under normal use or test conditions.

3. **Other Life Distribution Models**

Life distribution models also include distribution models such as lognormal distribution, gamma distribution, and extreme value distribution.

6.4.2.3 Acceleration Model and Acceleration Factor

1. **High Temperature Acceleration Model**

The high temperature acceleration model is often called the Arrhenius model, which assumes that the reaction rate is an exponential function of absolute temperature.

The reaction rate can be expressed by formula (6.16):

$$u_l = Ae^{-\frac{E_a}{K_B \times T_l}} \quad (6.16)$$

In the formula:

μ_l—The reaction rate under the condition of temperature stress T_l;

A—Frequency factor, constant (independent of temperature);

E_a—Activation energy (eV);

K_B—Boltzmann constant (8.6174×10^{-5} eV/K);

T_l—Absolute temperature (K) at the stress level l.

The acceleration factor is the ratio of the reaction rates in two different test environments, see formula (6.17):

$$AF = \frac{u_a}{u_u} = \frac{A \times e^{-\frac{E_a}{K_B} \cdot \frac{1}{T_a}}}{A \times e^{-\frac{E_a}{K_B} \cdot \frac{1}{T_u}}} = e^{\left[\frac{E_a}{K_B} \times \left(\frac{1}{T_u} - \frac{1}{T_a}\right)\right]} \quad (6.17)$$

In the formula:

T_u—The absolute temperature under normal use or test environmental conditions;

T_a—The absolute temperature under the environmental conditions of the accelerated test.

The failure rate under accelerated stress conditions is shown in formula (6.18):

$$\lambda(T_a) = \lambda(T_u) \cdot AF = \lambda(T_u) \times e^{\left[\frac{E_a}{K_B} \times \left(\frac{1}{T_u} - \frac{1}{T_a}\right)\right]} \quad (6.18)$$

An example of using the Arrhenius model is that the failure rate/h at 25 1×10^{-8} °C (298 K) determines the failure rate in the test λ,which is a function of the absolute temperature *T*. The Arrhenius reaction model is shown in Fig. 6.25.

2. Temperature and Humidity Acceleration Model and Acceleration Factor

The temperature-humidity acceleration model assumes that the reaction rate is the product of an exponential function of absolute temperature and a power function of relative humidity.

The reaction rate can be expressed by formula (6.19):

$$u_l = Ae^{-\frac{E_a}{K_B T_l}} \cdot RH_l^n \quad (6.19)$$

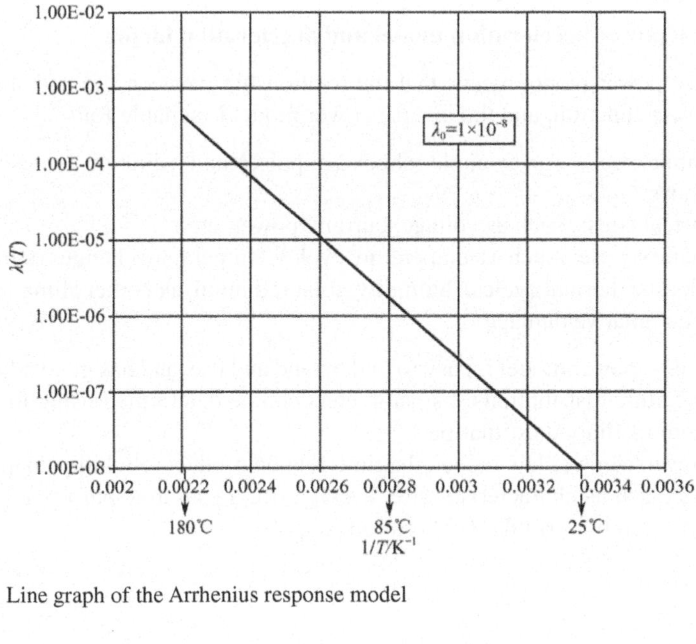

Fig. 6.25 Line graph of the Arrhenius response model

In the formula:

μ_l—The reaction rate under the conditions of temperature stress T (K) and relative humidity stress %;

E_a—The activation energy, in units of eV, the empirical value is between 0.6 and 2.51;

A—The frequency factor;

K_B—Boltzmann constant (8.6174×10^{-5}eV/k);

T_l—The absolute temperature (K);

RH_l—Relative humidity (%);

n—Power exponent.

The acceleration factor can be deduced as shown in formula (6.20):

$$AF = e^{\frac{Ea}{K_B}\left(\frac{1}{T_u}-\frac{1}{T_a}\right)} \cdot \left(\frac{RH_a}{RH_u}\right)^n \tag{6.20}$$

In the formula:

E_a—Activation energy, in units of eV, the empirical value is between 0.6 and 2.51;

A—The frequency factor;

K_B—Boltzmann constant (8.6174×10^{-5}eV/k);

T_u—The absolute temperature (K) under reference conditions;

T_a—The absolute temperature (K) under accelerated conditions;

RH_u—Relative humidity (%) under reference conditions;

RH_a—Relative humidity (%) under accelerated conditions;

n—Power exponent.

3. **Inverse power acceleration model and acceleration factor**

The inverse power model means that the relationship between life and stress is an inverse power function, and the inverse power model is suitable for:

(1) Dynamic stress, for example, shock (impulse) and vibration (sinusoidal and random);
(2) Electrical stress, such as voltage, current, power, etc.;
(3) Climatic stresses, such as temperature cycles, temperature changes (temperature shocks and thermal cycles), humidity, solar radiation, and other climatic stresses with cumulative damage.

The inverse power model is easy to understand and use, and has good adaptability to various failure distributions. Its parameters can be determined using the method of maximum likelihood estimation.

In the inverse power law model, the time-related product reliability characteristic parameters (such as characteristic life, average life, mean time before failure, etc.) can be expressed by formula (6.21) as follows:

$$L(S) = C^{-1} \times S^{-m} \tag{6.21}$$

In the formula:
S—Stress magnitude;
C—Undetermined constant ($c > 0$);
m—Undetermined parameters related to stress;
$L(s)$—Life or specified time period (as a function of stress).

Considering that the lifetime is inversely proportional to the reaction rate, the lifetime inverse power model becomes a power exponential model when the reaction rate is used to represent it.

The acceleration factor of the inverse power model is shown in formula (6.22):

$$AF = \frac{u_a}{u_u} = \frac{L_u}{L_a} = \frac{C^{-1} \times S_u^{-m}}{C^{-1} \times S_a^{-m}} = \left(\frac{S_a}{S_u}\right)^m \tag{6.22}$$

In the formula:
AF—Stress acceleration in the inverse power model;
L_u—Life characteristic value under actual environmental conditions (function related to actual service stress);
L_a—Characteristic value of life under accelerated test conditions (function related to test stress);
S_u—Stress value under actual environmental conditions;
S_a—Stress value under accelerated test conditions;
m—Inverse power exponent.

4. **Other accelerated models**

Other acceleration models include those applicable to temperature cycling, random vibration, sinusoidal vibration, temperature-vibration, temperature-cycle-vibration, temperature-humidity-vibration, and other typical stress tests.

6.4.3 *Method for Determining Accelerated Test Conditions*

6.4.3.1 Determination of Reference Conditions

According to the environmental control requirements of the installation site of the medical electronic linear accelerator and the environmental conditions of the actual use of the electrical equipment site, the benchmark conditions are determined as the benchmark for the evaluation of the acceleration factor.

For electrical equipment directly exposed to the indoor atmosphere, the temperature reference can be determined as 20–30 °C, and 25 °C is recommended; if necessary, the relative humidity can be determined as 50–75%RH, and 60%RH is recommended.

For the electrical equipment inside the chassis, the temperature reference can be determined as 30–60 °C, and 40 °C is recommended. The reference temperature can also be determined according to the actual measurement results of the local ambient temperature of the electrical equipment.

6.4.3.2 Determination of Test Stress

1. **Choice of Stress Type**

The electrical equipment of the medical electron linear accelerator is mainly subjected to temperature and humidity stress. High temperature, temperature cycle, temperature and humidity and their combination can be selected as the acceleration stress of the electrical equipment. If necessary, the vibration stress and the combination of the above stress can be added as the acceleration stress stress.

This standard mainly adopts the high temperature aging accelerated test method and conducts quantitative evaluation.

2. **Selection of Stress Levels**

Accelerated test stress should be selected appropriately.

When the acceleration model parameters and acceleration factors are unknown or not determined in advance, no less than 3 stress levels shall be selected to carry out the accelerated test.

When the acceleration model parameters or acceleration factors are known or determined in advance, one stress level can be selected to carry out the accelerated test.

3. **Determination of Stress Magnitude**

When multiple sets of stresses are used to carry out accelerated tests, first determine the highest stress value, then determine the lowest stress value, and finally determine the intermediate stress value.

Carrying out accelerated tests at the highest stress value shall not cause a change in the failure mechanism. The maximum stress value can be based on the working limit found in the previous reliability enhancement test (step test), and a certain margin is reserved. The recommended value is to relax the working limit by 10 to 15 basic unit values. Under the condition of no reliability enhancement test (step test), the maximum stress value can also leave a margin of 20 to 30 basic units on the basis of the investigation and analysis of the subjects.

The minimum working stress value is recommended to be the specification limit value of the sample machine or the highest stress value verified by the environmental test, and a margin of 10 basic unit values can be left.

The intermediate stress value is determined by interpolation and rounding between the lowest working stress value and the highest working stress value. The principle of interpolation is to keep the reciprocals of each adjacent stress point equidistant. When there are group stresses, the intermediate stress value l interpolation See formula (6.23) for the method:

$$\begin{cases} \Delta = \frac{\left(\frac{1}{T_{al}} - \frac{1}{T_{ah}}\right)}{l-1} \\ \frac{1}{T_k} = \frac{1}{T_{al}} - (k-1)\Delta\, k = 2, 3, \cdots \end{cases} \tag{6.23}$$

In the formula:

T_{al}—The minimum stress level group temperature determined by the accelerated test;

T_{ah}—The temperature of the highest stress level group determined by the accelerated test;

l—Number of accelerated test stress level groups;

Δ—The difference between the reciprocals of the stress levels of adjacent groups;

T_k—The corresponding temperature of k-th acceleration test, in which $k = 1, 2, 3, \cdots, l$.

A certain interval should be kept between each group of stresses. Among them, the interval of temperature stress should be kept above 10 °C, the interval of humidity stress should be kept above 10%RH, and the interval of electrical stress should be kept above 10%.

6.4.3.3 Requirements for the Sample Machine

1. **Subject to Sample Machine Status**

Before the accelerated test, the technical state of the sample machine should be basically solidified, and it has passed the necessary functional performance test, environmental stress screening, environmental test, and reliability test.

Where possible, before the accelerated test, the same batch of prototypes has undergone reliability enhancement tests and improvement measures have been taken to improve the environmental resistance.

The prototypes used for accelerated testing can be screened for environmental stress before the accelerated testing to eliminate failures, and then used for accelerated testing.

2. **The Number of Sample Machines**

When the acceleration model parameters or acceleration factors are unknown, at least three sets of accelerated tests need to be carried out. The number of samples required for each group of accelerated life tests is usually 10–30, and a total of 30–90 samples are required for the three groups; The number of prototypes is usually 3 to 5, and a total of 9 to 15 prototypes are required for the three groups.

When the method of estimating the acceleration factor by accelerated modeling is adopted, the number of prototypes required for a group of accelerated tests is only 1 to 10.

Increasing the number of prototypes can shorten the evaluation time of reliability indicators (such as MTBF), but cannot shorten the evaluation time of life indicators, but both can enhance the representativeness and credibility of accelerated tests.

6.4.3.4 Testing Requirements

1. **Detection Timing**

Before and after the test, conduct a comprehensive functional inspection and performance test on the sample machine under laboratory environmental conditions.

During the test, test the sample machine according to the test timing specified in the test cycle. When it is necessary to restore the sample machine to normal temperature for testing, sufficient and fixed recovery time shall be ensured to allow the sample machine to return to normal temperature.

2. **Test Items**

Testing items are often determined based on product technical conditions. Before and after the test, the sample machine shall be fully inspected. In the test, the inspection should focus on the parameters representing the life characteristics of the sample machine. The method of determining the characteristic parameters of life is as follows:

(1) Through analysis, select key parameters representing product performance;
(2) According to the long-term testing and inspection experience, select parameters with time-deteriorating characteristics;
(3) Test as many product performance parameters as possible within the possible testing time and testing workload;
(4) Consider time and workload constraints for manual testing, and consider monitoring parameters as much as possible for automatic testing methods.

3. **Detection Cycle and Times**

When the acceleration model parameters or acceleration factors are unknown, according to the planned test time and the principle of equal-period testing, the number of testing cycles for the accelerated life test shall not be less than 5, and the number of testing cycles for the accelerated degradation test shall not be less than 10.

When using accelerated modeling to estimate the acceleration factor, the testing cycle of the accelerated test should be consistent with the actual regular testing cycle of the product.

When determining the inspection period, the convenience of the inspection work arrangement should also be considered, and a fixed inspection cycle is usually adopted.

The number of inspections can be determined based on the test time and inspection cycle, and the inspection cycle can be adjusted appropriately to obtain the required number of inspections.

4. **Testing Instrument Requirements**

In the accelerated degradation test, the detection work should eliminate the detection error as much as possible. Measures such as fixed fixtures, test instruments, test cables, test personnel, and recovery time can be used to reduce test errors by using high-precision test instruments and taking the average value through multiple tests. Special attention should also be paid to taking the average value of multiple tests before and after the test.

6.4.3.5 High Temperature Accelerated Aging Test Case

1. **Determine the Baseline Conditions**

For electrical equipment directly exposed to the indoor atmosphere, the temperature reference can be determined as 20–30 °C, and the relative humidity can be determined as 50–75%RH if necessary.

For the electrical equipment inside the chassis, the temperature reference can be determined as 30–60 °C, and the reference temperature can be determined according to the actual measurement results of the local ambient temperature of the electrical equipment.

The reference temperature can be determined according to the actual measurement results of the local ambient temperature of the electrical equipment.

2. **Select Accelerated Stress**

Using a group of accelerated tests, the recommended temperature stress is +55 ± 80 °C reasonably given by combining the investigation of the material temperature resistance range and the reliability enhancement test..

3. **Modeling Evaluation Acceleration Factors**

According to the types and quantities of components of electrical equipment and the basic failure rate and activation energy parameters of each type of components, the acceleration factor model of the whole electrical equipment can be established AF_s as shown in formula (6.24):

$$AF_s = \frac{\sum_{i=1}^{m} N_i \lambda_{iu} AF_i}{\sum_{i=1}^{m} N_i \lambda_{iu}} = \frac{\sum_{i=1}^{m} N_i \lambda_{iu} e^{\frac{E_{ai}}{K_B}\left(\frac{1}{T_u} - \frac{1}{T_a}\right)}}{\sum_{i=1}^{m} N_i \lambda_{iu}} \tag{6.24}$$

In the formula:

N_i—The quantity of the i-th type components, $i = 1, 2, \ldots$, m;

λ_{iu}—Failure rate of the i-th type components;

E_{ai}—Activating energy of the i-th type components, with the unit of eV, and the empirical value is between 0.6 and 2.51;

K_B—Boltzmann constant (8.6174×10^{-5}eV/k);

T_u—Absolute temperature (K) under normal use or test conditions;

T_a—Absolute temperature (K) under accelerated test conditions;

λ_s—The failure rate of the whole machine.

Among them, the types and quantities of components are determined by the research and development party; the failure rate of each type of components is firstly derived from the reliability statistical analysis results of existing products, and secondly, it can refer to standard data; the activation energy is preferentially calculated using the accumulated accelerated test data statistics The results of the analysis can be followed by standards and results of literature surveys.

4. **Number of Samples**

This standard adopts the acceleration modeling method to obtain the acceleration factor in advance, and conducts a quantitative evaluation by carrying out a group of acceleration tests. The number of prototypes required is 1 to 10.

5. **Test Items**

Before and after the test, conduct a comprehensive functional inspection and performance test on the sample machine under laboratory environmental conditions.

During the test, at least the main functional performance of the sample machine should be tested, and the items that cannot be tested should be explained.

6. **Detection Cycle and Test Cycle**

When the electrical equipment can carry out online automatic detection synchronously during the test, the detection cycle is determined according to the characteristics of the online detection system, and the test cycle is determined to be 100 h. In a test cycle, the online automatic detection data is extracted every 10 h. Return to normal temperature for 1 detection.

When the electrical equipment must be taken out of the test box for off-line testing, the testing period is specified as 100 h, the testing time is controlled to be completed within 20 h, and the testing period is 120 h.

6.4.4 *Acceleration Test Failure Definition and Statistics*

6.4.4.1 Failure Definition

If any of the following situations occurs in the accelerated test of the modulator sample machine, it will be judged as a failure:

(1) The sample machine cannot work or some functions are lost;
(2) The test results of the parameters of the sample machine exceed the allowable range of the specifications (regulations);
(3) The mechanical, structural parts or components of the test machine are loosened, cracked, broken or damaged.

6.4.4.2 Classification of Failure Consequences

Divide failures into two categories according to their consequences:

(1) Serious failure—an event that directly leads to shutdown, resulting in failure to start up, fail to operate normally, fail to realize basic and main functions, technical indicators are out of tolerance to unacceptable, may lead to serious consequences or fail to comply with safety regulations, and must be shut down for processing failure;
(2) General failures—the prototype has a failure alarm or symptom, some functions are lost, and the technical indicators exceed the standard, but the prototype is not shut down, does not need to be shut down, can operate normally, can continue to be used normally, and can complete basic and main functions.

6.4.4.3 Classification of Failure Nature

All failures that appear in the reliability evaluation are divided into correlated failures and non-correlated failures.

Non-associated failures refer to the failures that have been proven not to be used according to the specified conditions, mainly including:

(1) Failures caused by test equipment, test instruments and supporting conditions guarantee not meeting the requirements;
(2) The test stress that does not meet the requirements is applied or the failure is determined to be caused by overstress;
(3) Man-made failures caused by improper handling, operation, testing and maintenance of the sample machine;
(4) Dependent failures caused by independent failures, failures occurring beyond the specified life span, etc.

The failures other than non-related failures are all related failures. The related failures mainly refer to the failures caused by the problems of the sample machine itself. Combined with the characteristics of the life evaluation test, the related failures mainly include:

(1) Failures caused by improper design, process and assembly of the sample machine;
(2) Failures caused by improper design, manufacture and selection of parts and components;
(3) Obvious wear-and-tear failures such as aging, corrosion, and wear appear in the sample machine.

6.4.4.4 Determination of the Principle of Failure Statistics

The statistical principles for determining the number of failures are as follows:

(1) If a related or serious failure occurs, it will be recorded as a judged failure;
(2) The occurrence of the same associated serious failures shall be separately recorded as one judged failure;
(3) For every 5 associated general failures, it is recorded as 1 judged failure.

According to the classification of failure nature and consequences, the total number of judged failures is:

$$r = r_1 + r_2/5 \tag{6.25}$$

In the formula:
r—The number of judged failures;
r_1—The number of associated failures with serious consequences;
r_2—Consequence general associated failure number.

6.4.5 *Rapid Verification Method of Electrical Equipment Reliability Index*

6.4.5.1 Determination of Reliability Index Requirements

Before carrying out the accelerated test to evaluate the reliability index of electrical equipment, the reliability index of electrical equipment should be clarified.

The typical reliability index of electrical equipment is the Mean Time Between Failures (MTBF), and the minimum acceptable value of each electrical equipment reliability index (MTBF) can be determined according to the distribution of the overall reliability index of the medical electron linear accelerator θ_1.

6.4.5.2 Selection of the Statistical Scheme

To carry out accelerated tests to verify the reliability indicators of electrical equipment, a statistical scheme should be selected first to determine the test time. It is recommended to use a timed censored test scheme, see Table 6.10. The test subject can select a statistical plan based on factors such as product quality, risk tolerance, and test cost.

Table 6.10 Timed censored protocol

Plan serial number	Features of the program			Censoring time T (θ_1 multiplies m)	Judgment failure number r	
	Risk nominal value/%		Discrimination ratio $D = =\theta_0/\theta_1$		Refused (≥)	Accepted (≤)
	θ	θ				
1	30	30	3.37	1.20	1	0
2	30	30	2.22	2.44	2	1
3	30	30	2.00	3.70	3	2
4	30	30	1.72	4.76	4	3
5	30	30	1.62	5.89	5	4
6	20	20	7.22	1.61	1	0
7	20	20	3.63	2.99	2	1
8	20	20	3.00	4.30	3	2
9	20	20	2.79	4.28	3	2
10	20	20	2.40	5.51	4	3
11	20	20	2.17	6.72	5	4
12	10	10	21.85	2.30	1	0
13	10	10	7.32	3.89	2	1
14	10	10	4.83	5.32	3	2
15	10	10	3.83	6.68	4	3
16	10	10	3.29	7.99	5	4

6.4.5.3 Determination of the Accelerated Test Time

1. **Determining the Total Time of the Accelerated Test**

According to the value of m given in Table 6.10, the total accelerated test time t_{ta} requirement can be found in formula (6.26):

$$t_{ta} = \frac{m \times \theta_1}{\mathrm{AF}} \tag{6.26}$$

In the formula:

m—The multiple relationship between the test time and the minimum acceptable value in the statistical scheme;θ_1.

θ_1—Minimum acceptable value of Mean Time Between Failures (MTBF);

AF—Acceleration coefficient under accelerated test conditions;

t_{ta}—The total unit hours required for all prototypes under accelerated test conditions.

2. **Determining the Time for a Single Accelerated Test**

After determining the number of tested products (n) and the acceleration factor AF, the single accelerated test time t_{sa} can be obtained from formula (6.27):

$$t_{\mathrm{sa}} = \frac{t_{\mathrm{ta}}}{n} = \frac{m \times \theta_1}{n \times \mathrm{AF}} \tag{6.27}$$

In the formula:
n—The number of prototypes put into the test;
t_{sa}—Planned test time for a single prototype under accelerated test conditions.

6.4.5.4 Statistics on the Effective Accelerated Test Time of a Single Prototype

In life evaluation, it is not allowed to accumulate the effective verification time of each prototype as the total effective verification time; in reliability evaluation, it is allowed to accumulate the effective accelerated test time of each prototype as the total effective accelerated test time.

For reliability and life evaluation, it is necessary to count the effective accelerated test time of a single prototype. The effective verification time of a single prototype is the sum of its determinable normal operation time, and it can also be its total verification time minus the invalid verification time. The statistical principles are as follows:

(1) If the prototype does not fail during the test, the entire test time is valid verification time;
(2) If the prototype fails during the test, the time spent running with the failure cannot be used as the effective verification time;
(3) When a failure of a sample machine is found in the verification test, the invalid verification time is the period between the end of the test when the last test result of the failure sample machine was normal and the start time of the test corresponding to the failure found in this test time.

6.4.5.5 Conversion Equivalent Test Time

1. **Conversion of Equivalent Test Time for a Prototype at a Certain Moment**

After the necessary point in time and the failure of the moment point statistics effective acceleration test time, according to the acceleration factor and acceleration test the actual time $\hat{t}_{ta}$, calculated (failure) corresponding to the moment of the equivalent test time $\hat{t}_{te}$, (failure) corresponding to the moment of the equivalent test time $\hat{t}_{te}$ is equal to the acceleration test time $\hat{t}_{ta}$ and the product of the acceleration factor is shown in the formula (6.28):

$$\hat{t}_{tek} = \mathrm{AF} \cdot \hat{t}_{tak} \tag{6.28}$$

In the formula:

$\hat{t}_{tak}$—The cumulative effective accelerated test bench time of the prototype at the moment when the k-th prototype fails under the accelerated test conditions;

$\hat{t}_{tek}$—The equivalent (under normal use or test conditions) test time of accumulating effective accelerated test time up to the time when the prototype fails.

2. **The Equivalent Test Time Conversion of All Prototypes at the End of the Test**

When the test is over, the calculation of the cumulative equivalent test time of all prototypes is shown in formula (6.29):

$$\hat{t}_{te} = \mathrm{AF}\sum_{k=1}^{n} \hat{t}_{tak} \tag{6.29}$$

In the formula:

$\hat{t}_{ta}$—Under the accelerated test conditions, the accumulated effective accelerated test bench time at the end of the k-th prototype test;

$\hat{t}_{te}$—Cumulative equivalent (under normal use or test conditions) test time for all prototypes.

6.4.5.6 Determination of the Principle of Failure Statistics

The statistical principles for determining the number of failures are as follows:

(1) If a related or serious failure occurs, it will be counted as a judged failure;
(2) The occurrence of the same related serious failure shall be counted separately as one judgment failure;
(3) For every 5 associated general failures, it is recorded as one judged failure.

According to the classification of failure nature and consequences, the total number of judged failures is:

$$r = r_1 + r_2/5 \tag{6.30}$$

In the formula:

r—The number of judged failures;

r_1—The number of associated failures with serious consequences;

r_2—Consequence general associated failure number.

6.4.5.7 Reliability Index Evaluation

Using the cumulative equivalent test time at the corresponding moment $\hat{t}_{te}$, the cumulative number of responsible failures r, and the lower confidence limit C (usually $C = 1\text{-}\beta$), the minimum acceptable value of the Mean Time Between Failures corresponding to the accelerated test can be evaluated.

When the test is passed according to the timed censored statistical test plan, the lower confidence limit of the lowest acceptable value of the Mean Time Between Failures is shown in formula (6.31):

$$\theta_{L,C} = \frac{2\hat{t}_{te}}{\chi^2_{\beta}(2r+2)} \tag{6.31}$$

In the formula:

$\hat{t}_{te}$—Cumulative equivalent (under normal use or test conditions) test time for all prototypes;

r—Accumulative judgment failure number of all prototypes;

β—User risk;

C—Confidence, $C = 1 - \beta$.

When the timed censored statistical test scheme fails, the lower confidence limit of the lowest acceptable value of the Mean Time Between Failures is shown in formula (6.32):

$$\theta_{L,C} = \frac{2\hat{t}_{te}}{\chi^2_{\beta}(2r)} \tag{6.32}$$

In the formula:

$\hat{t}_{te}$—Cumulative equivalent (under normal use or test conditions) test time for all prototypes;

r—Accumulative judgment failure number of all prototypes;

β—User risk;

C—Confidence, $C = 1 - \beta$.

6.4.6 Quick Verification Method for Lifetime Indicators of Electrical Equipment

6.4.6.1 Life Index Requirements

Before carrying out the accelerated test to evaluate the life index of electrical equipment, the life index of electrical equipment should be clarified.

The typical life index of electrical equipment is the service life. The service life unit of the medical electron linear accelerator and its equipment can be calendar year, power-on time, working time, high-voltage beam output time, and the number of people treated. Wherein, the power-on time includes standby time and working time, and the high-voltage beam output time is the time for treating patients with high-voltage beam output during the working period.

When multiple life indicators are used, the first-come-first-served principle is usually adopted to determine the lifespan, and each indicator should be reasonably matched.

6.4.6.2 Selection of Engineering Experience Coefficients

In the life verification and evaluation process, the engineering experience coefficient k is related to the life index verification time, and the life index verification time is usually the engineering experience coefficient k multiplied by the life index time.

Usually, the value of k is between 1.0 and 1.5, and the typical value is 1.2. For objects with a long lifetime index and a long verification period, the value of k can be 1.0.

6.4.6.3 Accelerated Test Time

According to the selected engineering experience coefficient k and acceleration factor AF, the accelerated test time t_{ta} requirement can be obtained as shown in formula (6.33):

$$t_{ta} = \frac{k \cdot l}{\mathrm{AF}} \tag{6.33}$$

In the formula:

k—Engineering experience coefficient, k preferably 1.0–1.5, usually 1.2;

l—Life index requirements;

AF—Acceleration factor;

t_{ta}—Test time required for all prototypes under accelerated test conditions.

6.4.6.4 Conversion of Equivalent Test Time

At the necessary time point and the time point of the failure, after counting the effective accelerated test time of the k -th sample machine, the $\hat{t}_{tak}$ equivalent test time at the corresponding moment (failure) can be calculated according to the acceleration factor and the actual time of the accelerated test $\hat{t}_{tek}$, (failure) The equivalent test time at the corresponding moment is equal to $\hat{t}_{te}$ the product of the accelerated test time and the acceleration factor $\hat{t}_{ta}$, see formula (6.34):

$$\hat{t}_{tek} = \mathrm{AF} \cdot \hat{t}_{tak} \tag{6.34}$$

In the formula:

$\hat{t}_{tak}$—Accelerated test bench time accumulated by the prototype at the moment when the *kth prototype fails under accelerated test conditions;*

$\hat{t}_{tek}$—The equivalent (under normal use or test conditions) test time of the accelerated test time accumulated up to the time when the prototype fails.

When carrying out the accelerated test to evaluate the life, the equivalent test time of multiple prototypes cannot be accumulated for life evaluation.

6.4.6.5 End of Life Determination

In the life test, considering the nature and consequences of the failure, combined with maintenance engineering, the end-of-life criteria are determined as follows:

(1) The related failure with serious consequences of the failure of the sample machine, the failure cannot be repaired, and it is determined that the service life of the sample machine is terminated;
(2) For the associated failure with serious consequences of the failure of the sample machine, the failure can be repaired, but the maintenance cost is unacceptable, and it is determined that the service life of the sample machine is terminated;
(3) If the life of the sample machine is terminated due to unrelated failures, the sample machine will not be used as a sample for life evaluation.

6.4.6.6 Evaluation of Life Index

Using the equivalent test time $\hat{t}_{tek}$ and engineering experience coefficient at the corresponding moment k, the observation life corresponding to the accelerated test of a single prototype can be evaluated, see formula (6.35):

$$\hat{l}_i = \frac{\hat{t}_{tek}}{k} = \frac{\hat{t}_{tak} \cdot \mathrm{AF}}{k} \tag{6.35}$$

In the formula:

$\hat{t}_{tek}$—The equivalent (under normal use or test conditions) test time of the accumulative effective accelerated test time up to the time when the prototype fails;

k—Engineering experience coefficient, k preferably 1.0–1.5, usually 1.2;

$\hat{t}_{tak}$—The accumulative effective acceleration test bench time of the k -th prototype at the time of the failure of the prototype under the accelerated test conditions;

AF—Acceleration factor;

$\hat{l}_k$—The life observation value of *the k-th* prototype.

Using the observed life of each prototype, the average life of this type of prototype can be estimated, see formula (6.36):

$$\hat{l} = \frac{\sum_{i=1}^{n} \hat{l}_i}{n} \tag{6.36}$$

In the formula:
$\hat{l}_k$—The life observation value of the *k-th* prototype;
n—The number of prototypes;
$\hat{l}$—The average lifespan of n prototypes.

6.5 Durability Evaluation Test Technology of Structural Parts

6.5.1 Salt Spray Test for Metal Structural Parts

6.5.1.1 Purpose and Application

Salt spray test is mainly used to examine the ability of metal structural parts to resist the effects of salt spray.

1. **Test Purposes**

(1) Determine the effectiveness of the protective and decorative layers of the material;
(2) Determine the influence of salt deposits on the physical and electrical properties of equipment.

2. **Application**

(1) Evaluate the quality and effectiveness of the equipment and its material protective covering, locate potential problem areas, find quality control defects and design defects, etc.;
(2) Optimize materials and evaluate equipment;
(3) Equipment mainly exposed to the atmosphere with high salt content.

6.5.1.2 Environmental Effects

1. **Corrosion Effect**

Salt spray environments can cause the following corrosive effects on equipment:

(1) Corrosion caused by electrochemical reactions;
(2) Accelerated stress corrosion;
(3) Salt ionizes in water to form an acidic or alkaline solution.

2. **Electrical Effect**

Salt spray environments can cause the following electrical effects on equipment:

(1) Salt deposits can cause damage to electrical equipment;
(2) Generate a conductive covering layer;
(3) Corrosion of insulating materials and metals.

3. **Physical Effect**

The salt spray environment may cause the following physical effects on the equipment:

(1) Blockage or jamming of moving parts of mechanical parts and assemblies;
(2) Blistering of the coating due to electrolysis.

6.5.1.3 Determination of Test Conditions

1. **Saline Solution**

The concentration of saline solution is generally 5%.

2. **Test Duration**

This experiment recommends the use of alternating 24 h salt spray and 24 h dry in two states for a total of 96 h test procedure. Experience has shown that this alternating approach and test time provides salt spray test results that are closer to the true exposure situation than continuous spraying for 96 h and have greater potential for damage because of the higher corrosion efficiency from the wet to dry state.

3. **Temperature**

The test temperature in the spray stage is 35 ± 5 °C, which does not simulate the actual exposure temperature.

4. **Wind Speed**

During the test, the wind speed in the test chamber should be kept as zero as possible.

5. **Sedimentation Rate**

Adjust the sedimentation rate of the salt mist to ensure that the collection volume of each collector in a horizontal collection area of 80 cm^2 (10 cm in diameter) is 1-3 mL of solution per hour.

6. **Orientation of the Specimen**

The orientation of the specimen in the salt spray test shall be placed according to its intended orientation in storage, transportation or use.

6.5.1.4 Information Requirements

1. **Pre-experiment Information**

(1) The scope of visual inspection and performance inspection of the test piece, and the description of including or excluding these scopes;
(2) The concentration of the salt solution;
(3) The resistivity of water and the type of water.

2. **Information in Test**

(1) The record of the temperature change with time in the test chamber;
(2) Sedimentation rate of salt solution (mL/(80 cm ^{2} ·h));
(3) pH value of salt spray.

3. **Post Test Information**

(1) The scope of visual inspection and performance inspection of the test piece, and the description of including or excluding these scopes;
(2) Test variables: pH value of salt spray and sedimentation rate of salt solution (mL/(80 cm ^{2} ·h));
(3) Detection results of corrosion effects, electrical effects and physical effects;
(4) Observations for failure analysis.

6.5.1.5 Test Requirements

1. **Test Equipment**

(1) Test chamber

All parts in contact with the test piece must not cause electrochemical corrosion, and the condensate must not drip on the test piece; any test solution that has been in contact with the test box or the test piece must not return to the salt solution tank; the test box should have drains. The air outlet ensures the pressure level.

(2) Salt solution tank

Use materials that do not react with salt solutions, such as glass, plastic, and rubber.

(3) Saline solution injection system

The salt solution is filtered and delivered to the test chamber, where the atomizer produces a dispersed, fine and moist dense mist.

(4) Salt mist collector

At least 2 salt spray collectors are used to collect salt solution samples. One is placed at the edge of the test piece closest to the nozzle and the other is also placed at the edge of the test piece but farthest from the nozzle.

2. **Test Control**

After the compressed air removes oil and dirt, it should be preheated and humidified. The purpose of preheating is to compensate for the cooling effect of compressed air expanding to atmospheric pressure. Table 6.11 shows the recommended compressed air pressure and corresponding preheating temperature requirements.

3. **Test Interruption**

(1) Under test interruption. In the event of an unplanned test interruption that results in test conditions below specified values and out of tolerance, a complete visual inspection of the test piece shall be performed and a technical assessment of the effect of the test interruption on the test results shall be made. Stabilize the specimen under the test conditions and restart the test from the point of interruption.
(2) The test is interrupted. In the event of an unplanned test interruption that results in test conditions that are higher than specified and outside the tolerances, the test conditions shall be stabilized within the tolerances and maintained at this level until a full visual inspection and technical evaluation can be performed to confirm the test the impact of the interruption on the test results. If it is confirmed that the effect of the interruption is negligible, the test conditions before the interruption should be re-stabilized and the test should be continued from the moment when the tolerance was exceeded. Otherwise restart the test with a new test piece.

Table 6.11 Compressed air pressure and corresponding preheating temperature requirements

Air pressure/ kPa	Preheating temperature (before atomization)/ °C
83	46
96	47
110	48
124	49

6.5.1.6 Test Preparation

1. **Specimen Pre-treatment**

The surface of the contaminated test piece should be pre-treated to ensure that the surface of the test piece is free of contaminants such as oil, grease or dirt, as they can cause the surface water film to break. Any cleaning method should not use corrosive solvents, should not use solvents that form a corrosion layer or protective layer on the surface of the test piece, and should not use abrasives other than pure magnesium oxide. The pretreatment of the specimen should be as little as possible.

2. **Preparation of Test Solution**

The salt used in this test is sodium chloride. This sodium chloride in dry state shall not contain more than 0.1% sodium iodide and shall not contain more than 0.5% total impurities. Sodium chloride with anti-caking agents should not be used because of the corrosion inhibitor effect.

In general, 5% sodium chloride solution should be prepared as follows:

Dissolve 5 parts by weight of sodium chloride in 95 parts by weight of water, and adjust and maintain the specific gravity of the saline solution by adjusting temperature and concentration. In order to keep the pH value of the sedimentation salt solution collected in the test chamber between 6.5 and 7.2 at a temperature of 35 ± 5 °C, the pH value can only be adjusted with dilute chemically pure hydrochloric acid or sodium hydroxide. The measurement of pH value can adopt electrochemical method or colorimetric method.

3. **Test Chamber Operation Check**

If the test box has not been used within 5 days before the test or the nozzle is not blocked, all test parameters of the test box should be adjusted under no-load conditions before the test starts to meet the requirements of this test. Guarantee the test conditions for at least 24 h, or keep the test conditions until the normal operation status and salt mist deposition rate are confirmed. In order to ensure the normal operation of the test chamber, the sedimentation rate of the salt mist should still be detected after 24 h. The temperature of the test chamber should be continuously monitored and recorded, or monitored every 2 h until the test starts.

4. **Initial Detection**

Before the test, all test pieces should be tested under standard atmospheric conditions to obtain baseline data. Testing should be carried out in the following steps:

(1) Record the atmospheric conditions in the laboratory.
(2) Carry out a comprehensive visual inspection of the test piece, paying attention to the following:

- High stress areas;
- Parts where dissimilar metals are in contact;

- Electrical and electronic components—especially circuit elements that are close together, uncoated or exposed;
- Metal surface;
- Enclosed areas where condensation has occurred or is likely to occur;
- Surfaces or components with coating or surface anti-corrosion treatment;
- Cathodic protection system;
- Mechanical systems malfunctioning due to blockage or coverage by salt deposits;
- Electric and thermal insulator.

(3) Record the inspection results.
(4) Install the test piece in the test box and meet the required technical status.

6.5.1.7 Test Procedure

The test steps are as follows:

(1) Adjust the temperature of the test chamber to 35 °C, and keep the test piece under this condition for at least 2 h before spraying.
(2) Spray salt spray for 24 h or the time stipulated in relevant documents. During the entire spraying period, the salt mist sedimentation rate and the pH value of the sedimentation solution are measured at least once every 24 h to ensure that the salt solution sedimentation rate is (1–3) mL/(80 $cm^2 \cdot h$).
(3) Dry the specimen for 24 h or the time specified in the relevant documents under the condition of standard atmospheric temperature (15–35 °C) and relative humidity not higher than 50%. During drying, it is not possible to change the technical state of the test piece or to adjust its mechanical state.
(4) At the end of the drying period, unless otherwise specified, the test piece should be reset in the salt spray test chamber and repeat (2) and (3) at least once.
(5) Carry out physical and electrical performance testing, and record the test results. If it is helpful for the subsequent corrosion inspection, the test piece can be gently rinsed with running water under standard atmospheric conditions, and then tested and recorded.

6.5.1.8 Result Analysis

(1) Physics. Salt deposits can cause clogging or binding of mechanical parts or assemblies. Any salt deposits produced by this experiment may represent the result of the expected environment.
(2) Electrical. After the 24 h drying period, residual moisture can lead to electrical failures. Consideration should be given to correlating such failures with failures in actual use.
(3) Corrosion. Analyze the effect of corrosion on the normal function and structural integrity of the specimen in terms of short-term and potential long-term effects.

6.5.2 *Solar Radiation Test for Non-Metallic Structural Parts*

6.5.2.1 Purpose and Application

The solar radiation test is mainly used to investigate the ability of the equipment to withstand direct solar radiation.

1. **Test Purposes**

(1) Determine the thermal effect of direct solar radiation on equipment;
(2) Determine the photochemical effect of direct solar radiation on the equipment.

2. **Application**

It is used to evaluate the ability of the equipment exposed directly to the solar radiation environment in the hot season during the life cycle to withstand the thermal effect or photochemical action produced by the solar radiation.

This test cannot simulate all natural climate and environmental conditions, and is not suitable for the simulation of uniform thermal effects in a closed environment, nor for indirect thermal effects in sheltered areas or under covered storage conditions.

6.5.2.2 Environmental Effects

1. **Thermal Effect**

Different from the thermal effect produced by high temperature, the thermal effect of solar radiation is directional and produces thermal gradients. In solar radiation tests, the absorption or reflection of heat depends mainly on the roughness and color of the irradiated surface. Variations in solar irradiance cause different materials and components to expand or contract at different rates, creating severe stress and compromising structural integrity.

2. **Photochemical Reaction**

In general, the rate of photochemical reactions increases with temperature, so the full spectrum should be used to fully simulate the photochemical effects of solar radiation, resulting in:

(1) Discoloration of fabrics and plastics;
(2) Coating cracking, powdering and discoloration;
(3) Photochemical reactions caused by shorter wavelength radiation lead to cracking of natural rubber, synthetic rubber and polymers.

6.5.2.3 Test Procedure

This experiment includes two test procedures: procedure circular test; procedure—steady state test. Due to different considerations, the solar radiation load and loading time used are different.

1. **Procedure I—Round Robin Test**

Focusing on the thermal effect produced by solar radiation, the test piece is exposed to the actual maximum level of solar radiation simulated in the world, and 24 h is a cycle.

This procedure should be used to test the temperature response of equipment to solar radiation when the equipment is exposed to outdoor hot climates and no degradation in performance is expected during and after exposure. Use this procedure when equipment is subject to non-uniform heating, or when the magnitude or mechanism of heating due to solar radiation is unknown.

2. **Procedure II—Steady State Test**

Focusing on the photochemical effect of accelerated solar radiation, it exposes the specimen to an enhanced solar radiation load (about 2.5 times the normal magnitude), with a 24-h cycle to accelerate the realization of The photochemical effect can only be accumulated for a long time, and the actual acceleration rate is related to the characteristics of the material.

The photochemical effect usually occurs after the surface of the equipment receives a large amount of sunlight, and the impact of long-term solar radiation on the equipment is detected. The 4 h non-radiation period in each 24 h cycle is to make the physical and chemical state of the specimen return to the "normal state" under the non-radiation condition, during which the specimen will also be subjected to a certain degree of thermal stress.

6.5.2.4 Determination of Test Conditions

1. **Daily Cycle**

(1) The peak condition of cycle A_1 is 1120W/m^2, and the test temperature is 49 °C, which represents the hottest condition in the world;
(2) The peak condition of cycle A_2 is 1120W/m^2, and the test temperature is 44 °C, which represents less severe conditions, and its location has high temperature and moderately low humidity accompanied by high-intensity solar radiation;
(3) The peak condition of cycle A_3 is 1120W/m ^{2}, and the test temperature is 39 °C, which represents less severe conditions, and the area where it is located experiences moderately high and moderately low humidity conditions for at least part of the year.

2. **Test Duration**

(1) **Procedure I**

A minimum of 3 cycles and a maximum of 7 cycles were performed, with a cycle time of 24 h each, during which the maximum response temperature was required to be reached.

(2) **Procedure II**

Alternate between thermal stress and the so-called "dark" process. To simulate 10 days of natural exposure, 4 cycles are acceptable; to simulate occasional outdoor use, 10 cycles are recommended; and for gear that is continuously exposed to outdoor conditions, a minimum of 56 cycles is recommended.

3. **Test Piece Work**

When specimen work is required, the requirements are as follows:

(1) Adopt the working mode with the maximum energy consumption (produce the most heat);
(2) If the change of voltage will affect the heat dissipation or thermal response of the test piece, indicate the change range of the input voltage of the test piece;
(3) Introduce the cooling medium normally used during equipment use.

6.5.2.5 Information Requirements

1. **Pre-experiment Information**

(1) Humidity conditions included in the program I daily cycle (when applicable);
(2) Work requirements of the test piece;
(3) The spectrum of the radiant lamp;
(4) Temperature measurement method.

2. **Information in Test**

(1) Records of temperature and irradiance changes over time in the test chamber;
(2) The record of the temperature change of the test piece with time;
(3) pH value of salt spray.

3. **Post Test Information**

(1) The position of the temperature sensor on the test piece;
(2) The temperature of the test piece and the number of exposure cycles;
(3) Identification of radiation lamps.

6.5.2.6 Test Equipment Requirements

1. **Basic Requirements**

(1) Be able to maintain and monitor the temperature, wind speed and irradiance required by the test;
(2) In order to minimize or eliminate radiation reflection from the inner surface of the test chamber, the volume of the test chamber is usually at least 10 times the volume of the outer shell of the test piece.

2. **Base**

The base on which the test piece is mounted may be a raised bracket or a base with specified characteristics.

3. **Solar Radiation Lamp**

(1) Solar radiation lamps include heating radiation lamps or radiation lamps simulating the solar spectrum;
(2) Use the maximum irradiance of (1120 ± 12) W/m2 to ensure that the specimen receives uniform radiation, and the deviation of the irradiance measured on the upper surface of the specimen does not exceed 10% of the required value;
(3) When the radiation lamp is directly facing the test piece, and the entire surface of the test piece facing the radiation lamp is irradiated, the measured value of 1120W/m2 theoretically includes all the radiation received by the test piece, including the radiation from the test chamber wall radiant reflection, tank wall reflection, and any long-wave infrared radiation scattered by the tank wall;
(4) The radiation lamp should be placed at least 0.76 m away from the surface of the test piece.

6.5.2.7 Test Control Requirements

1. **Temperature**

Ensure that the air temperature in the test chamber is consistent with the air temperature in the vicinity of the test piece.

2. **Surface Contamination**

During the test, ensure that the test piece is clean. Dust and other surface contaminants can significantly change the absorption characteristics of the irradiated surface.

3. **Gauge**

Use a pyranometer, pyrheliometer, or other suitable device to measure the applied radiant energy over time.

Pyranometer requirements:

(1) Spectral range: 0.280–2.500 μm;
(2) Azimuth response error: ±1%;
(3) Cosine response error: ±1%;
(4) Non-linear error: <1.5%;
(5) Tilt error: <1.5%;
(6) Working temperature: —40–80 °C;
(7) Sensitivity: ± 2% (–10–40 °C).

6.5.2.8 Test Interruption Requirements

1. **Under Test Interruption**

After any interruption of the test, it shall be re-stabilized to the specified value and the test shall be resumed from the point of interruption.

2. **Over Test Interruption**

After any interruption of the overtest, the test piece should be thoroughly inspected to verify the influence of the overtest, and the test should be repeated with a new test piece.

6.5.2.9 Test Procedure

1. **Procedure I**

(1) Adjust the air temperature of the test chamber to the minimum value of the temperature cycle without irradiation;
(2) Control the irradiance and dry bulb temperature of the test chamber, measure and record the temperature of the specimen during the whole test period;
(3) If the test piece is required to work, the test piece is in the working state when the cycle temperature reaches the peak value. For the one-time use test piece, it is necessary to install a temperature sensor on the key part of the test piece to determine the time and value of the temperature peak., make the specimen work when the cycle temperature reaches the peak value;
(4) Adjust the air temperature of the test chamber to standard atmospheric conditions and maintain it until the temperature of the test piece is stabilized;
(5) Carry out a comprehensive visual inspection of the test piece;
(6) Carry out work inspection on the test piece;
(7) Compare the data before and after the experiment.

2. **Procedure II**

(1) Adjust the air temperature of the test chamber to the temperature specified in the technical documents;
(2) Adjust the irradiance of the radiation lamp to $(1120 \pm 12)\ W/m^2$ or the value specified in the product specification;
(3) Keep these conditions for 20 h, measure and record the temperature of the test piece;
(4) Turn off the radiation lamp for 4 h. If necessary, the working test is carried out when the temperature of the test piece is the highest during the non-radiation period of each cycle;
(5) At the end of the last radiation cycle, return the specimen to standard atmospheric conditions;
(6) Perform visual inspection and work inspection on the test piece, and record the results.

6.5.2.10 Results Analysis

1. **Procedure I**

Under the temperature peak conditions and after returning to the standard atmospheric conditions, the performance and characteristics of the test specimens must not change to meet the requirements of the product specification.

2. **Procedure II**

Changes in the performance and characteristics of the test piece (such as color or other surface conditions) cannot appear to fail to meet the requirements of the product specification.

6.6 Statistical Evaluation of Usability in Field Operations

The usability and reliability level reflect the actual usability and reliability level of a product. Therefore, combining the on-site operation to carry out the usability statistical evaluation and obtain the real level and failure information of a series of usability and related parameters can provide the research and development unit with a basis for improving products. Information support can also provide information support for the research and development unit to develop new products in the future to determine indicators and implement improvements.

At present, China's research and development institutions generally lack effective quality information. The main reason is that there is no information collection mechanism, lack of good information collection methods, lack of active awareness and clear goals for information collection, and the same is true in the medical equipment industry. In the end, there is a lack of effective information for research and development demonstration, improvement implementation, and determination of service life, which can only be determined by patting the head, which often leads to contradictions in various technical decisions.

6.6.1 Terms and Definitions

Availability: It is a comprehensive parameter, which is a comprehensive embodiment of reliability parameters, maintainability parameters, and support parameters, involving Mean Time Between Failures (MTBF), Mean Time To Repair (MTTR), Mean Preventive Maintenance Time (MPMT), and delays parameters such as time. In order to give readers a clearer understanding of the connotation of availability and its related parameters, we first understand the definitions of related terms.

Maintainability: The ability of the product to maintain or return to the specified state when it is maintained according to the specified procedures and methods under the specified conditions and within the specified time. Maintainability reflects the possibility of completing maintenance under specified constraints (maintenance conditions, maintenance time, maintenance procedures, and maintenance methods). The specified conditions include maintenance level (hospital site, regional maintenance center, manufacturer), maintenance organization and site (such as use place, special repair workshop, maintenance base, factory, etc.) and corresponding personnel and facilities, equipment, tools, spare parts, Support resources such as technical data. The prescribed procedures and methods refer to the types, steps and methods of maintenance work stipulated in the technical documents. Maintainability is a design feature of a product, an inherent attribute given to a product during design. Maintainability directly affects the maintenance workload and difficulty of the product. Maintainability can be described by qualitative and quantitative characteristics. The qualitative characteristics of maintainability affect the number of customer service personnel, technical level and professional type, maintenance test equipment, maintenance man-hours and costs, etc. Quantitative properties of maintainability include maintenance time parameters and maintenance man-hour rate parameters, such as Mean Time to Repair (MTTR), Mean Preventive Maintenance Time (MPMT), Mean Downtime (MDT) and Maintenance Man-hours per Hour (MMH/OH)wait.

Supportability: The design characteristics of equipment and the ability of planned support resources to meet operational requirements or user needs.

Availability: The degree to which a product is in a working or usable state at any time when it is needed and begins to perform a task. The probability measure of availability is called availability. Availability refers to the ability of a product to be in a state that can perform specified functions within a specified time interval and under specified conditions under the premise that external resources are guaranteed. Availability is closely related to reliability, maintainability and supportability.

Mean Time Between Failures: The ratio of the total number of product life units to the total number of failures under specified conditions and within a specified period of time. It is a basic reliability parameter of repairable products. failure refers to the state that the product cannot perform the specified function, including loss of function, out-of-tolerance performance, structural damage, etc.

Mean Time To Failure: The ratio of the total number of product life units to the total number of failed products under specified conditions and within a specified period of time. It is a basic reliability parameter of non-repairable products. Product repairable and non-repairable are relative. Usually, the test object is the corresponding level. For example, in a certain equipment test, the failure of the equipment is due to the failure of a component. From the equipment level, the component can be replaced, and the equipment can be Repaired; for example, in a component test, the component failure is due to bonding failure, and the component is not repairable. For repairable test objects, MTTF can also be used to express its mean time to first failure. For irreparable test subjects, MTTF can also be used to express their lifetime.

Mean Time Between Serious Failures: The ratio of the total time of product missions to the total number of serious failures in a specified series of mission profiles. It is a reliability parameter related to the task. The life profile refers to the sequential description of all events and environments experienced by a product during the period from delivery to end of life or out of use. A task profile is a sequential description of the events and environments experienced by a product during the time it takes to complete a specified task. A critical failure is a failure that prevents the product from performing its specified tasks.

Average preventive maintenance time: The average value of preventive maintenance time for a specified object within a specified time interval, that is, for all preventive maintenance events that occur on the object within this time interval, the sum of the preventive maintenance time and the preventive maintenance time The ratio of maintenance times.

Preventive maintenance: through systematic inspection, detection and elimination of product failure symptoms, all activities carried out to keep it in the specified state, including pre-maintenance, scheduled maintenance, condition-based maintenance and failure detection, etc. Predictive maintenance refers to the identification, monitoring and elimination activities taken to address the root cause of the failure. Scheduled maintenance refers to the maintenance carried out according to the pre-arranged content when the product is used to a predetermined interval. Condition-based maintenance refers to regular or continuous monitoring of products, and targeted maintenance when signs of functional failure are found. Preventive maintenance time is the time spent performing preventive maintenance on a product. Annual repair time is the total time a product is in repair repair time within a year. Monthly repair time refers to the total time the product is in repair repair state within one month.

Mean time to repair: A basic parameter of product maintainability, which is a design parameter. Its measurement method is: under the specified conditions and within the specified period, the product is at the specified maintenance level, the ratio of the total repair maintenance time to the total number of failures of the repaired product at this level.

Restorative maintenance: All activities performed to restore a product to a specified state after a failure occurs, including failure location, failure isolation, disassembly, replacement, assembly, adjustment, and testing, etc. The entire activity is also called repair. Corrective maintenance time is the time spent performing corrective maintenance on a product. Annual repair time is the total time a product is in repair repair time within a year. Monthly repair time refers to the total time the product is in repair repair state within one month.

Mean time to repair: The ratio of the total time on product missions to the total number of critical failures in a specified series of mission profiles. It is a reliability parameter related to the task. Maintenance refers to all activities performed to maintain or restore the product to the specified state, usually including preventive maintenance and corrective maintenance. Maintenance time refers to the time spent in downtime for maintenance, excluding improvement time and delay time. The annual average repair time refers to the total time that the product is in repair state in a year. Monthly repair time refers to the total time the product is in repair state within a month.

Delayed time: the time delayed by failure to guarantee the product in time due to guarantee resource supply or management reasons. Guaranteed resource delay time refers to the time delayed in guaranteeing the product due to waiting for the required guarantee resources, such as the time delayed in waiting for spare parts, customer service personnel, guarantee equipment, information and appropriate environmental conditions. Management delay time refers to the delay time due to failure to guarantee the product in time due to management reasons.

Availability: In a specified time interval, the ratio of the time that the product is in a usable state to the specified time interval. Availability includes inherent availability, reachable availability and usage availability. Inherent availability (A_i) is an availability parameter related only to working time and corrective maintenance time. Its measurement method is the ratio of the Mean Time Between Failures of the product to the sum of the Mean Time Between Failures and the mean time to repair. Availability (A_a) is an availability parameter related only to working time, corrective maintenance time and preventive maintenance time. Its measurement method is: the ratio of the working time of the product to the sum of working time, corrective maintenance time and preventive maintenance time. Availability (A_o) is an availability parameter related to working time and non-working time. Its measurement method is the ratio of the working time of the product to the sum of the working time and the non-working time. Usually, in addition to the working time, corrective maintenance time and preventive maintenance time, it also includes (management and guarantee) delay time.

Boot rate: The probability that the device can be booted normally when it is in good condition. The actual start-up rate is the ratio of the time that the equipment is in the actual running state to the time it should be working. The expected working time can be defined as the typical working interval expected by typical users, and different types of users may define different expected working hours. For example, when a medical electron linear accelerator works in a hospital, the working hours can usually be defined as the normal working hours of the working day; while when it is in a professional diagnosis and treatment institution, the working hours may be determined as 24 h a day throughout the year. The start-up rate refers to the probability that the prototype can be started up in a good state, and is usually measured by the ratio of the start up time to the start up time. When calculating the bootable time, only the time when the machine cannot be turned on due to machine reasons is included, and the time when the machine is not turned on due to external factors (such as power outages, water outages, holidays, relocation, etc.) during normal operation is ignored. The maximum boot rate is the maximum boot rate that can be obtained when the non-start time caused by external factors can be completely ignored (that is, the machine is normal when the external factors occur).

6.6.2 Determination of Evaluation Conditions

1. **Evaluation Time**

For the diagnosis and treatment equipment that has been delivered to the hospital, the cycle of availability evaluation is recommended to be 1 year.

For machines that have not been delivered to the hospital, evaluation can be carried out in the computer room of the production unit. According to the schedule cycle requirements, the evaluation time can be shortened by increasing the intensity of use. Generally, it is recommended not to be less than 1 month, and 3 months is recommended, otherwise the cycle is too short. May lead to evaluation results relative to the actual preference.

2. **Evaluation Site**

For the diagnostic and treatment equipment that has been delivered to the hospital, when there are multiple users in use, when selecting the evaluation location, it should be combined with the manufacturer's expected sales area to cover typical climate characteristics as much as possible, such as cold and dry areas, hot and humid areas, and plateaus. Low-pressure areas, coastal high-salt areas, etc.

3. **Evaluate the Computer Room**

The computer room used in the evaluation should meet the planning requirements of the computer room, including requirements for space, shielding, power supply, ventilation, and environmental control, so as to ensure the normal operation of medical equipment.

6.6.3 Equipment Operation Requirements

6.6.3.1 Switching Machine Requirements

When evaluating the machines that have been delivered to the hospital, the on/off operation can be performed according to the actual use of the hospital, and no additional on/off measures are required.

When evaluating a machine that has not been delivered to the hospital, before conducting the usability evaluation, it is necessary to estimate the number of times the medical electron linear accelerator is expected to be switched on and off in one year of use based on the user's actual switching habits during use. Before the evaluation, the number and cycle of switching on and off should be agreed, and the switching on and off operation and inspection should be carried out according to the relevant agreement. The agreed on and off times should be combined with the running time of the machine and the frequency of on and off in the actual use of the user.

6.6.3.2 Running Status Configuration

Hospital computer room operating status configuration: When evaluating a machine that has been delivered to a hospital, it is not necessary to additionally configure the operating status of the machine according to the normal use process of the hospital.

Factory computer room operating status configuration: When evaluating machines that have not been delivered to hospitals, their operating status and configuration ratio should be determined based on the typical life history of the equipment.

First of all, the annual unavailable state time of the medical electron linear accelerator should be evaluated by combining the annual preventive maintenance frequency and downtime, the annual corrective maintenance failure frequency and downtime, and the unavailable downtime caused by non-machine reasons. Then, deduct the unavailable state time from the total time to calculate the available state time for the whole year. Secondly, according to the available state time of the year combined with the usage scenarios, the standby time and working time are further estimated. Finally, according to the working time combined with the frequency of use, estimate the high-voltage working time and filament working time.

Through the above process, the annual accumulated unavailable time, available time, power-on standby time, power-on working time, high-voltage working time and their proportions to the total time can be calculated. Determine the ratio of the power-on working state and the high-voltage working state in the usability evaluation process. When the evaluation time needs to be shortened, the proportion of time in the working state can be increased, but it should not be higher than the time corresponding to the machine's maximum bootable rate. Maintenance work should be carried out in strict accordance with the specified cycle and requirements during the startup process.

The time of various states of the machine should be recorded, including unavailable state time (usually divided into preventive maintenance downtime, corrective maintenance downtime, non-machine downtime), available state working time (usually divided into complete machine And the power-on time of each system, the working time in normal state, the working time in special state), these time records are essential for the statistics of availability and various related indicators.

Taking the medical electron linear accelerator as an example, the daily state record table is shown in Table 6.12, and the statistics are 1-time in unavailable state and 2-time in available state. For 1-unavailable state time, further subdivide and count 1–1 abnormal unavailable state time caused by machine reasons, 1–2 normal unavailable state time caused by non-machine reasons, and 1–3 start-up preparation state time. 2-Available state time is further subdivided into statistics: 2–1 partial power-on standby time, 2–2 start-up working time, 2–3 high-voltage working time, 2–4 filament working time (acceleration tube, magnetron/speed adjustment Tube).

Table 6.12 Medical electron linear accelerator daily status record form (example)

	1—Unavailable state time			2—Available state time				
Hour Between Part	1–1 Caused by machine reasons Abnormal unavailable state time		1–2 Normal unavailable state time caused by non–machine reasons	2–1 Partial power–on standby time	2–2 Full boot working time	2–3 Open high pressure working time	2–4 Filament time	
	1–1–1 Preventive Maintenance Downtime	1–1–2 Corrective Maintenance Downtime					Accelerator tube	– Magnetron – Klystron

6.6.3.3 Use Mode Configuration

In the actual use process of the hospital, the user adopts the relevant use mode according to the actual needs, and there is no need to configure the use mode, but the statistical evaluation results of the usability may be biased due to the single mode of use by the user.

When conducting statistical evaluation in the computer room of the research and development enterprise, the use mode configuration should be combined with various actual use scenarios of medical equipment, and the type of use mode and configuration ratio should be determined to fully and comprehensively assess various use modes.

Taking the medical electron linear accelerator as an example, the usage mode includes the type of treatment object, the number of treatment and positioning movement operation. Treatment object types include real patients and simulated body membranes. According to the typical number of patients that can be treated by the medical electron linear accelerator every day, the total time required for each patient's treatment and the typical time of high-voltage output beam therapy, the proportion of the high-voltage output beam treatment time can be calculated. According to the characteristics, quantity and corresponding treatment plan of the treatment objects, the number and time of setting up during one day's treatment can be estimated.

Configuration of hospital clinical use mode of medical electron linear accelerator: When carrying out annual usability evaluation in combination with the actual use process of the hospital, real patients should be used as treatment objects, and corresponding positioning operations and high-voltage radiation therapy should be completed according to the corresponding treatment plan, without additional Configure the machine usage mode and strictly record the actual usage mode of the machine operation.

Configuration of the use mode of the factory computer room of the medical electron linear accelerator: during the usability evaluation of the factory computer room during the development process, the simulated body membrane can be used as the treatment object. The number of treatments determines the number of simulated treatments, completes the equivalent number of setup operations and the equivalent time of high-voltage radiation therapy, and equivalently carries out the quality control and observation of radiation quality in clinical use.

6.6.4 Requirements for the Design of Prototype Running Cycle

In order to standardize the operation and maintenance of the prototype in the process of availability evaluation, before testing, it is necessary to formulate the operation cycle diagram of the prototype. The following content is used as a reference when formulating the cycle diagram.

Inspection before the first run: After the prototype has been installed, debugged, and tested to confirm that it meets the requirements for use, the prototype should be inspected and tested according to the user's acceptance conditions under the organization of the evaluation agency. After confirming that the prototype is normal, it will officially enter the usability evaluation stage.

Routine low-voltage power-on and preparation: routine low-voltage power-on, turn on the power supply of the control system (as the starting point of the cycle), complete the equipment warm-up, and make the equipment reach the state of treating patients (that is, the ready state).

Normal use: Simulate the whole process of patient treatment, including reception of diagnosis and treatment plans, patient positioning, implementation of diagnosis and treatment, and patient unloading.

Routine shutdown: shut down according to the normal process designed for the whole machine performed after routine shutdown and is only carried out during availability evaluation under factory conditions. Artificially disconnect all the system network power, which is used to simulate the situation that the network power is completely disconnected due to initial installation, power outage, regular maintenance, etc. When conducting usability evaluation, determine the number of non-routine shutdowns according to the evaluation cycle. When the evaluation cycle is not less than 1 year, the non-routine shutdown is once a month; when the evaluation cycle is not less than 6 months, the non-routine shutdown is every two weeks. When the evaluation period is not less than 3 months, non-routine shutdown once a week.

Clinical quality control (QA) of equipment: According to the requirements of daily inspection, weekly inspection, monthly inspection and annual inspection stipulated in clinical quality control (QA), equipment inspection is carried out, and the inspection results are recorded.

Regular maintenance: During the evaluation process, regular maintenance should be carried out according to the equipment maintenance requirements or manuals provided by the equipment manufacturer.

6.6.5 Evaluation Conduct and Information Collection

6.6.5.1 Operation of the Equipment

When evaluating at the manufacturer's site, the simulated operating state and working mode of the equipment shall be completely or as consistent as possible with the real operating state and working mode. The daily operating intensity can be appropriately increased according to the extension of working hours to shorten the evaluation time. Form 6–13 should be strictly filled during equipment use, and Form 6–14 should be strictly filled during equipment shutdown.

6.6.5.2 Preventive Maintenance

During the use of the equipment, the daily maintenance work of the equipment should be completed in strict accordance with the requirements of the manufacturer, and records should be made.

6.6.5.3 Failure Classification, Recording and Handling

1. **Classification of Failure Consequences**

Generally, it can be divided into serious failure and general failure.

Severe failures—events that directly lead to downtime, resulting in failure to start up, fail to operate normally, fail to realize basic and main functions, and technical indicators to be out of tolerance to unacceptable, which may lead to serious consequences or fail to comply with safety regulations, and must be shut down for processing; In the clinical mode, non-resettable interlocks are judged as serious failures, which require immediate corrective maintenance; resettable interlocks, if they occur too frequently and cause downtime for maintenance, should also be judged as serious failures.

General failures—prototypes have failure alarms or symptoms, some functions are lost, and technical indicators exceed the standard, but the prototypes are not shut down, do not need to be shut down, can operate normally, can continue to be used normally, and can complete basic and main functions. For example, in the clinical mode, if the resettable interlock does not cause downtime for maintenance, it will be judged as a general failure.

2. **Classification of Failure Nature**

Generally, it can be divided into correlated failures and non-correlated failures.

Non-associated failures refer to the failures that have been proven not to be used according to the specified conditions, mainly including:

(1) Failures caused by test equipment, test instruments and supporting conditions guarantee not meeting the requirements;
(2) The test stress that does not meet the requirements is applied or the failure is determined to be caused by overstress;
(3) Man-made failures caused by improper handling, operation, testing and maintenance of the sample machine;
(4) Dependent failures caused by independent failures, failures caused by use beyond the specified life span, etc.

The failures other than non-correlated failures are all related failures. The related failures mainly refer to the failures caused by the problems of the sample machine itself. The related failures mainly include:

(1) failures caused by improper design, process and assembly of the sample machine;
(2) failures caused by improper design, manufacture and selection of parts and components;
(3) failures caused by software errors;
(4) Failures caused by improper operation, maintenance and maintenance procedures specified by the manufacturer.

3. **Broken Record**

In the event of a serious failure, report for repair if necessary. The record should include the time point when the failure occurred, when it is determined that the equipment status is unavailable (the start time of this unavailability), record the time of repair report (the start of the after-sales response time for this failure); when the manufacturer's customer service personnel arrive at the scene, record the customer service The first visit time (the end of the after-sales reflection time of this failure); when the customer service personnel repairs the equipment and is checked and tested by the user organization, it is determined that the equipment status is restored to usable (the end time of this unavailability), and the restored usable time should be filled in.

For general failures, use Table 6.15 to record and give regular feedback on the problems that affect the use and cause abnormal status.

6.6.5.4 Recording and Calculation Requirements

1. **Record Requirements**

Inspection records before the first run: Prototype test records (including test items, qualification criteria, test methods and test results).

Routine low-voltage power-on and preparation records: low-voltage power-on time (accurate to minutes).

Normal use records: Depending on the configuration of the equipment, the data required to be recorded is different, but at least it should include the number of patients treated, the cumulative time of high voltage on and the cumulative time of filament.

Routine shutdown record: routine shutdown time (accurate to minutes).

Non-routine shutdown records: non-routine shutdown time (accurate to minutes) and cumulative number of non-routine shutdowns.

Equipment clinical quality control (QA) records: In addition to all clinical quality control records, at least the cumulative high-pressure time and cumulative filament time should be recorded.

Regular maintenance records: In addition to all maintenance records of each manufacturer, at least the cumulative high-pressure time and cumulative filament time should be recorded.

2. **Time Calculation Requirements**

Service Response Time: From the moment when the failure is reported by the user to the moment when the customer service personnel arrives at the scene.

Failure repair time: From the time when the customer service first visits the door to the time when the service is restored. It includes the time from the start of failure detection to the completion of the calibration process (including the time of maintenance scope confirmation and maintenance method confirmation) as the time of this corrective maintenance, that is, the time for failure detection and isolation, maintenance preparation time, replacement of failure parts/Repair time, repair adjustment and calibration time, cleaning site time and other components.

Preventive maintenance time: The preventive maintenance time is from the moment when the preventive maintenance is started to the time when the preventive maintenance is completed. Time spent on preventive maintenance is not counted as downtime nor due work time in the calculation of availability.

Downtime: The sum of service response time and failure repair time, that is, the time between the end of failure repair and the time of repair. During on-site evaluation, if the failure is recovered within 10 h, the downtime is not included in the statistics of the uptime rate. If the failure is restored after more than 10 h, the failure repair time minus 10 h will be counted as downtime.

6.6.6 Selection of Statistical Dimensions

The statistical time range is recommended to use the year as the statistical period.

The scope of statistical objects can include a single device and all such devices of the same manufacturer and model.

Statistical indicators include:

(1) The annual shutdown times, downtime, failure times, maintenance times, maintenance time and their average value of the equipment;
(2) Availability, start-up rate, stop-down rate and their average value of equipment;
(3) Mean time between downtime, mean time between serious failures and their average value;
(4) Average service response time, average failure repair time, average preventive maintenance time, average downtime and their average values.

6.6.7 *Usability Information Statistics*

6.6.7.1 Time Information Statistics

Check the completeness and accuracy of the information in Table 6.13. First of all, clearly stipulate the calendar time that the equipment should work in the corresponding statistical interval and the specified working time period every day. Calculate the following information for the equipment in the year according to Table 6.13:

(1) The sum of working hours (T);
(2) The sum of usage time (every end usage time—start usage time) (T_u);
(3) The sum of the high-voltage opening time (T_{uh});
(4) The sum of working hours of individual components (T_{da});
(5) Sum of downtime (T_{nd});
(6) The sum of downtime times (N_{nd});
(7) The sum of the number of patients treated (N_p).

If necessary, downtime can be further divided into downtime that affects normal work and downtime that does not affect normal work Table 6.14.

6.6.7.2 Failure Information Statistics

Check the completeness and accuracy of the information in Table 6.15, based on the following information of the equipment in the calculation year (or specified statistical interval):

(1) The sum of the number of severe failures (N_{fc});
(2) The sum of general failure times (N_{fn});

Table 6.13 Equipment use record form

Use agency				Placement						
Device name				Equipment Model Specifications						
Device ID				Installation date						
Manufacturer name				Record personnel information						
Number	Number	Low–Voltage Power–On Time	Shutdown Time	Filament Time/ h	High Pressure Time/ h	Whether Shutdown	Occur Failure	Treat Number	State	Illustrate
	YYYY/MM/DD	Time: –:–	Time:–:–			☐ yes ☐No	☐ yes ☐ no		☐ use ☐QA ☐Maintenance	

Table 6.14 Equipment downtime record form

Use agency					Placement			
Device name					Equipment Model Specifications			
Device ID					Installation date			
Supplier name					Customer Service Information			
Correspond date	Stop number	Downtime reason	Unavailable start time	Repair time	Customer service for the first time door time	Repair frequency	Recover available time	Affect should work hours/ h
YYYY/ MM/DD		☐ failure shutdown ☐ Preventive mainte- nance ☐ Other reasons	YYYY/ MM/DD Time:–:–	YYYY/ MM/DD Time:–:–	YYYY/MM/DD Time:–:–		YYYY/MM/DD Time:–:–	

(3) The sum of failure times (N_f), $N_f = N_{fc} + N_{fn}$;
(4) The sum of the number of failures in the open high voltage (N_{fh});
(5) Statistics of individual component failures, such as accelerator tubes, modulators, magnetrons, electron gun power supplies, etc.

6.6.7.3 Maintenance Information Statistics

Check the completeness and accuracy of the information in Table 6.15, based on the following information of the equipment in the calculation year (or specified statistical interval):

(1) The sum of preventive maintenance times (N_{mp});
(2) The sum of preventive maintenance time (T_{mp});
(3) The sum of maintenance times (N_m), $N_m = N_{mp} + N_{mt}$;
(4) The sum of maintenance time (T_m), $T_m = T_{mp} + T_{mt}$.

6.6.7.4 Stop Information Statistics

Check the correspondence between all downtime events in the "Equipment Usage Record Form " and "Equipment Downtime Record Form", confirm the completeness of the "Equipment Downtime Record Form", track and supplement the missing downtime records, and clearly list those that cannot be supplemented. Calculate the following information in the "Equipment Shutdown Record Form" within the year (or specified statistical interval):

(1) The sum of the number of stoppages for preventive maintenance (N_{dp});
(2) The sum of preventive maintenance downtime (T_{dp});
(3) Number of shutdowns for failure maintenance (N_{dm});
(4) The sum of downtime for failure maintenance (T_{dm});
(5) The sum of the number of downtimes caused by the machine (N_{dd}), $N_{dd} = N_{dp} + N_{dm}$;
(6) The sum of the downtime caused by the machine (T_{dd}), $T_{dd} = T_{dp} + T_{dm}$;
(7) The sum of the number of shutdowns (N_d), $N_d = N_{dd} + N_{dh}$;
(8) Sum of downtime (T_d), $T_d = T_{dd} + T_{dh}$ (recovery availability time of each downtime event—unavailability start time).

6.6.8 *Usability Index Evaluation*

6.6.8.1 Reliability Index Statistics

According to time information statistics and failure information statistics, the following indicators can be evaluated:

(1) Mean Time Between Failures (MTBF): Divide the sum of the times (T_u) by the sum of the number of failures (N_f), that is, MTBF = T_u / N_f;
(2) Mean Time Between Serious Failures (MTBCF): Divide the sum of times (T_u) by the number of serious failures (N_{fc}), that is, MTBCF = T_u / N_{fc};
(3) Mean time between general failures (MTBNF): use the sum of time (T_u) divided by the sum of general failure times (N_{fn}), that is, MTBNF = T_u / N_{fn};
(4) Average time between failures in high voltage and high voltage (MTBF-HM): the sum of high voltage and high voltage (T_{uh}) divided by the number of failures in high voltage and high voltage (N_{fh}), that is, MTBF—HM = T_{uh} / N_{fh};
(5) The average working time between failures of a single component (such as accelerating tube, klystron, etc.): the total working time of a single component divided by the number of failures of a single component, that is, MTBF (da) = $T_{da}/Nf_{(da)}$.

Note: The sum of the use time can be calendar time, working time, and high-voltage open time.

6.6.8.2 Shutdown Parameter Evaluation

Based on the outage statistics, the following metrics can be evaluated:

(1) Mean Time Between Downtime and Failure (MTBDF-D): Divide the sum of time (T_u) by the sum of downtimes due to equipment failure (N_{dd}), that is, MTBDF-D = T_u / N_{dd};
(2) Mean time between downtimes (MTBDF): divide the sum of times (T_u) by the sum of downtimes (N_d), that is, MTBDF = T_u / N_d;
(3) The number of patients treated at the average downtime and failure interval (MPBDF-P): the total number of patients treated (N_p) divided by the sum of the number of downtime and failures due to equipment reasons (N_{dd}), that is, MTBDF-P = N_p / N_{dd}.

Table 6.15 Equipment failure and maintenance information record sheet

Use agency				Placement			
Device name				Equipment Model Specifications			
Device ID				Installation date			
Supplier name				Service staff information			
Corresponding date	Failure serial number	Symptoms	Failure consequences	Failure Cause Analysis	On-site repair Compound	Follow-up prevention improvement measures	Whether it occurs repeatedly
			☐Serious failure ☐General failure				☐ yes ☐No

6.6.9 *Usability Evaluation Report*

The usability evaluation report of the medical electron linear accelerator shall be issued within the specified statistical dimension, the main contents are as follows:

(1) Evaluation purpose;
(2) Evaluation basis;
(3) Evaluation time, place, and number of prototypes;
(4) Overview of the use, failure and maintenance of the prototype;
(5) Availability evaluation results;
(6) Reliability evaluation results;
(7) Maintenance support evaluation results;
(8) Document verification and evaluation results;
(9) Physical verification and evaluation results;
(10) Evaluation conclusion;
(11) Questions and suggestions.

References

1. Grgg k.hobbs. highly-accelerated life test-halt, screening technology seminar notes, available from hobbs engineering, Westminster, co.1988.
2. *General Requirements for Equipment Reliability Work* [S]. National Military Standard of the People's Republic of China GJB450A- 2004. Released with the approval of the General Armament Department of the Chinese People's Liberation Army, 2004.
3. *Reliability, Maintainability and Support Terminology* [S]. National military standard of the People's Republic of China GJB451A- 2005. Released with the approval of the General Armament Department of the Chinese People's Liberation Army, 2005.
4. *Failure Tree Analysis Guide* [S]. National Military Standard of the People's Republic of China GJB/Z768A- 1998. Approved by the National Defense Science, Technology and Industry Committee, 1998.
5. *Guidelines for Failure Mode, Effect and Hazard Analysis* [S]. National Military Standard of the People's Republic of China GJB/Z 1391- 2006. Approved and issued by the General Armament Department of the Chinese People's Liberation Army, 2006.
6. *Failure Mode and Effects Analysis (FMEA) Procedure* [S]. National Standard of the People's Republic of China GB/T 7826- 2012. Issued by the General Administration of Quality Supervision, Inspection and Quarantine of the People's Republic of China, 2012.
7. *Test Method for Failure Rate of Electronic Components* [S]. National Military Standard of the People's Republic of China GB/T 1772- 1979. Issued by the State Administration of Standards, 1979.
8. *Sampling Plan and Procedure for Failure Rate of Military Electronic Components* [S]. National Military Standard of the People's Republic of China GJB 2649A- 2011. Approved and issued by the General Armament Department of the Chinese People's Liberation Army, 2011.
9. *Destructive Physical Analysis of Military Components* [S]. National Military Standard of the People's Republic of China GJB 4027A- 2006. Approved by the General Armament Department of the Chinese People's Liberation Army, 2006.
10. *Electronic Equipment Reliability Prediction Manual* [S]. National Military Standard of the People's Republic of China GJB/Z 299C- 2006. Released with the approval of the General Armament Department of the Chinese People's Liberation Army, 2006.
11. *Reliability Model Establishment and Reliability Prediction* [S]. National Military Standard of the People's Republic of China GJB 813- 1990. Released with the approval of National Defense Science, Technology and Industry Committee, 1990.
12. *Electronic Equipment Non-Working State Reliability Prediction Manual* [S]. National Military Standard of the People's Republic of China GJB/Z 108A- 2006. Released with the approval of the General Armament Department of the Chinese People's Liberation Army, 2006.
13. *Baseline Conditions for Failure Rate and Transformation Stress Model* [S]. National Standard GB/T 7289- 2017 of the People's Republic of China. Released by the General Administration of Quality Supervision, Inspection and Quarantine of the People's Republic of China, 2017.

X. Li et al., *Reliability Engineering Technology of Digital Diagnosis and Treatment Equipment*, https://doi.org/10.1007/978-981-99-5522-0

14. *Electronic Equipment Reliability Prediction Model and Data Booklet* [S]. National Standard GB/T 37963- 2019 of the People's Republic of China. Released by the State Administration for Market Regulation, 2019.
15. Ruitang L. Failure Analysis and Examples of Mechanical Parts[M]. Harbin: Harbin Institute of Technology Press; 2014.

SPRINGER NATURE

GPSR Compliance

The European Union's (EU) General Product Safety Regulation (GPSR) is a set of rules that requires consumer products to be safe and our obligations to ensure this.

If you have any concerns about our products, you can contact us on ProductSafety@springernature.com

In case Publisher is established outside the EU, the EU authorized representative is:

Springer Nature Customer Service Center GmbH
Europaplatz 3
69115 Heidelberg, Germany

The manufacturer's authorised representative in the EU is Springer Nature Customer Service Centre GmbH, Europaplatz 3, 69115 Heidelberg, Germany. If you have any concerns regarding our products, please contact ProductSafety@springernature.com

Printed and bound by CPI Group (UK) Ltd, Croydon, CR0 4YY
30/09/2026
02225314-0017